CANCER ETIOLOGY, DIAGNOSIS AND TREATMENTS

CERVICAL CANCER

SCREENING METHODS, RISK FACTORS AND TREATMENT OPTIONS

CANCER ETIOLOGY, DIAGNOSIS AND TREATMENTS

Additional books in this series can be found on Nova's website
under the Series tab.

Additional e-books in this series can be found on Nova's website
under the e-book tab.

OBSTETRICS AND GYNECOLOGY ADVANCES

Additional books in this series can be found on Nova's website
under the Series tab.

Additional e-books in this series can be found on Nova's website
under the e-book tab.

CANCER ETIOLOGY, DIAGNOSIS AND TREATMENTS

CERVICAL CANCER

SCREENING METHODS, RISK FACTORS AND TREATMENT OPTIONS

LAURIE ELIT

EDITOR

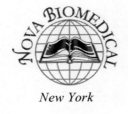

New York

For permission to use material from this book please contact us:
Telephone 631-231-7269; Fax 631-231-8175
Web Site: http://www.novapublishers.com

NOTICE TO THE READER

Library of Congress Cataloging-in-Publication Data

ISBN: 978-1-62948-062-6

Library of Congress Control Number: 2013948182

Published by Nova Science Publishers, Inc. † New York

The test of progress is not whether we add to the abundance of those who have much. It's whether we provide enough to those who have little.

Franklin D. Roosevelt

This book is dedicated to women through-out the world affected by HPV related diseases. In countries like Kenya and Mongolia, women present with bloody foul smelling vaginal discharge. The treatment for advanced staged cervical cancer is pelvic radiation therapy but this is not uniformly available because of a lack of resources (like only 1 radiation machine in the country) or geographic barriers to access of care. As if this travesty was not enough, these women often die in excruciating pain because anti-inflammatory or narcotic medications are not available. In contrast, in high resource settings, there are other women who because of screening will be diagnosed with cancer and they will get treatment. In some cases their treatment leaves them with life long complications, but they will survive their encounter with lower genital tract disease. For those women diagnosed with preinvasive disease, the treatment is less debilitating but anxiety provoking all the same. This book is dedicated to all these women.

Contents

Contents

Preface

Laurie Elit

Department of Obstetrics and Gynecology, Division of Gynecologic Oncology,
McMaster University, Hamilton, Canada
Scientific Lead for the Ontario Cervical Screening Program, Cancer Care Ontario

There is this about a story, when we get caught up in a story, we don't know how it is going to end. Nor do we know who else is going to be part of the story. Nothing in a skillfully told story is predictable. But also, nothing is without meaning-every detail, every word, every name, every action is part of the story.

Eugene Peterson, The Pastor

Globally, cervical cancer is the second leading cause of death for women with cancer. This story is a tragedy. In part this is because cervical cancer affects women usually a decade sooner than other cancer when that woman is in the midst of her reproductive career and in her prime of her employment career. While screening with the Pap test or other more recently evaluated tests has resulted in low cervical cancer rates in high resource countries, the lack of screening options in low resource countries means that many women present with symptoms reflective of advanced disease and so low chance of survival even with aggressive treatment. In 2008, Professor zur Hausen was award the Nobel prize for physiology or medicine for his part in this story. His work in cervical cancer is where he discovered the role of the human papilloma virus. Subsequently, vaccines have been developed which if delivered prior to sexual debut, can prevent the occurrence of at least 70% of cervical cancer. Unfortunately the high cost of the vaccine and the low to mediocre uptake of the vaccine in many jurisdictions are two areas that require intensive effort in order that the world sees the benefit of this incredible breakthrough. Currently both prevention using the HPV vaccine and screening using one of the tests available (Pap test, Visual Inspection with Acetic Acid, or careHPV^{TM}) are recommended to provide optimal prevention against developing cervical cancer.

If you don't know where you are going, you may go somewhere else.

Laurence J. Peter

In contrast to this quote, in this book, our objective is is to improve knowledge and strategies for optimizing care delivery for women affected by preinvasive and invasive cervical disease. We strive toward a world that is not only without small pox and soon poliomyelitis. Would it not be an incredible dream to have a world without oncogenic HPV related diseases like cervical cancer. However, to get to that future, we must travel on the bridge known as "dreams". And that is this generation's role in the cervical cancer story.

I would like to thank the chapter authors for their contributions to this work on Cervical Cancer: Screening Methods, Risk Factors and Treatment Options. Their efforts bring to you the reader various perspectives on the cervical cancer story. It is told from the vantage of high, medium and low resource settings. It is also told by authors who represent various generations and disciplines of health care providers and researchers. The chapter contents are described below.

Chapter

1. HPV infects cells and results in cytological and molecular changes. This process is discussed in words and pictorially
2. The strengths and weakness of various cervical screening methodologies are discussed. Their application to high and low resource settings is presented.
3. The exciting opportunity that telemedicine offers for both cytology and colposcopy in geographically isolated settings is presented.
4. Planning and implementing an organized cervical screening program and the assessment of quality indicators as a means of evaluation is outlined. Examples of this process are provided from the Millenium Challenge Mongolia health project on a national cervical cancer prevention, early detection, case management, follow-up and palliative care program.
5. The risk factors associated with persistent and recurrent HSIL and persistent LSIL are evaluated in a population from La Paz hospital, Madrid.
6. Developing quality indicators for assessing a screening or diagnostic program is discussed. The process of developing colposcopy indicators is provided as an example of using the Delphi method.
7. Given that HPV is the agent causing precancerous and cancerous lesions of the cervix, anti-HPV treatment is needed to deal with such lesions. Although the HPV vaccine is very efficacious when provided prior to sexual debut. Currently treatment for pre-cancers still involve topical agents (ie., podophyllin), ablation, or immunomodulators (ie., imiquimod). Novel agents in development are discussed.
8. Early stage cervical cancer can be treated surgically. The role of the vagina in assessment and operability is discussed. The various surgical options depending on stage, the woman's desire for fertility and the surgical team's experience are reviewed.
9. Role of neoadjuvant chemotherapy for locally advanced disease is reviewed.
10. The role of surgically staging women to define more advanced disease is outlined including options for management of metastatic and/or recurrent disease with chemotherapy and targeted therapies.

11. The prevalence and prognosis of positive para-aortic nodal disease in cervical cancer is discussed. Evaluation of women with clinically early stage cervical cancer using novel techniques like CT/PET can help define those with para-aortic nodal disease. Strategies to treat this disease using extended field radiation with or without chemotherapy is discussed.

12. The benefits that standard chemotherapy agents can bring in advanced or metastatic cervical cancer are discussed. A rationale for and current knowledge of the role for novel angiogenic target agents like bevacizumab, epidermal growth factor receptor inhibitors like cetuximab, activators of AMP Kinase, Insulin-like growth factor inhibition, mTOR inhibitors, cyclooxygenase inhibitors, and histone deacetylase and DNA methylation inhibition are elaborated upon.

13. The special situation of a woman found to be pregnant during the diagnosis of pre-invasive or invasive cervical cancer; the diagnosis and management principles are reviewed.

14. The chapter provides an review of topics in identifying and managing preinvasive and invasive disease.

In: Cervical Cancer
Editor: Laurie Elit

ISBN: 978-1-62948-062-6
© 2014 Nova Science Publishers, Inc.

Chapter I

Cervical Cancer: A Cytological and Molecular Overview

A. C. Freitas,[1] A. P. A. D. Gurgel,[1] B. S. Chagas[1] and J. C. Silva Neto[2]

[1]Department of Genetics, Federal
University of Pernambuco, Brazil
[2]Department of Histology and Embryology,
Federal University of Pernambuco, Brazil

Abstract

Cervical cancer is the third leading cause of cancer in women worldwide, with 529.800 new cases and 275.100 deaths in 2008. The highest incidence and mortality caused by cervical cancer occur in developing countries. In contrast, the incidence and mortality of cervical cancer in developed countries decreased due to organized cytological screening programs. Persistent infection caused by Human Papillomaviruses (HPV) plays a critical role in the development of cervical lesions. HPV is a small, non-enveloped, double-stranded genome virus that can cause both benign and malignant lesions in epithelial tissues. High-risk HPV (HR-HPV) infection is necessary but not sufficient to cause cervical cancer. This statement can be confirmed by the observation that a large number of women infected with HPV will never develop cervical disease. Thus, other genetic and environmental factors must be involved in its development. In this context, several studies have been carried out concerning to genetic variability of HPV, in an attempt to demonstrate that there is a relationship between specific variants and cervical cancer. Genetic variability in L1 gene of HR HPV might affect immune response. Moreover, DNA variability in E5, E6 and E7 oncoproteins can be more efficient in cell transformation. In addition, genetic variability in viral transcriptional factor E2 and long control region (LCR) might alter the expression of viral genes. Therefore, this chapter will discuss the cytological aspects of cervical lesions and cervical cancer, as well as, genetic variability of HR-HPV that might be involved in high risk phenotype for cervical cancer.

Keywords: Human Papillomavirus; abnormal cytology; cervical cancer; HPV variants

Introduction

Cervical cancer is an important problem of public health worldwide. It represents 9% of the cases of female cancer and is considered as the third largest cause of death in women worldwide, with over 529,800 new cases and 275,100 deaths per year [1]. When compared to more developed countries, its incidence is approximately two times higher in less developed countries. Developed countries have reduced the number of cases of cervical cancer by 80% as a result of programs for the detection and treatment of precancerous lesions, such as Papanicolaou smear (Pap test). In contrast, in developing countries, it is difficult to perform clinical screening of precancerous lesions since their National Health System have limited financial resources [2].

The Human Papillomavirus (HPV) is a DNA virus belonging to the family *Papillomaviridae* [3]. This type virus infects the skin or mucous cells in epithelial tissue through microlesions, being the sexual contact their primary transmission form [4, 5]. Currently, over 120 HPV types have been described, as well as subtypes and variants based on the differences between the genotypes sequences of nucleotide [6, 7]. HPV can be classified as high-risk HPV (HR-HPV) and low-risk HPV (LR-HPV), according to the degree of severity of cervical lesions [8]. The LR-HPV includes types that are found in genital warts (HPV-6, 11, 42, 43 and 44) while the viral types of HR-HPV are associated with different degrees of squamous intraepithelial lesions of the cervix, vagina, vulva, penis and development of cervical carcinoma (HPV-16, 18, 31, 33, 34, 35, 39, 45, 51, 52, 56, 58, 59, 66, 68 and 70) [9–12].

Advances in tumor virology have shown that HPV infection has an important function in the development of cervical cancer. However, HPV infection is not sufficient to produce neoplastic transformation. Therefore, viral genetic factors are important in the risk of progression of HPV infection to neoplasia. In this context, several studies have shown a natural genetic diversity of HPV types [13–15]. These intratype variants may differ biologically and etiologically, and have been carried out an attempt to demonstrate that there is a relationship between specific variants and cervical cancer [16–19]. Moreover, this fact can contribute to the differences in the incidence of cervical cancer worldwide [20].

This chapter will discuss about cytological as well as molecular aspects regarding cervical lesions and cervical cancer.

Cytologycal Aspects

Normal Cells in Cervical Cytology

With regard to superficial squamous cells, these are the largest cells found in normal cervical smears (Figure 1A). They are located in the superficial layer of the vaginal epithelium and represent the last stage of maturation. They are prevalent in pre-ovulation and ovulation, estrogen therapy, and functioning ovarian tumors. On the outermost part of the squamous epithelial layer, there are anucleate (or phantom) cells with a superficial squamous cell format. The Intermediate squamous cells are characterized by the form a thicker squamous epithelial multilayer (Figures 1B, 1C).

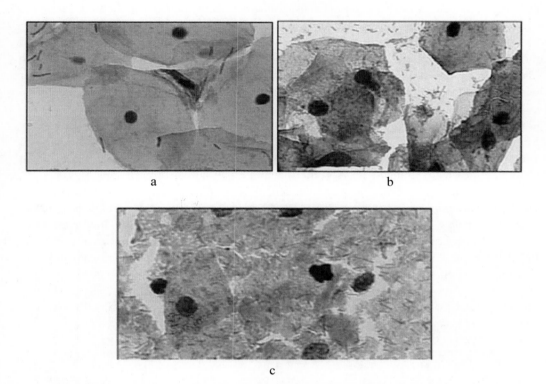

Figure 1. superficial squamous cells (A). Intermediate cells without cytolosis (B) and with cytolosis (C) (Papanicolaou).

Their presence is common in cervical smears and mainly occur in response to an adrenocortical and progestagen stimulus (during the post-ovulatory phase, pregnancy or menopause). They can be seen in Papanicolaou staining which appears as a yellowish tint in the most central region of the cytoplasm, and are indicative of glycogen concentration, a glucose polymer that serves as a food supply for Döderlein bacilli (Lactobacillus). When the bacilli consume the polymer, they trigger cytolysis, which is characterized by naked nuclei and fragments of cytoplasm.

In the basal and parabasal squamous cells, the presence of deep cells in cervicovaginal smears of normal women are rare, except in cases of atrophy or abnormal conditions. Basal cells are the deepest layer of the stratified epithelial cells where effective mitotic activity can be found. Parabasal cells are larger than basal cells and rarely display mitotic activity. They are often present in the following: an absence of maturation of the epithelium in post-menopausal women, estrogen deficiency, lactation, pre-puberty, and post-radiation treatment (Figures 2A, 2B). The reserve cells are responsible for the maintenance of the epithelium and are located in the region between the basal membrane and the glandular cells. It is difficult to see them in cervical smears. Since they are multipotent, they have the capacity to become squamous or columnar cells. When stimulated, they can multiply and thus cause hyperplasia of reserve cells. Studies based on immunohistochemistry with cytokeratins indicate that they are similar to basal cells. Their main cytomorphological features include small, overlapping cells that are round or oval and, occasionally triangular, and which are smaller than parabasal cells. Their cytoplasm is basophilic, sparse or absent and they have vacuoles.

The nucleus is round or oval, and hyperchromatic with small chromocentres and moderately granular chromatin. Multinucleation is rare. They can be confused with histiocytes, small neuroendocrine cells, carcinoma and endometrial cells. They often appear when there is treatment with tamoxifen. Concerning to the endocervical glandular cells, except during menstruation, they are the most common glandular cells in cervical smears, especially when the collection is performed with an endocervical brush (cytobrush). They form the endocervical columnar epithelium (endocervix) and can be classified into ciliated and secretory cells, or producers of the mucous. The glandular cells can be visualized in patterns of cervical cytology smears in the shape of a palisade or "honeycomb" (Figures 2C, 2D). The endometrial and stromal glandular cells is unusual in normal cervical smears except during menstruation or shortly afterwards (first 12 days of the menstrual cycle). When present in postmenopausal women or women over 40 years of age, they must be reported because of the risk of neoplasm. The following conditions can give rise to their appearance: use of the IUD, hormonal therapy, menstruation, pregnancy, postpartum, dysfunctional bleeding, chronic endometritis, endometriosis, chronic and acute endocervicitis, recent endometrial procedure, endometrial polyp, submucous myoma, hyperplasia, endometrial carcinoma. These cells vary with the stages of the menstrual cycle and the level of preservation. If well preserved, they appear grouped in three-dimensional and closely bound patterns.

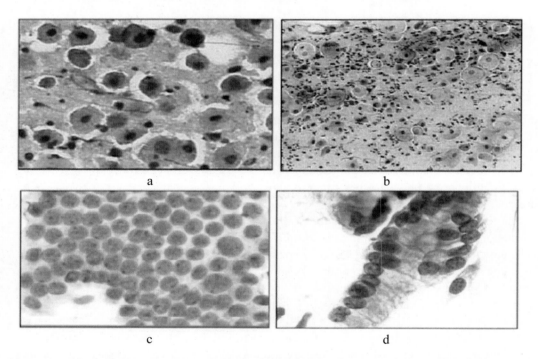

Figure 2. Deep Layer of Cells: basal and parabasal cells (atrophy) (A, B). Endocervical glandular cells, cellular "beehive" pattern (C) and palisade (D) (Papanicolaou).

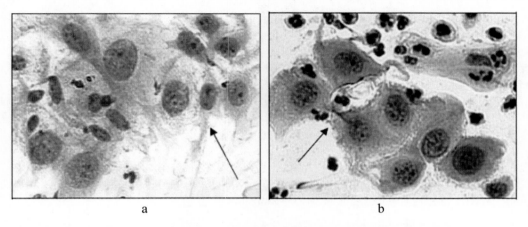

Figure 3. Cells in immature squamous metaplasia (A, B). Check intercellular bridges (Papanicolaou).

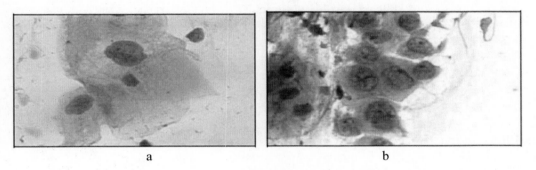

Figure 4. ASC-US (A). ASC-H represented by atypical squamous metaplasia "with a high nucleus/ cytoplasm ratio and variations in size and shape (B) (Papanicolaou).

The cells in squamous metaplasia is considered when the physiological phenomenon which may become more evident in certain pathological states involving injury to epithelial tissue.

These cells originate from the reserve cells hyperplasia, and when the cell change is complete are called "mature" or "immature" metaplasia if the alteration is incomplete. Cytomorphological features occur when in the "immature" form cytoplasmic projections are called intercellular bridges (aracniforms). There are possible vacuoles and dense cytoplasm. The nucleus is round with fine homogeneous chromatin, and small nucleoli (Figures 3A, 3B).

Atypias and Intraepithelial Lesions

Atypical squamous cells of undetermined significance (ASC-US) is used when no causative agent is present and it is still possible to detect discrete cytomorphological changes that overlap in inflammation. This is mainly because there is no inflammatory agent present, but the changes are not enough to characterize an intraepithelial lesion. Thus its subtle changes mainly affect the nuclear volume. The nuclear chromatin pattern is homogeneous and coarse with the presence of one or more nucleoli evident in the squamous cells (Figure 4A).

With regard to the atypical squamous cells not excluding squamous high-grade lesions (ASC-H), the changes are confused with high-grade lesions and are represented by cells in atypical immature squamous metaplasia. They are suggestive of HSIL, but there is a lack of criteria to allow a definitive interpretation to be made. ASC-H is noted in 30 to 40% of cases of HSIL lesions (Figure 4B).

Squamous Intra-Epithelial Lesions (SIL)

According to the Bethesda System, squamous non-invasive lesions are classified as Intra-epithelial lesions of Low-grade Squamous (LSIL), squamous intraepithelial lesions of high-grade (HSIL) and HSIL with features arousing suspicions of invasion.

Intra-Epithelial Squamous Lesions of a Low-Grade (LSIL)
In the presence of koilocytes. cell with irregular perinuclear vacuole that does not stain and with mature hyperchromasia should be described as LSIL + HPV (Figure 5). Approximately 57% of the cases of CIN-I regress spontaneously and only 11% progress to CIN-II and III. Squamous cell carcinoma may develop in 0.3% of cases with CIN-I. In the absence of koilocytes the atypia will only be described as LSIL.

Squamous Intraepithelial Lesions of High-Grade (HSIL)
This encompasses the classification of cervical intraepithelial neoplasia II and III (CIN II and III). The cytomorphological changes found in HSIL are the same as those in LSIL but more pronounced with some additional features and more immature cells (Figure 6).

HSIL with Suspicious Invasive Features
Changes consistent with HSIL that have greater intensity, for example, enhanced cellular and nuclear pleomorphism, with no keratinization or tumor diathesis.

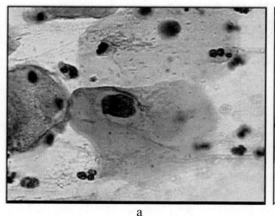 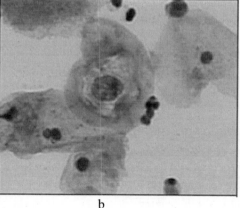

a   b

Figure 5. Only LSIL: Note the raisin-like nuclei. (A). LSIL+HPV, HPV cytopathic effect (koilocytosis). Great perinuclear halo, bi or multinucleation, some nuclei increased in size, hyperchromatic coarse chromatin and discrete changes in the nuclear contour (B) (Papanicolaou).

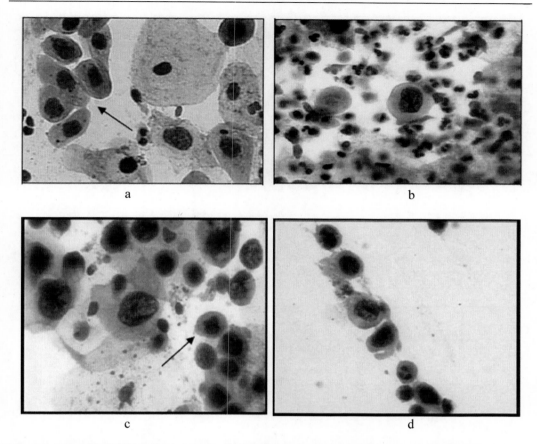

Figure 6. Intraepithelial High Grade Lesions (HSIL). Hyperchromatic nuclei, increased volume and subtle changes in the nuclear contour. There is still the presence of mature and abundant cytoplasm when HSIL/NIC-II(A, B). Single cells (C), and cells in single file is also common in advanced lesions HSIL / CIN III (D) (Papanicolaou).

Moreover, epithelial cell necrosis, micronucleoli or macronucleoli with a strong presence or absence of inflammatory cells and blood are observed. These smears may appear with a light and clear background. This classification is corroborated by the microinvasion charts diagnosed in the histology (Figure 7).

Atypical Endocervical Glandular Cells

The atypical endocervical glandular cells shown changes exceed the reactive or reparative changes, but show no changes in situ or invasive adenocarcinoma.

Their main features are as follows: Presence of some characteristics of adenocarcinoma in situ; mild hyperchromasia; clusters of endocervical cells in the monolayer; increase by approximately 3x the nucleus of a glandular endocervical cell that is round or oval; loss of polarity nucleolus-small-cytoplasm-columnar, vacuolated, distinct edges; close relationship between nucleus/cytoplasm; Mitosis-possible (Figure 8).

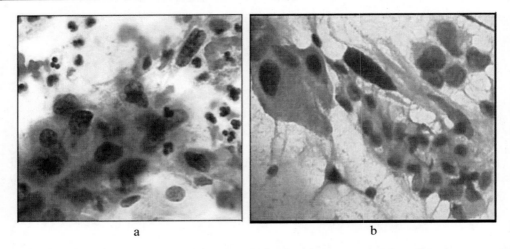

Figure 7. Intraepithelial High Grade Lesions (HSIL). This does not rule out the possibility of invasion (A, B). Immature cells with a lack of t cytoplasm, high nucleus/cytoplasm ratio, cariomegalia, hyperchromasia, abnormal nuclear shape and nucleoli. Absence of tumor diathesis (Papanicolaou).

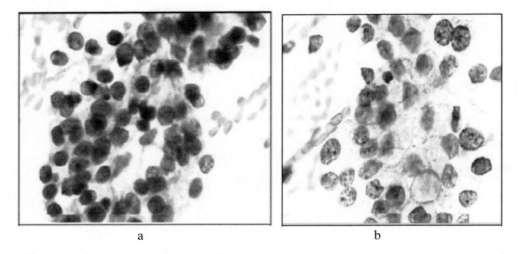

Figure 8. Atypical endocervical cells (A, B). Grouping plan anisonucleose discrete evident nucleoli, coarse chromatin and mild hyperchromasia (Papanicolaou).

Atypical Features Endocervical Cells (Neoplastic)

In this category, it is not yet possible to characterize in situ or invasive adenocarcinoma. In these cells there are only a few changes suggestive of a more advanced lesion (Figure 9).

Atypical Features in Endometrial Glandular Cells

The atypical features observed in endometrial glandular cells can be present in smears collected during the menstrual period, in atypical endometrial hyperplasia, endometritis, endometrial polyps, hormonal therapy and changes of Arias-Stella. Cytological abnormalities are characterized by cells arranged in small clusters (5-10 cells), cohesive, scant cytoplasm, occasionally vacuolated, slightly enlarged nuclei with hyperchromasia and moderate/ occasional /small nucleoli.

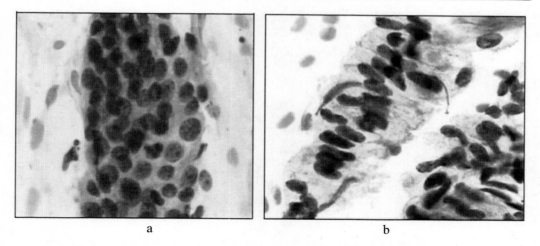

a   b

Figure 9. Atypical endocervical cells, favor neoplastic (A, B). Endocervical cells in full clusters, two-dimensional, anisonucleose, enlarged nuclei, elongated and overlapping. Slight change in contour, hyperchromasia and evident nucleoli (Papanicolaou).

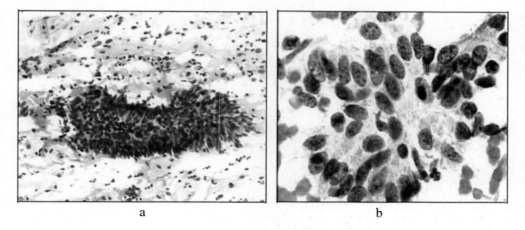

a   b

Figure 10. Adenocarcinoma in situ. Nuclei arranged in plumage "Feathering" (A) and "Rosettes" (B), hyperchromatic and rod-shaped (long) (Papanicolaou).

Adenocarninoma Endocervical in Situ (AIS)

Some studies have shown that there is a link between this type of injury and infection caused by HPV16 and 18, especially 18. Due to the sensitivity of cervico-vaginal cytology, the incidence of invasive adenocarcinoma is higher than the AIS. On some occasions, the criteria can be very subjective and confuse the cytologist. The main features are hyperchromasia, stick nuclei, and groupings in the form of feathers and rosettes (Figure 10).

Squamous Carcinoma (Invasive)

The squmanous carcinoma is characterized by the invasion of adjacent stroma through the disruption of the basal membrane, mainly affecting the ectocervix. The cytomorphological features are almost the same as in the lesions observed in HSIL but more pronounced with the presence or absence of tumor diathesis and the characteristics of the tumor itself (Figure 11).

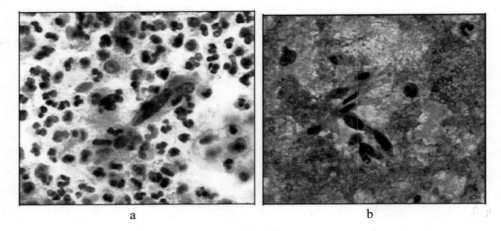

Figure 11. Squamous cell carcinoma (A, B). Plemorphic nucleus, spindle cells, irregular chromatin. The background of the tumor diathesis characterizes the smear as "dirty" (B) (Papanicolaou).

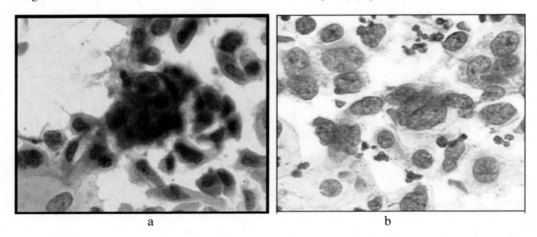

Figure 12. Squamous keratinized. Celular specimen with bizarre opaque nuclei and orangeophilic cytoplasm (A). Non-keratinized carcinoma (B) (Papanicolaou).

The squamous carcinomas are classified into: keratinizing, large non-keratinizing cells and small cells. The characteristics of keratinizing invasive carcinoma can be clearly distinguished into large non-keratinized and small non-keratinized cells. The non-keratinizing carcinoma large cell represents approximately 70% of the cervical tumors. Unlike keratinizing carcinoma, they do not have sheet clusters and pearl-cornea. The cells vary from round to oval. They mainly appear in the areas of metaplasia (Figure 12).

Endocervical Adenocarcinoma

Endocervical adenocarcinoma represents approximately 25-30% of cervical carcinomas and is associated with the use of oral contraceptives and HPV18 infections. In most cases, they are asymptomatic. Often the presence of atypical squamous cells is derived from squamous components coexisting with squamous adenocarcinoma or partly in squamous differentiation (Figure 13). In some studies, it was found that approximately half of adenocarcinoma in situ lesions have a squamous intraepithelial lesion that can be largely linked to HSIL.

Endometrial Adenocarcinoma

Endometrial adenocarcinoma represents approximately 80% of adenocarcinomas, with the highest incidence in postmenopausal women. The average age of diagnosis is about 60 years. They are asymptomatic and the Pap test is not an appropriate methodology for screening, because its sensitivity varies from 40-70% depending on the technique used to collect. Moreover, it is recommended for endometrial aspiration or biopsy that increases the specificity to 99% (Figure 14).

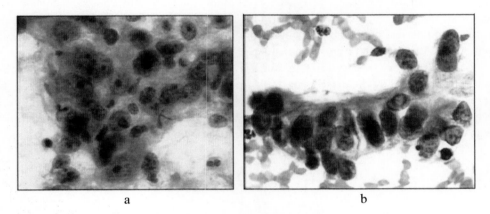

a   b

Figure 13. Endocervical adenocarcinoma (A, B). Loosely cohesive, nuclear atipia (hyperchromatic and pleomorphic nuclei with irregular chromatin), macronucleoli. (Papanicolaou).

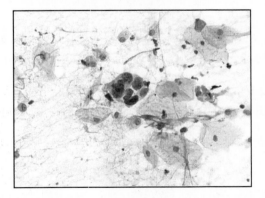

Figure 14. Endometrial adenocarcinoma (Papanicolaou). Source: Frappart L, Fontanière B, E Lucas, R. Sankaranarayanan Histopathology and cytopathology of the uterine cervix - digital atlas. IARC, Lyon, 2004. Available at: http://screening.iarc.fr/atlashisto.php?lang=1.

Cervical Cancer and Human Papillomavirus

According to the World Health Organization (WHO), persistent infection caused by Human Papillomavirus (HPV) is the main risk factor for developing cervical cancer, where it is estimated that about 98% of cervical tumors are associated with HPV [5, 21]. The contribution of HPV infection in cervical pathogenesis is related to HPV type and period of virus replication in the epithelial cells of the cervix transformation zone [22, 23]. The relationship between HPV types and cervical cancer was established from epidemiological and functional studies [8, 24], where the virus was detected in more than 99.7% of squamous cell carcinoma [25, 26] and in 94-100% of cervical adenosquamous carcinomas [27, 28]. Actually, more than 120 HPV types have been identified [7] and about 40 types affecting the genital tract, with HPV-16 responsible for 50 to 60% of cervical cancer cases, followed by HPV-18 (10-12%), and HPV 31 and 45 (5.4% each) [24, 29].

The host can combat HPV infection spontaneously, causing transient or subclinical abnormalities [30]. However, in some cases of carcinogenic HPV infection, the lesions do not regress, and may persist for extended periods. The long period between infection and the appearance of cervical carcinoma explains why this type of cancer is uncommon in women younger than 25 years with progressive incidence between 40 and 50 years old [31].

The natural history of cervical carcinoma is divided into the following phases: the first phase is characterized by the presence of HPV infection; the second phase is characterized by the presence of morphological alterations in the epithelial cervical cells, which cause intraepithelial lesions; and the third phase is characterized by the presence of the lesion through the basement membrane of the epithelium, leading to invasive carcinoma [32].

Classification

Initially, *Papillomavirus*es were originally classified with Polyomavirus in the family *Papovaviridae* for presenting similar characteristics, such as icosahedral capsid composed of 72 pentamers, capsid non-enveloped and double-stranded circular DNA. However, the capsid and viral genome of Papillomavirus are larger than the Polyomavirus. Hence, the two groups of viruses have been classified by the International Committee on Taxonomy of Viruses (ICTV) as two distinct families such as Polyomaviridae *(Polyomavirus)* and *Papillomaviridae* (including Papillomavirus) [6].

A new HPV type is defined by the presence of less than 90% of identity compared to established prototypes in L1 gene sequence, associated with the cloning and sequencing of its complete genome [3, 6]. In addition, the term subtype is used to identify HPV genomes with L1 nucleotide sequences that differ between 2-10% from the closest type, and the variants differ less than 2% in nucleotide sequence of L1, and 5% in LCR [6, 15].

Actually, there are more than 120 HPV types divided into five genera: *Alphapapillomavirus* (Alfa), *Betapapillomavirus* (Beta), *Gammapapillomavirus* (Gama), *Mupapillomavirus* (Mu) and *Nupapillomavirus* (Nu) [3, 6]. The two main HPV genera are the Alpha and Beta, with approximately 90% of HPVs characterized belonging to one of these two genera [33].

Among the five genera, there are about forty HPV types, which infect the genital tract, 15 of them considered as high-risk HPV types (HPV-16, HPV-18, HPV-31, HPV-33, HPV-35, HPV-39, HPV-45, HPV-51, PV-52, HPV-56, HPV-58, HPV-59, HPV-68, HPV-73 and HPV-82), six are considered with low-risk HPV types (HPV-6, HPV-11, HPV-42, HPV-44, HPV-

51, HPV-81 and HPV-83) and three types are considered as intermediate-risk HPV (HPV-26, HPV HPV-66 and -53) [8].

HPVs infections are considered of great medical importance due its relationship with genital and mucosal cancers, mainly the virus that belongs to the Alpha genus. The cervical cancer is often associated with HPV types that are found in the species 5, 6, 7, 9 and 11 [34, 35]. HPV-16, most commonly associated with cervical cancer, is a member of the species Alpha-9, HPV-18, the next type most commonly associated with cervical cancer, is a member of the species Alpha-7, and HPV-6 and HPV-11, which cause cutaneous warts, is a member of the species Alpha-10 [2]. Papillomaviruses that belonging to the Beta genus are typically associated with skin infections, such as patients with inherited epidermodysplasia verruciformis (EV) or in immunocompromised patients, these viruses may be associated with the development of skin cancer [36]. Other HPV types belonging to the three genera, Gamma, Mu and Nu, and cause cutaneous papillomas and warts, which usually do not progress to cancer [6].

Viral Genome Organization

Human Papillomaviruses are small non-enveloped viruses, presenting an icosahedral capsid, with 72 capsomeres and 52-55 nm in diameter, where is deposited the circular double-stranded DNA, constituting approximately 8 kb (8000 bp) [4, 37–39]. The HPV genome can be divided into three regions: the noncoding regulatory region (Upstream Regulatory Region - URR) or long control region (LCR); the early region (E) and the late region (L) [40].

The regulatory region LCR or URR comprises approximately 1 kb and is located between the regions L1 and E6 genes. In this region, there are enhancer and repressor sequences of the viral transcription, and the sequence of replication origin [11] (Figure 15).

The region E is formed by genes: E1, E2, E4, E5, E6 and E7, which are expressed immediately after infection of the host cell with the virus [4, 41]. The region L is formed by L1 and L2 genes, which are expressed late [4].

The Open Reading Frames (ORFs) E1 and E2 are responsible for encoding proteins essential for replication of extrachromosomal DNA, as well as to perform the viral infection cycle [42]. The E2 ORF encodes transcriptional regulatory proteins which is complexed with E1 protein and interacts with specific binding sites in LCR [4], where can inhibit transcription of the early region genes or increase the transcription of genes E [42] (Figure 15). One characteristic of HPV-associated cervical carcinoma is the loss of the expression of viral E2 protein [43]. The E4 protein is expressed in later stages of infection when the viruses are being formed.

Furthermore, the E4 protein is not known to have properties transformants. However, the E4 protein plays an important role for the viral maturation and replication [21, 42]. E5 protein is a hydrophobic protein membrane-associated which is responsible for the regulation of epidermal growth receptor, resulting in the stimulation of cell growth [4].

Moreover, E5 is suppressed in carcinoma cervix cells, which indicates that this protein may not be essential in maintaining of the malignant transformation of the host cell [42].

E6 and E7 are considered as the main HPV genes, by encode oncoproteins that allow replication of the virus immortalization and transformation of the host cell [42].

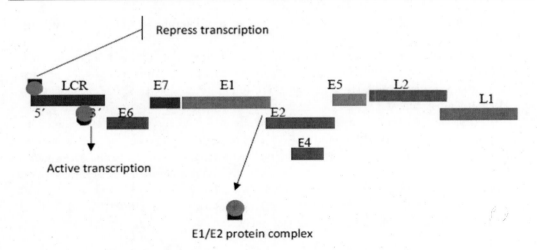

Figure 15. HPV-16 genome showing early genes E1, E2, E4, E5, E6 and E7, late genes L1, L2 and LCR. The E1/E2 complex bound into specific regions LCR allows repress the expression of E6 and E7 oncogenes or the activation of viral DNA replication.

The late region containing the genes which are expressed after viral infection [42]. The L1 gene is responsible for encoding the major viral capsid protein, while the L2 gene encodes the secondary protein of the viral capsid [40]. The L1 protein is highly conserved [42, 44]. The L2 protein is more internally and is involved in encapsidation of the viral genome, the viral capsid stability and transport of HPV nuclear genome [44].

Viral Infection Cycle

Although the HPV present a small genome, the gene expression pattern is complex, which makes its infectious cycle dependent of keratinocyte differentiation of the epithelium [45]. The cervix is covered by two epithelium denominated endocervix (secretory columnar epithelium) and ectocervix (squamous non-keratinized). The viral infection begins in the basal cells of the squamous epithelium by a breakage of stratified epithelium, as microdamage or abrasions, which occur on the skin or mucosa by direct contact such as the sexual contact or during birth [45] (Figure 16). Briefly, the HPV entry into the basal membrane cells occurs through the receptor binding heparan sulfate proteoglycans (HSPGs). After the binding, structural changes occur and the virus is transferred to a still unknown second receptor. These changes allow begin the uncoating programme, which includes the cleavage of site within the exposed N-terminus of L2.

After the entry of the virus in the host cell, occurs the acidification of the endocytic vesicles, leading to viral uncoating [46] (Figure 16). Subsequently, the HPV genome is established as extrachomosomal elements in the nuleus and copy number is increased to approximately 50-100 copies per cell. When these infected cells divide, viral DNA is distributed equitably between daughter cells.

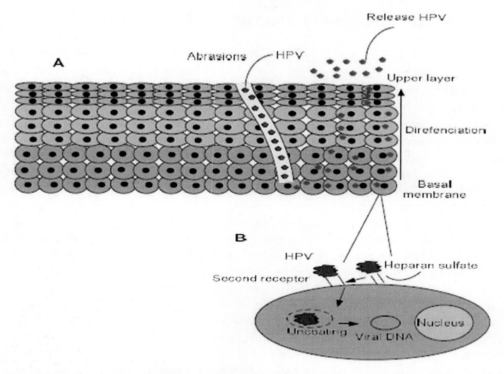

Figure 16. HPV cycle infection. A- HPV introduces into epithelium through microabrasions and infects the basal membrane cells. Afterwards, the early genes and late viral genes are expressed according to the cells differentiation from the basal membrane until upper layer. Finally, the viruses are released. B- HPV entry into basal membrane cells occurs through the HSPGs receptor. Subsequently, several conformational changes allow the recognition of the second receptor, internalizing of viral particle and viral uncoating.

One of infected cells migrates away from the basal layer toward the uppermost layer of the epithelium in order to monitor the process of cell differentiation of keratinocytes, while the other daughter cell continues to divide in the basal layer and provides a reservoir of viral DNA for subsequent cell divisions (Figure 16) [47-49].

During the stage of cell division occurs a minimal viral gene expression, particularly the expression of oncogenes E6 and E7. When the infected cell finished the stage of cell division and begins to differentiate, the virus activates the oncogenes E6 and E7, and starts the stage expression.

In the epithelium superficial layers to occur the last stages of the cycle, which corresponds to the assembly of virions, where L1 and L2 proteins are expressed and several thousand copies of the viral genome suffer encapsidation [40]. The nonstructural E4 protein is also expressed in this stage, facilitating the disruption of the cytoplasmic cytoskeleton to release the virions [45].

The infection may develop in any location of the female genital mucosa, however, the carcinogenic process development occurs most frequently in the epithelium transformation zone [41]. The time of infection until the release of viral particles is approximately three weeks, corresponding to the time required for the differentiation and desquamation of the basal keratinocyte [40].

Oncogenesis by Humam Papillomavirus

The primary transforming activity of HR-HPV is promoted by the oncoproteins E6 and E7 [50], which functionally inactivate the products of two important tumor suppressor genes, TP53 and pRb, respectively. Both oncoproteins induce proliferation, immortalization and malignant transformation of the infected cells [51].

The p53 protein has the ability to perceive different stresses that cells can undergo, for example, exposure to ultraviolet (UV), with consequent damage to the DNA. Thus, this protein is responsible for activating genes mechanism repair of the DNA or signal for apoptosis. When present in the cell, the E6 viral oncoprotein recruits the association protein to E6 (E6-AP), a cellular polypeptide that has ubiquitin ligase activity, and this recruitment results in ubiquitination and degradation of p53 [47]. Without the p53 protein, the cell loses the ability to perceive and repair possible DNA damage, having an increase in the frequency of mutations, chromosomal rearrangements and aneuploidy. The accumulation of these events enables the development of a neoplastic phenotype resulting in cancer. Additionally, the E6 oncoprotein inhibits the kinases degradation of the SRC family by E6-AP, stimulating the mitotic activity [8] and also activates telomerase, an enzyme responsible for the replication of telomeric DNA at the ends chromosome [48].

The retinoblastoma protein (pRb) has the function to perform the inhibition of cell cycle progression, since it is capable of preventing the transcription factor E2F promotes transcription of genes necessary for DNA replication in S phase. Hence, the pRb protein plays a negative regulation of the cell cycle through specific phosphorylation dependent cycle, where the dephosphorylated pRb is able to inhibit cell cycle progression by specific binding to E2F. Once phosphorylated by cyclin-dependent kinases (CDK), the connection between pRb and E2F does not occur, and this results directly in stimulating the transcription of genes that are responsible for DNA replication during S phase of the cell cycle.

The association of the viral oncoprotein E7 with the protein pRb prevents its binding to the E2F factor, resulting in continuous progression to the S phase of the cell cycle and became a stimulus for proliferation of infected cells [52]. In addition to pRb, E7 interacts with two other family members' pRb, p107 and p130, which also negatively regulate the transcription factor E2F [51]. Moreover, E7 is efficient in the complex formation cyclins A and E, interacts with complex cyclin-kinase and cancels activity of cyclin kinases inhibitors dependent (CKIs) such as p21 and p27, which are important regulators during differentiation epithelium [53, 54].

The physical state of the HPV DNA into the host cell is indicative of the pathological course of infection [51]. An important difference between types of HPV high and low risk is integrating its DNA into the host genome [4]. Oncogenic High-risk HPVs have a higher tendency to integrate genomics, whereas oncogenic low-risk HPVs is preferentially retained in episomal form [55].

The integration of the HPV genome occurs due to cleavage in the region of the E1/E2 genes, resulting in the loss of the E1 gene and E2 gene disruption. Thus, the integration annuls the inhibitory action of E2 protein on viral promoter of the oncogenes E6 and E7, resulting in high levels of expression of the same, which probably contributes to cell transformation and eventually results in tumor formation [42, 56].

Although E6 and E7 are oncoproteins most widely studied, E5 oncoprotein has shown importance in relation to formation of cervical neoplasia by cooperating with the E6 and E7 oncoproteins in promoting hyperproliferation of infected cells to malignant progression [57]. The action of the oncoprotein E5 supports tumor progression in early stages of disease, since the oncogene E5 is deleted after the process of integration of the viral genome is not necessary to maintain the transformed phenotype.

HPV Genetic Variants

Genetic variations in the HPV sequence have been associated with different risk for cancer progression. In several studies, the functional significance of HPV polymorphism was investigated as key events for the induction of cervical intraepithelial neoplasia (CIN) and the progression from CIN to cancer [58–60].

As reviewed by Bernard et al. [12], genetic and epidemiological studies show the existence of natural variations in the HPV genome. Differents variants of HPV-16 and HPV-18 co-evolved with African, Caucasian and Asian human phylogenetic branches. HPV-16 variants have been clessified into four major lineages based upon common phylogenetic patterns of single nucleotide polymorphisms: European Asian, including the sublineages European (EUR), and Asian (As), African 1 (AFR1), African 2 (AFR2) and Asian American/North American (AA/NA), including the sublineages Asian American 1, Asian American 2 and North American [61, 62]. HPV-18 variants are grouped in European (E), Asian-American (AA) and Africa (Af) groups [63, 64].

The names of the lineages abd sublineages originate from the geographical origin of the populations in which they were initially isolated. With regard to HPV-31 variants, it is suggested that these variants do not exhibit the same patterns of co-evolution with human ethnic groups as seen in HPV16 and HPV18 [14, 65, 66].

Humam Papillomavirus Type 16

Several studies about genetic variability of HPV-16 have been performed in the E6 gene, which codes an important viral oncoprotein. In these studies, it was investigated the association between E6 HPV-16 variations, viral persistence and progression of cervical neoplasia [16, 67, 68].

Studies conducted by Zehbe et al. [69] with Swedish women indicated that invasive cancers were more associated with E6 HPV-16 variants than with the prototype, where the most frequent E6 variation identified was L83V (at residue 83). This polymorphism was detected in 88% of invasive cervical carcinoma (ICC) and 44% of cervical intraepithelial neoplasia III (CIN) [69].

Grodzki et al. [70] identified a similar association in studies conducted with French women, where was found an elevated odds ratios of infection persistence and progression in women infected with the variation at residue 83.

The E6 oncoprotein interacts with a cellular protein p53 and alteration of the levels or activity of this protein could have a major impact on tumorigenesis, as mentioned earlier.

Variations within the E6 gene leading to changes in amino acid can change the biological or immunogenic properties of the encoded protein [71, 72]. With respect to the E6 functional activity, studies have showed that amino acid changes can alter their ability to abrogate serum/calcium-dependent differentiation, induce p53 degradation in vitro and regulate tumorigenesis by Notch signaling and oncogenic Ras [73].

Cento et al. (2009) identified several mutations in high-grade lesions patients from Italy, and among them, the N127H mutation was most interesting, since the N127 residue is considered necessary for the binding of the E6 protein to p53, a change at this position may affect the activity of the oncoprotein E6 [74]. In Indonesia, de Boer et al. [75] have found a high frequency of mutations. Among those, the nucleotide variation A276G in the E6 ORF promotes the amino acid change N58S of E6 protein in patientes with cervical intraepithelial neoplasia (CIN) and cervical cancer.

Analysis of the E7 oncogene indicates that the E7 ORF is very stable. Identified variations occurring within the E7 ORF in most instances do not affect amino acids sequences or the amino acid changes are located in regions considered not important for the transforming activity of the E7 oncoprotein [76, 77]. Cento et al. [77], in their study, identified a change at position 31, replacing Ser with Arg, and this change should alter the phosphorylation of E7 oncoprotein by Casein Kinase II (CKII) [74]. Another study reported a change in the nucleotide position 647 in the HPV-16 E7 ORF, with asparagine to serine mutation at position 29 (N29S) [75]. This mutation is likely to be significant because of its location in an immunoreactive region [69]. Furthermore, this mutation in E7 was significantly more frequent in carcinomas (70%) compared to the control group (33%) or CIN III group (50%) [78].

Nucleotide sequence variation within L1 gene can play an important role in the structure of the viral capsid, in the immune recognition, and in the viral neutralization and it is important in the interference in vaccine strategies [79]. For instance, the variation His202 within L1 protein can assemble into virus-like particles (VLPs) more efficiently than its prototype Asp202 [80]. In addition, variations in the 83-97 residues of the L1 gene have an impact on the yield of the L1 protein [81]. Several studies have been reported variants within HPV16 L1 gene [13, 61, 75, 77, 80, 82–91].

These studies have been performed in complete or partial sequence of L1 gene. Some of these described variants are nonsynonimous variants and are embedded within hypervariable immunodominant regions BC, DE, EF, FG, HI loops of L1 protein. Moreover, some of these variants are embedded within T-cell or B-cell epitopes binding region [92]. With regard to the vaccine strategies, the cross-protective efficacy vaccine could be different due to the nucleotide change within epitope regions [93]. However, despite the importance of the viral polymorphisms in the structure and biological function of the L1 protein of HPV-16, there are no studies demonstrating a link between HPV L1 gene variants and carcinogenesis.

The LCR is the binding site of cellular and viral transcription factors. The entire LCR is divided into three segments: the 5′segment, central region and 3′segment. The 5′segment contains binding sites for represses viral oncoprotein. The central region possesses epithelial-specific enhancer and the 3′segment contains the binding sites for replication and the p97 promoter.

Hence, variability in the nucleotide sequence of LCR can alter the expressions of E6 and E7 oncogenes as well as the viral replication of DNA. Several studies have reported nucleotide variation within LCR [15, 63, 79, 81, 82, 86, 89, 91, 94–106].

The variation G7521A within HPV-16 LCR has been found in some studies of cervical cancer [79, 82, 91, 96, 107]. The G7521A variant is located in the YY1 binding site and this variation can increase the p97 promoter activity three to six-fold [103].

Furthermore, other studies have demonstrated that non-European variants within LCR are related to the increase of promoter activity and, subsequently expression of E6 and E7 oncogenes. For instance, the variants AA or NA showed 3-fold increase in the promoter activity when compared to prototype sequence [107]. These results agreed with other studies that indicate the relationship between non- European variants and progression to lesion [16, 17, 59, 61, 67–69, 83, 108–110].

The E2 proteins of HPV are transcriptional transactivator proteins with very high affinities for their binding sites [111]. The E2 nucleotide sequence is divided into three domains: transactivation domain; hinge domain and; DNA binding domain. Therefore, variants within E2 gene can alter the DNA replication as well as the expression of early genes. In addition, the variants of E2 gene can alter the binding sites for transcriptional cell factors, which can alter the viral activity. In this context, several studies have reported variants within E2 gene in the tree domains [97, 112–117]. Moreover, variants or epigenetic factor within E2 and LCR can alter the expression of E6/E7 oncoproteins. For instance, the involvement of E2 binding site methylation in presence of intact E2, leading to loss of E2 repressor activity in CaCx [96].

Humam Papillomavirus Type 18

Studies suggest that HPV-18 variants are associated with different levels of oncogenic potential and persistence and histological tumor types [89, 118–121]. Much less is known about the clinical importance of HPV-18 variants, although it is the second most common HPV infection detected in cervical cancer and is the type most strongly associated with adenocarcinoma of the cervix [34, 122, 123]. Studies suggest that certain HPV-18 variants are more probable to be identified in adenocarcinomas and others in squamous cell carcinomas [119, 124]. In a study performed in Brazil, Villa et al. [17] identified a tendency for an increased risk of high-grade cytologic abnormalities associated with non-European variants, compared with European variants.

The study of genetic variability of E6 ORF carried out by Cerqueira et al. [125] revealed an amino acid alteration N129K. This change was also identified by de Boer et al. [124] in all HPV-18 African variants from Dutch, Indonesian and Surinamese patients. Codon 129 is highly conserved within oncogenic HPV genotypes.

Though, studies have demonstrated that this change in E6 ORF did not affect its capacity in promoting p53 degradation [125, 126].

In the case of E7, few changes have found, probably because it is known to be a more conserved ORF. de la Cruz Hernandez et al. [126] identified changes at positions 640, 751, 770, 806, 865 and 864 of E7 ORF, the latter leading to one amino acid change at position 92 (N92S), which does not discard the possibility of an altered E7 function.

Variants within L1 gene of HPV-18 are having been described in different population. Some of these variants are embedded within L1 binding epitope regions or in external loops. The knowledgemnt of these variants are important to vaccines strategies, due the quadrivalent and bivalent vaccine licenced are prevent HPV-18.

The major capsid L1 protein is target to neutralize antibody response. Therefore, variants within L1 nucleotide sequence can be important to immune response and viral strategies, since HPV-18 VLPs are used in bivalent and quadrivalent licensed vaccines. In the L1 coding region, the variants A to G transition at nucleotide 5503, C5701G, C6470G, C6625G, C6842G are reported in two studies [63, 127]. These variants are near to the L1 C-terminal domain, which may affect immune responses to HPV-18 capsid protein [63, 88].

With regard to the LCR, Cerqueira et al. [125] found A41G and T104C variations within HPV-18 LCR. These variations seem to be able to achieve a high activity of the E6/E7 p97 promoter by modulating Sp1 and YY1 activities. The studies that found specific HPV-18 variants were associated to cervical cancer in different populations, such as the variation C for T at nucleotide 104 are embedded into YY1 binding site. Moreover, non-European variants are also related to persistence, progression and oncogenicity in HPV-18. Villa et al. [17] showed that non-European variants tended to persist more frequently than European variants with regard to the risk of persistence for non-oncogenic HPV [17]. Moreover, the transcriptional activities in LCR was found also altered in 2.64-8.18 in LCR variants when compared to prototype sequence [128].

Humam Papillomavirus Type 31

Nucleotide and amino acid analysis were performed to E6 ORF of HPV-31, where it was identified the presence of nucleotide variations at positions 141, 190, 213, 368, 413 [65], 178, 297 [14], 321 [65] and 537 [66]. Mutations at positions 190, 368, 413 and 537 caused amino acid changes at codons 64 (T to A), 123 (K to R), 138 (A to V) and 144 (R to G), respectively [65,66]. Studies about the clinical relevance of HPV-31 variants are limited [66]. The observed genetics variations at positions 190 (A190G), 368 (A368G), 413 (C413T) and 537 (G537G) were located in T-cell and/or B-cell epitope site [65, 66]. These variations may influence the viral peptides presentation to T-cell, being this a key mechanism for the control of infection and development of cervical lesions. The recognition of T-cell determinants by T cells (principally T helper cells) contributes to the cell-mediated immune response against infectious organisms, as T cells cooperate with B cells in the induction and maintenance of an effective antibody response and contribute to the maturation of cytotoxic T cells by interacting with macrophages [129]. Considering the genetic variations of E7 ORF, it was detected nucleotide changes at positions 67, 111, 136, 184 [65] and 580, 592 [66]. Mutations at positions 67, 136 and 184 were classified as non-synonymous, causing amino acid changes at codons 23 (H to Y) 46 (E to Y) and 62 (K to E), respectively [65]. The observed genetics variations at positions 67 (C67T), 136 (G136A), 184 (A184G) were located in T-cell and/or B-cell epitope site [65]. With regard LCR of HPV-31, analysis revealed the G7449A, G7457A, C7474T, G7525A and T7575C variations are embedded in binding sites for the transcriptional factors, which potentially can affect the expression of early genes [102].

Humam Papillomavirus Type 33

The differential risk for cancer development associated to viral variants is not well documented to HPV-33, with scarce data.

Published study has explored the variability of this genotype [130], but no precise information on the prevalence of the different variants in lesion has been provided. did not reveal ethnic or geographical clustering as observed previously for HPV-16 and -18 [102].

Several studies have been reported variation within LCR, E6, E7 and L1 gene of HPV-33 [85, 98, 104, 131–133]. HPV-33 variants were significantly more frequently observed in CINs I/II than in CIN III/ICCs [134]. According to Khouadri et al. [98] the L83V variation at nucleotide 355 has been identified in HPV-16 at nucleotide 350 [98]. In HPV-16, this variation was associated in some studies with HSILs [69, 135], however in the study performed by Khouadri et al [98] the L83V variation was not associated with HPV persistence or the risk of HSILs [104]. In addition, HPV33 E6 variants were more frequently observed in CINs I/II than in CIN III/ICCs in a Japanese population [134]. The findings suggest the involvement of HPV-33 E6 variants in carcinogenesis process. Non–prototype variants within LCR of HPV-33 were significantly associated to HSILs in the Brazilian and Canadian populations [98]. The C7732G variation, which results in the loss of a putative binding site for the cellular upstream stimulatory factor, was significantly associated to HSILs [98]. The presence of a 78-base pair deletion in HPV-33 and the presence of nonsynonymous E7 variations in HPV-35 were associated to persistence [136]. These studies also suggested the involvement of LCR in the carcinogenesis and showed the relationship between non-prototype variants and high grade lesion.

Humam Papillomavirus Type 58

For HPV-58, the date for the risk of developing cervical cancer in association with viral variants is still scarce [102, 132, 134, 137–140]. Published studies have explored the variability of this genotype, but no accurate information on the prevalence of the different variants in lesion has been provided.

HPV-58 was reported to have a high frequency in East Asian, Central and South American. The HPV-58 did not reveal ethnic or geographical clustering as observed in HPV-16 and -18 [102]. Among HPV58-positive women, a study demonstrated that the occurrence of E7 C632T (T20I) and E7 G760A (G63S) variants showed a positive association with the severity of neoplasia [140], with OR higher than 6.5-fold [137]. However, no significant association was found between the E6 and E7 mutations of both HPV types and the cytological lesion found. Xin et al. [134], has found DNA sequence alterations at three nucleotide positions of the HPV-58 E6 ORF (C187T, C307T and C367A). However, E6 variation was found only at residue 86 with asparagine acid (D) being replaced with glutamic acid (E). The D86E variant was detected only in one CIN III case [134]. Still with respect to variation E6 ORF, Raiol et al. [86] examined eight isolates and all had the same sequence pattern with one variation at position 307 (C to T), as reported previously [14, 134]. In a study carried out by Cento et al. [102], were identified 13 nucleotide variations, however, no significant associations were found between the specifics variations identified and the cytological cervical lesions. With respect to E7 ORF, Cento et al. [102] identified 12 nucleotide substitution. The G41R is located at the end of the N-terminal unstructures domain of E7 protein, while the G at position 63 (G63S) is the initial amino acid of the β-2 sheet and this variation was more frequently present in CIN II/III and has been associated with an increased oncogenic risk [137].

With regard the HPV-58 LCR, a significant association was found between T7207A, C7284G, T7345C, T7369G, T431G and T7483G and abnormal cervical cytology [102]. Some mutations found in the LCR of HPV 58 are embedded into transcription binding sites, which can affect the transcription of the oncogenic genes [102].

References

[1]   Jemal, A., Bray, F., Center, M. M., Ferlay, J., Ward, E., Forman, D. Global cancer statistics. *CA Cancer J. Clin.* 2011, Mar. 1, 61, 69–90.

[2]   Hoory, T., Monie, A., Gravitt, P., Wu, T-C. Molecular Epidemiology of Human Papillomavirus. *J. Formos. Med. Assoc.*, 2008 Mar., 107, 198–217.

[3]   Bernard, H-U., Burk, R. D., Chen, Z., Van Doorslaer, K., Hausen, H., zur de Villiers, E-M. Classification of papillomaviruses (PVs) based on 189 PV types and proposal of taxonomic amendments. *Virology*, 2010 May 25, 401, 70–79.

[4]   Scheurer, M. E., Tortolero-Luna, G., Adler-Storthz, K. Human papillomavirus infection: biology, epidemiology, and prevention. *Int. J. Gynecol. Cancer Off. J. Int. Gynecol. Cancer Soc.*, 2005 Oct. 15, 727–746.

[5]   Baseman, J. G., Koutsky, L. A. The epidemiology of human papillomavirus infections. *J. Clin. Virol. Off Publ. Pan. Am. Soc. Clin. Virol.*, 2005 Mar., 32, Suppl. 1, S16–24.

[6]   De Villiers, E-M., Fauquet, C., Broker, T. R., Bernard, H-U., zur Hausen, H. Classification of papillomaviruses. *Virology*, 2004 Jun. 20, 324, 17–27.

[7]   Rombaldi, R. L., Serafini, E. P., Mandelli, J., Zimmermann, E., Losquiavo, K. P. Perinatal transmission of human papilomavirus DNA. *Virol. J.*, 2009, 6, 83.

[8]   Zur, Hausen; H. Papillomaviruses and cancer: from basic studies to clinical application. *Nat. Rev. Cancer*, 2002 May 2, 342–350.

[9]   Badaracco, G., Venuti, A., Morello, R., Muller, A., Marcante, M. L. Human papillomavirus in head and neck carcinomas: prevalence, physical status and relationship with clinical/pathological parameters. *Anticancer Res.*, 2000 Apr. 20, 1301–1305.

[10] Stevens, L. M. JAMA patient page. Papillomavirus. *Jama J. Am. Med. Assoc.*, 2002 May 8, 287, 2452.

[11] Burd, E. M. Human Papillomavirus and Cervical Cancer. *Clin. Microbiol. Rev.*, 2003 Jan. 1, 16, 1–17.

[12] Bernard, H-U., Calleja-Macias, I. E., Dunn, S. T. Genome variation of human papillomavirus types: phylogenetic and medical implications. *Int. J. Cancer J. Int. Cancer,* 2006 Mar. 1, 118, 1071–1076.

[13] Stewart, A. C., Eriksson, A. M., Manos, M. M., Muñoz, N., Bosch, F. X., Peto, J., et al. Intratype variation in 12 human papillomavirus types: a worldwide perspective. *J. Virol.*, 1996 May, 70, 3127–3136.

[14] Calleja-Macias, I. E., Villa, L. L., Prado, J. C., Kalantari, M., Allan, B., Williamson, A-L., et al. Worldwide genomic diversity of the high-risk human papillomavirus types 31, 35, 52, and 58, four close relatives of human papillomavirus type 16. *J. Virol.*, 2005 Nov., 79, 13630–13640.

[15] Prado, J. C., Calleja-Macias, I. E., Bernard, H-U., Kalantari, M., Macay, S. A., Allan, B., et al. Worldwide genomic diversity of the human papillomaviruses-53, 56, and 66, a group of high-risk HPVs unrelated to HPV-16 and HPV-18. *Virology*, 2005 Sep. 15, 340, 95–104.

[16] Xi, L. F., Critchlow, C. W., Wheeler, C. M., Koutsky, L. A., Galloway, D. A., Kuypers, J., et al. Risk of anal carcinoma in situ in relation to human papillomavirus type 16 variants. *Cancer Res.*, 1998 Sep. 1, 58, 3839–3844.

[17] Villa, L. L., Sichero, L., Rahal, P., Caballero, O., Ferenczy, A., Rohan, T., et al. Molecular variants of human papillomavirus types 16 and 18 preferentially associated with cervical neoplasia. *J. Gen. Virol.*, 2000 Dec., 81, 2959–2968.

[18] Hildesheim, A., Wang, S. S. Host and viral genetics and risk of cervical cancer: a review. *Virus Res.*, 2002 Nov., 89, 229–240.

[19] Lizano, M., De la Cruz-Hernández, E., Carrillo-García, A., García-Carrancá, A., Ponce de Leon-Rosales, S., Dueñas-González, A., et al. Distribution of HPV16 and 18 intratypic variants in normal cytology, intraepithelial lesions, and cervical cancer in a Mexican population. *Gynecol. Oncol.*, 2006 Aug., 102, 230–235.

[20] Calleja-Macias, I. E., Kalantari, M., Huh, J., Ortiz-Lopez, R., Rojas-Martinez, A., Gonzalez-Guerrero, J. F., et al. Genomic diversity of human papillomavirus-16, 18, 31, and 35 isolates in a Mexican population and relationship to European, African, and Native American variants. *Virology*, 2004 Feb. 20, 319, 315–323.

[21] Zur Hausen, H. Papillomavirus infections--a major cause of human cancers. *Biochim. Biophys. Acta*, 1996 Oct. 9, 1288, F55–78.

[22] Ter Harmsel, B., Smedts, F., Kuijpers, J., van Muyden, R., Oosterhuis, W., Quint, W. Relationship between human papillomavirus type 16 in the cervix and intraepithelial neoplasia. *Obstet. Gynecol.*, 1999 Jan., 93, 46–50.

[23] Hopman, E. H., Rozendaal, L., Voorhorst, F. J., Walboomers, J. M., Kenemans, P., Helmerhorst, T. J. High risk human papillomavirus in women with normal cervical cytology prior to the development of abnormal cytology and colposcopy. *Bjog. Int. J. Obstet. Gynaecol.*, 2000 May, 107, 600–604.

[24] Bosch, F. X., de Sanjosé, S. Chapter 1: Human papillomavirus and cervical cancer--burden and assessment of causality. *J. Natl. Cancer Inst. Monogr.*, 2003, 3–13.

[25] Walboomers, J. M., Jacobs, M. V., Manos, M. M., Bosch, F. X., Kummer, J. A., Shah, K. V., et al. Human papillomavirus is a necessary cause of invasive cervical cancer worldwide. *J. Pathol.*, 1999 Sep, 189, 12–19.

[26] Muñoz, N. Human papillomavirus and cancer: the epidemiological evidence. *J. Clin. Virol. Off Publ. Pan. Am. Soc. Clin. Virol.*, 2000 Oct., 19, 1–5.

[27] Van Muyden, R. C., ter Harmsel, B. W., Smedts, F. M., Hermans, J., Kuijpers, J. C., Raikhlin, N. T., et al. Detection and typing of human papillomavirus in cervical carcinomas in Russian women: a prognostic study. *Cancer* 1999 May 1, 85, 2011–2016.

[28] Zielinski, G. D., Snijders, P. J. F., Rozendaal, L., Daalmeijer, N. F., Risse, E. K. J., Voorhorst, F. J., et al.: The presence of high-risk HPV combined with specific p53 and p16INK4a expression patterns points to high-risk HPV as the main causative agent for adenocarcinoma in situ and adenocarcinoma of the cervix. *J. Pathol.*, 2003 Dec., 201, 535–543.

[29] Trottier, H., Franco, E. L. The epidemiology of genital human papillomavirus infection. *Vaccine*, 2006 Mar. 30, 24 Suppl. 1, S1–15.

[30] Bosch, F. X., Lorincz, A., Muñoz, N., Meijer, C. J. L. M., Shah, K. V. The causal relation between human papillomavirus and cervical cancer. *J. Clin. Pathol.*, 2002 Apr., 55, 244–265.

[31] Snijders, P. J. F., Steenbergen, R. D. M., Heideman, D. A. M., Meijer, C. J. L. M. HPV-mediated cervical carcinogenesis: concepts and clinical implications. *J. Pathol.*, 2006 Jan., 208, 152–164.

[32] Zeferino, L. C., Amaral, R. G. do., Dufloth, R. M. HPV e a neoplasia do colo do útero; HPV and the neoplasms uterine cervix. *Femina*, 2002 Aug., 30, 471–475.

[33] Muñoz, N., Castellsagué, X., de González, A. B., Gissmann, L. Chapter 1: HPV in the etiology of human cancer. *Vaccine*, 2006 Aug. 31, 24 Suppl. 3, S3 1–10.

[34] Muñoz, N., Bosch, F. X., de Sanjosé, S., Herrero, R., Castellsagué, X., Shah, K. V., et al. Epidemiologic Classification of Human Papillomavirus Types Associated with Cervical Cancer. *N Engl. J. Med.*, 2003, 348, 518–527.

[35] Schiffman, M., Herrero, R., Desalle, R., Hildesheim, A., Wacholder, S., Rodriguez, A. C., et al. The carcinogenicity of human papillomavirus types reflects viral evolution. *Virology*, 2005 Jun. 20, 337, 76–84.

[36] Pfister, H. Chapter 8: Human papillomavirus and skin cancer. *J. Natl. Cancer Inst. Monogr.*, 2003, 52–56.

[37] Bernard, H-U. Gene expression of genital human papillomaviruses and considerations on potential antiviral approaches. *Antivir. Ther.*, 2002 Dec., 7, 219–237.

[38] Nelson, L. M., Rose, R. C., Moroianu, J. Nuclear import strategies of high risk HPV16 L1 major capsid protein. *J. Biol. Chem.* 2002 Jun. 28, 277, 23958–23964.

[39] Dunne, E. F., Markowitz, L. E. Genital Human Papillomavirus Infection. *Clin. Infect. Dis.*, 2006 Sep. 1, 43, 624–629.

[40] Stanley, M. Prophylactic human papillomavirus vaccines: will they do their job? *J. Intern. Med.,* 2010 Mar. 1, 267, 251–259.

[41] Schiffman, M., Castle, P. E., Jeronimo, J., Rodriguez, A. C., Wacholder, S. Human papillomavirus and cervical cancer. *Lancet*, 2007 Sep. 8, 370, 890–907.

[42] Motoyama, S., Ladines-Llave, C. A., Luis Villanueva, S., Mauro, T. The role of human papilloma virus in the molecular biology of cervical carcinogenesis. *Kobe J. Med. Sci.*, 2004 Jan., 50, 9–19.

[43] Thierry, F., Benotmane, M. A., Demeret, C., Mori, M., Teissier, S., Desaintes, C. A genomic approach reveals a novel mitotic pathway in papillomavirus carcinogenesis. *Cancer Res.*, 2004 Feb. 1, 64, 895–903.

[44] Horvath, C. A., Boulet, G. A., Renoux, V. M., Delvenne, P. O., Bogers, J-P. J. Mechanisms of cell entry by human papillomaviruses: an overview. *Virol. J.,* 2010 Jan. 20, 7, 11.

[45] Doorbar, J. The papillomavirus life cycle. *J. Clin. Virol.*, 2005 Mar., 32, 7–15.

[46] Sapp, M., Day, P. M. Structure, attachment and entry of polyoma- and papillomaviruses. *Virology*, 2009 Feb. 20, 384, 400–409.

[47] Stubenrauch, F., Laimins, L. A. Human papillomavirus life cycle: active and latent phases. *Semin. Cancer Biol.*, 1999 Dec., 9, 379–386.

[48] Fehrmann, F., Laimins, L. A. Human papillomaviruses: targeting differentiating epithelial cells for malignant transformation. *Oncogene*, 2003 Aug. 11, 22, 5201–5207.

[49] McCance, D. J. Transcriptional regulation by human papillomaviruses. *Curr. Opin. Genet. Dev.*, 2005 Oct., 15, 515–519.

[50] McLaughlin-Drubin, M. E., Munger, K. Oncogenic Activities of Human Papillomaviruses. *Virus Res.*, 2009 Aug., 143, 195–208.

[51] Boulet, G., Horvath, C., Broeck, D. V., Sahebali, S., Bogers, J. Human papillomavirus: E6 and E7 oncogenes. *Int. J. Biochem. Cell Biol.*, 2007, 39, 2006–2011.

[52] Sandal, T. Molecular aspects of the mammalian cell cycle and cancer. *Oncologist*, 2002, 7, 73–81.

[53] Zur Hausen, H. Papillomaviruses causing cancer: evasion from host-cell control in early events in carcinogenesis. *J. Natl. Cancer Inst.*, 2000 May 3, 92, 690–698.

[54] Shin, M-K., Balsitis, S., Brake, T., Lambert, P. F. Human papillomavirus E7 oncoprotein overrides the tumor suppressor activity of p21Cip1 in cervical carcinogenesis. *Cancer Res.*, 2009 Jul. 15, 69, 5656–5663.

[55] Arends, M. J., Buckley, C. H., Wells, M. Aetiology, pathogenesis, and pathology of cervical neoplasia. *J. Clin. Pathol.*, 1998 Feb., 51, 96–103.

[56] Woodman, C. B. J., Collins, S. I., Young, L. S. The natural history of cervical HPV infection: unresolved issues. *Nat. Rev. Cancer*, 2007 Jan., 7, 11–22.

[57] DiMaio, D., Mattoon, D. Mechanisms of cell transformation by papillomavirus E5 proteins. *Oncogene*, 2001 Nov. 26, 20, 7866–7873.

[58] Asadurian, Y., Kurilin, H., Lichtig, H., Jackman, A., Gonen, P., Tommasino, M., et al. Activities of human papillomavirus 16 E6 natural variants in human keratinocytes. *J. Med. Virol.*, 2007 Nov., 79, 1751–1760.

[59] Zehbe, I., Lichtig, H., Westerback, A., Lambert, P. F., Tommasino, M., Sherman, L. Rare human papillomavirus 16 E6 variants reveal significant oncogenic potential. *Mol. Cancer,* 2011, 10, 77.

[60] Sichero, L., Sobrinho, J. S., Villa, L. L. Oncogenic potential diverge among human papillomavirus type 16 natural variants. *Virology*, 2012 Oct. 10, 432, 127–132.

[61] Yamada, T., Manos, M. M., Peto, J., Greer, C. E., Munoz, N., Bosch, F. X., et al. Human papillomavirus type 16 sequence variation in cervical cancers: a worldwide perspective. *J. Virol.*, 1997 Mar.,71, 2463–2472.

[62] Cornet, I., Gheit, T., Franceschi; Vignat, J., Burk, R. D., Sylla, B. S., et al. Human papillomavirus type 16 genetic variants: phylogeny and classification based on E6 and LCR. *J. Virol.*, 2012 Jun., 86, 6855–6861.

[63] Arias-Pulido, H., Peyton, C. L., Torrez-Martínez, N., Anderson, D. N., Wheeler, C. M. Human papillomavirus type 18 variant lineages in United States populations characterized by sequence analysis of LCR-E6, E2, and L1 regions. *Virology*, 2005 Jul. 20, 338, 22–34.

[64] Bernard, H-U. The clinical importance of the nomenclature, evolution and taxonomy of human papillomaviruses. *J. Clin. Virol. Off Publ. Pan. Am. Soc. Clin. Virol.*, 2005 Mar., 32 Suppl. 1:S1–6.

[65] Chagas, B. S., Batista, M. V. A., Guimarães, V., Balbino, V. Q., Crovella, S., Freitas, A. C. New variants of E6 and E7 oncogenes of human papillomavirus type 31 identified in Northeastern Brazil. *Gynecol. Oncol.*, 2011 Nov., 123, 284–288.

[66] Chagas, B. S., Batista, M. V. de A., Crovella, S., Gurgel, A. P. A. D., Silva Neto, J. da C., Serra, I. G. S. S., et al. Novel E6 and E7 oncogenes variants of human

papillomavirus type 31 in Brazilian women with abnormal cervical cytology. *Infect. Genet. Evol. J. Mol. Epidemiol. Evol. Genet. Infect. Dis.*, 2013 Feb. 10, 16C, 13–18.

[67]   Xi, L. F., Koutsky, L. A., Galloway, D. A., Kiviat, N. B., Kuypers, J., Hughes, J. P., et al. Genomic Variation of Human Papillomavirus Type 16 and Risk for High Grade Cervical Intraepithelial Neoplasia. *J. Natl. Cancer Inst.*, 1997 Jun. 4, 89, 796 –802.

[68]   Londesborough, P., Ho, L., Terry, G., Cuzick, J., Wheeler, C., Singer, A. Human papillomavirus genotype as a predictor of persistence and development of high-grade lesions in women with minor cervical abnormalities. *Int. J. Cancer,* 1996 Oct. 21, 69, 364–368.

[69]   Zehbe, I., Wilander, E., Delius, H., Tommasino, M. Human papillomavirus 16 E6 variants are more prevalent in invasive cervical carcinoma than the prototype. *Cancer Res.,* 1998 Feb. 15, 58, 829–833.

[70]   Grodzki, M., Besson, G.,Clavel, C., Arslan, A., Franceschi, S., Birembaut, P., et al. Increased risk for cervical disease progression of French women infected with the human papillomavirus type 16 E6-350G variant. *Cancer Epidemiol. Biomarkers Prev. Publ. Am. Assoc. Cancer Res. Cosponsored Am. Soc. Prev. Oncol.*, 2006 Apr. 15, 820– 822.

[71]   Ellis, J. R., Keating, P. J., Baird, J., Hounsell, E. F., Renouf, D. V., Rowe, M., et al. The association of an HPV16 oncogene variant with HLA-B7 has implications for vaccine design in cervical cancer. *Nat. Med.*,1995 May, 1, 464–470.

[72]   Zehbe, I., Mytilineos, J., Wikström, I., Henriksen, R., Edler, L., Tommasino, M. Association between human papillomavirus 16 E6 variants and human leukocyte antigen class I polymorphism in cervical cancer of Swedish women. *Hum. Immunol.*, 2003 May, 64, 538–542.

[73]   Chakrabarti, O., Veeraraghavalu, K., Tergaonkar, V., Liu, Y., Androphy, E. J., Stanley, M. A., et al.: Human papillomavirus type 16 E6 amino acid 83 variants enhance E6-mediated MAPK signaling and differentially regulate tumorigenesis by notch signaling and oncogenic Ras. *J. Virol.*, 2004 Jun., 78, 5934–5945.

[74]   Wise-Draper, T. M., Wells, S. I. Papillomavirus E6 and E7 proteins and their cellular targets. *Front Biosci. J. Virtual Libr.*, 2008, 13, 1003–1017.

[75]   De Boer, M. A., Peters, L. A. W., Aziz, M. F., Siregar, B., Cornain, S., Vrede, M. A., et al. Human papillomavirus type 16 E6, E7, and L1 variants in cervical cancer in Indonesia, Suriname, and The Netherlands. *Gynecol. Oncol.*, 2004 Aug., 94, 488–494.

[76]   Phelps, W. C., Münger, K., Yee, C. L., Barnes, J. A., Howley, P. M., Structure-function analysis of the human papillomavirus type 16 E7 oncoprotein. *J. Virol.*, 1992 Apr., 66, 2418–2427.

[77]   Cento, V., Ciccozzi, M., Ronga, L., Perno, C. F., Ciotti, M. Genetic diversity of human papillomavirus type 16 E6, E7, and L1 genes in Italian women with different grades of cervical lesions. *J. Med. Virol.*, 2009, 81, 1627–1634.

[78]   Song, Y. S., Kee, S. H., Kim, J. W., Park, N. H., Kang, S. B., Chang, W. H., et al.: Major Sequence Variants in E7 Gene of Human Papillomavirus Type 16 from Cervical Cancerous and Noncancerous Lesions of Korean Women. *Gynecol. Oncol.*, 1997 Agosto, 66, 275–281.

[79]   Pande, S., Jain, N., Prusty, B. K., Bhambhani, S., Gupta, S., Sharma, R., et al.: Human Papillomavirus Type 16 Variant Analysis of E6, E7, and L1 Genes and Long Control

Region in Biopsy Samples from Cervical Cancer Patients in North India. *J. Clin. Microbiol.,* 2008 Mar. 1, 46, 1060–1066.

[80]   Kirnbauer, R., Taub, J., Greenstone, H., Roden, R., Dürst, M., Gissmann, L., et al. Efficient self-assembly of human papillomavirus type 16 L1 and L1-L2 into virus-like particles. *J. Virol.,* 1993 Dec., 67, 6929–6936.

[81]   Chansaenroj, J., Theamboonlers, A., Junyangdikul, P., Swangvaree, S., Karalak, A., Poovorawan, Y. Whole genome analysis of human papillomavirus type 16 multiple infection in cervical cancer patients. *Asian Pac. J. Cancer Prev. Apjcp,* 2012, 13, 599–606.

[82]   Tornesello, M. L., Duraturo, M. L., Salatiello, I., Buonaguro, L., Losito, S., Botti, G., et al.: Analysis of human papillomavirus type-16 variants in Italian women with cervical intraepithelial neoplasia and cervical cancer. *J. Med. Virol.,* 2004 Sep., 74, 117–126.

[83]   Sichero, L., Villa, L. L. Epidemiological and functional implications of molecular variants of human papillomavirus. *Braz. J. Med. Biol. Res. Rev. Bras. Pesqui Médicas E Biológicas Soc. Bras. Biofísica Al,* 2006 Jun., 39, 707–717.

[84]   Sun, Z., Ren, G., Cui, X., Zhou, W., Liu, C., Ruan, Q. Genetic Diversity of HPV-16 E6, E7, and L1 Genes in Women With Cervical Lesions in Liaoning Province, China. *Int. J. Gynecol. Cancer,* 2011 Apr., 21, 551–558.

[85]   Ntova, C. K., Kottaridi, C., Chranioti, A., Spathis, A., Kassanos, D., Paraskevaidis, E., et al. Genetic Variability and Phylogeny of High Risk HPV Type 16, 18, 31, 33 and 45 L1 Gene in Greek Women. *Int. J. Mol. Sci.,* 2011 Dec. 22, 13, 1–17.

[86]   Raiol, T., Wyant, P. S., de Amorim, R. M. S., Cerqueira, D. M., Milanezi, N., von G Brígido, M de M., et al. Genetic variability and phylogeny of the high-risk HPV-31, -33, -35, -52, and -58 in central Brazil. *J. Med. Virol.,* 2009 Apr., 81,685–692.

[87]   Yue, Y., Yang, H., Wu, K., Yang, L., Chen, J., Huang, X., et al.: Genetic variability in L1 and L2 genes of HPV-16 and HPV-58 in Southwest China. *Plos One,* 2013, 8, e55204.

[88]   Frati, E., Bianchi, S., Colzani, D., Zappa, A., Orlando, G., Tanzi, E. Genetic variability in the major capsid L1 protein of human papillomavirus type 16 (HPV-16) and 18 (HPV-18). *Infect. Genet. Evol. J. Mol. Epidemiol. Evol. Genet. Infect. Dis.,* 2011 Dec., 11,2119–2124.

[89]   Sichero, L., Ferreira, S., Trottier, H., Duarte-Franco, E., Ferenczy, A., Franco, E. L., et al. High grade cervical lesions are caused preferentially by non-European variants of HPVs 16 and 18. *Int. J. Cancer J. Int. Cancer,* 2007 Apr. 15, 120, 1763–1768.

[90]   Wheeler, C. M., Yamada, T., Hildesheim, A., Jenison, S. A. Human papillomavirus type 16 sequence variants: identification by E6 and L1 lineage-specific hybridization. *J. Clin. Microbiol.,* 1997 Jan., 35, 11–19.

[91]   Shang, Q., Wang, Y., Fang, Y., Wei, L., Chen, S., Sun, Y., et al. Human Papillomavirus Type 16 Variant Analysis of E6, E7, and L1 Genes and Long Control Region in Identification of Cervical Carcinomas in Patients in Northeast China. *J. Clin. Microbiol.,* 2011 Jul. 1, 49, 2656–2663.

[92]   Pillai, M. R., Hariharan, R., Babu, J. M., Lakshmi, S., Chiplunkar, S. V., Patkar, M., et al. Molecular variants of HPV-16 associated with cervical cancer in Indian population. *Int. J. Cancer J. Int. Cancer,* 2009 Jul. 1, 125, 91–103.

[93]   Olsson, S-E., Kjaer, S. K., Sigurdsson, K., Iversen, O-E., Hernandez-Avila, M., Wheeler, C. M., et al. Evaluation of quadrivalent HPV 6/11/16/18 vaccine efficacy

against cervical and anogenital disease in subjects with serological evidence of prior vaccine type HPV infection. *Hum. Vaccin.*, 2009 Oct., 5, 696–704.

[94] López-Saavedra, A., González-Maya, L., Ponce-de-León, S., García-Carrancá, A., Mohar, A., Lizano, M. Functional implication of sequence variation in the long control region and E2 gene among human papillomavirus type 18 variants. *Arch. Virol.*, 2009 May 1, 154, 747–754.

[95] Veress, G., Szarka, K., Dong, X. P., Gergely, L., Pfister, H. Functional significance of sequence variation in the E2 gene and the long control region of human papillomavirus type 16. *J. Gen. Virol.*, 1999 Apr. 1, 80, 1035–1043.

[96] Bhattacharjee, B., Sengupta, S. HPV16 E2 gene disruption and polymorphisms of E2 and LCR: Some significant associations with cervical cancer in Indian women. *Gynecol. Oncol.*, 2006 Fevereiro, 100, 372–378.

[97] Eriksson, A., Herron, J. R., Yamada, T., Wheeler, C. M. Human papillomavirus type 16 variant lineages characterized by nucleotide sequence analysis of the E5 coding segment and the E2 hinge region. *J. Gen. Virol.*, 1999 Mar., 1; 80, 595–600.

[98] Khouadri, S., Villa, L. L., Simon, Gagnon; Koushik, A., Richardson, H., Ferreira, S., et al. Human Papillomavirus Type 33 Polymorphisms and High-Grade Squamous Intraepithelial Lesions of the Uterine Cervix. *J. Infect. Dis.*, 2006 Outubro, 194, 886–894.

[99] Cento, V., Rahmatalla, N., Ciccozzi, M., Lo Presti, A., Perno, C. F., Ciotti, M. Human papillomaviruses 53 and 66: clinical aspects and genetic analysis. *Virus Res.*, 2012 Jan., 163, 212–222.

[100] Nasir, L., Gault, E., Morgan, I. M., Chambers, G., Ellsmore, V., Campo, M. S. Identification and functional analysis of sequence variants in the long control region and the E2 open reading frame of bovine papillomavirus type 1 isolated from equine sarcoids. *Virology*, 2007 Aug. 1, 364, 355–361.

[101] Schmidt, M., Kedzia, W., Goździcka-Józefiak, A. Intratype HPV16 sequence variation within LCR of isolates from asymptomatic carriers and cervical cancers. *J. Clin. Virol. Off Publ. Pan. Am. Soc. Clin. Virol.*, 2001 Dec., 23, 65–77.

[102] Cento, V., Rahmatalla, N., Ciccozzi, M., Perno, C. F., Ciotti, M. Intratype variations of HPV 31 and 58 in Italian women with abnormal cervical cytology. *J. Med. Virol.*, 2011 Oct., 83, 1752–1761.

[103] Dong, X. P., Pfister, H. Overlapping YY1- and aberrant SP1-binding sites proximal to the early promoter of human papillomavirus type 16. *J. Gen. Virol.*, 1999 Aug., 80 (Pt 8), 2097–2101.

[104] Gagnon, S., Hankins, C., Money, D., Pourreaux, K., Franco, E., Coutlée, F. Polymorphism of the L1 capsid gene and persistence of human papillomavirus type 52 infection in women at high risk or infected by HIV. *J. Acquir. Immune Defic. Syndr.*, 1999 2007 Jan. 1, 44, 61–65.

[105] Kämmer, C., Tommasino, M., Syrjänen, S., Delius, H., Hebling, U., Warthorst, U., et al. Variants of the long control region and the E6 oncogene in European human papillomavirus type 16 isolates: implications for cervical disease. *Br. J. Cancer*, 2002 Jan. 21, 86, 269–273.

[106] Pittayakhajonwut, D., Angeletti, P. C. Viral trans-factor independent replication of human papillomavirus genomes. *Virol. J.*, 2010, 7, 123.

[107] Kämmer, C., Warthorst, U., Torrez-Martinez, N., Wheeler, C. M., Pfister, H. Sequence analysis of the long control region of human papillomavirus type 16 variants and functional consequences for P97 promoter activity. *J. Gen. Virol.*, 2000 Aug. 1, 81, 1975–1981.

[108] Ho, C-M., Yang, S-S., Chien, T-Y., Huang, S-H., Jeng, C-J., Chang, S-F., Detection and quantitation of human papillomavirus type 16, 18 and 52 DNA in the peripheral blood of cervical cancer patients. *Gynecol. Oncol.*, 2005 Dec., 99, 615–621.

[109] Schiffman, M., Rodriguez, A. C., Chen, Z., Wacholder, S., Herrero, R., Hildesheim, A., et al. A Population-Based Prospective Study of Carcinogenic Human Papillomavirus Variant Lineages, Viral Persistence, and Cervical Neoplasia. *Cancer Res.*, 2010 Avril, 70, 3159 –3169.

[110] Burroni, E., Bisanzi, S., Sani, C., Puliti, D., Carozzi, F. Codon 72 polymorphism of p53 and HPV type 16 E6 variants as risk factors for patients with squamous epithelial lesion of the uterine cervix. *J. Med. Virol.*, 2013 Jan., 85, 83–90.

[111] Steger, G., Corbach, S. Dose-dependent regulation of the early promoter of human papillomavirus type 18 by the viral E2 protein. *J. Virol.*, 1997 Jan. 1 71, 50–58.

[112] Tsakogiannis, D., Ruether, I. G. A., Kyriakopoulou, Z., Pliaka, V., Theoharopoulou, A., Skordas, V., et al. Sequence variation analysis of the E2 gene of human papilloma virus type 16 in cervical lesions from women in Greece. *Arch. Virol.*, 2012 May 1, 157, 825–832.

[113] Azizi, N., Brazete, J., Hankins, C., Money, D., Fontaine, J., Koushik, A., et al. Influence of human papillomavirus type 16 (HPV-16) E2 polymorphism on quantification of HPV-16 episomal and integrated DNA in cervicovaginal lavages from women with cervical intraepithelial neoplasia. *J. Gen. Virol.*, 2008 Jul. 1, 89, 1716 –1728.

[114] Graham, D. A., Herrington, C. S. HPV-16 E2 gene disruption and sequence variation in CIN 3 lesions and invasive squamous cell carcinomas of the cervix: relation to numerical chromosome abnormalities. *Mol. Pathol.*, 2000 Aug. 1, 53, 201–206.

[115] Giannoudis, A., Duin, M., van, Snijders, P. J. F., Herrington, C. S. Variation in the E2-binding domain of HPV 16 is associated with high-grade squamous intraepithelial lesions of the cervix. *Br. J. Cancer*, 2001 Apr., 84, 1058–1063.

[116] Casas, L., Galvan, S. C., Ordoñez, R. M., Lopez, N., Guido, M., Berumen, J. Asian-American variants of human papillomavirus type 16 have extensive mutations in the E2 gene and are highly amplified in cervical carcinomas. *Int. J. Cancer*, 1999, 83, 449–455.

[117] Watts, K. J., Thompson, C. H., Cossart, Y. E., Rose, B. R. Sequence variation and physical state of human papillomavirus type 16 cervical cancer isolates from Australia and New Caledonia. *Int. J. Cancer J. Int. Cancer*, 2002 Feb. 20, 97, 868–874.

[118] Altekruse, S. F., Lacey, J. V. Jr; Brinton, L. A., Gravitt, P. E., Silverberg, S. G., Barnes, W. A. Jr; et al. Comparison of human papillomavirus genotypes, sexual, and reproductive risk factors of cervical adenocarcinoma and squamous cell carcinoma: Northeastern United States. *Am. J. Obstet. Gynecol.*, 2003 Mar., 188, 657–663.

[119] Burk, R. D., Terai, M., Gravitt, P. E., Brinton, L. A., Kurman, R. J., Barnes, W. A., et al. Distribution of human papillomavirus types 16 and 18 variants in squamous cell carcinomas and adenocarcinomas of the cervix. *Cancer Res.*, 2003 Nov. 1, 63, 7215–7220.

[120] Schlecht, N. F., Burk, R. D., Palefsky, J. M., Minkoff, H., Xue, X., Massad, L. S., et al. Variants of human papillomaviruses 16 and 18 and their natural history in human immunodeficiency virus-positive women. *J. Gen. Virol.*, 2005 Oct., 86, 2709–2720.

[121] Xi, L. F., Koutsky, L. A., Hildesheim, A., Galloway, D. A., Wheeler, C. M., Winer, R. L., et al. Risk for high-grade cervical intraepithelial neoplasia associated with variants of human papillomavirus types 16 and 18. *Cancer Epidemiol. Biomarkers Prev. Publ. Am. Assoc. Cancer Res. Cosponsored Am. Soc. Prev. Oncol.*, 2007 Jan., 16, 4–10.

[122] Beskow, A. H., Engelmark, M. T., Magnusson, J. J., Gyllensten, U. B. Interaction of host and viral risk factors for development of cervical carcinoma in situ. *Int. J. Cancer J. Int. Cancer,* 2005 Nov. 20, 117, 690–692.

[123] Teshima, H., Beaudenon, S., Koi, S., Katase, K., Hasumi, K., Masubuchi, K., et al. Human papillomavirus type 18 DNA sequences in adenocarcinoma and adenosquamous carcinoma of the uterine cervix. *Arch. Gynecol. Obstet.*,1997, 259, 169–177.

[124] De Boer, M. A., Peters, L. A. W., Aziz, M. F., Siregar, B., Cornain, S., Vrede, M. A., et al. Human papillomavirus type 18 variants: histopathology and E6/E7 polymorphisms in three countries. *Int. J. Cancer J. Int. Cancer*, 2005 Apr. 10, 114, 422–425.

[125] Cerqueira, D. M., Raiol, T., Véras, N. M. C., Von Gal Milanezi, N., Amaral, F. A., De Macedo Brígido, M.,et al. New variants of human papillomavirus type 18 identified in central Brazil. *Virus Genes* 2008, 37, 282–287.

[126] De la Cruz-Hernández, E., García-Carrancá, A., Mohar-Betancourt, A., Dueñas-González, A., Contreras-Paredes, A., Pérez-Cardenas, E., et al. Differential splicing of E6 within human papillomavirus type 18 variants and functional consequences. *J. Gen. Virol.,* 2005, 86, 2459 –2468.

[127] Shen, M., Ding, X., Li, T., Chen, G., Zhou, X. Sequence variation analysis of HPV-18 isolates in southwest China. *Plos One*, 2013, 8, e56614.

[128] Sichero, L., Franco, E. L., Villa, L. L. Different P105 Promoter Activities among Natural Variants of Human Papillomavirus Type 18. *J. Infect. Dis.,* 2005 Mar. 1,191, 739–742.

[129] Comerford, S. A., McCance, D. J., Dougan, G. JP: Identification of T- and B-cell epitopes of the E7 protein of human papillomavirus type 16. *J. Virol.*, 1991 Setembro, 65:4681–4690.

[130] Chen, Z., Schiffman, M., Herrero, R., DeSalle, R., Anastos, K., Segondy, M., et al.: Evolution and Taxonomic Classification of Human Papillomavirus 16 (HPV16)-Related Variant Genomes: HPV31, HPV33, HPV35, HPV52, HPV58 and HPV67. *Plos One* 2011 Maio;6:e20183.

[131] Cornut, G., Gagnon, S., Hankins, C., Money, D., Pourreaux, K., Franco, E. L., et al.: Polymorphism of the capsid L1 gene of human papillomavirus types 31, 33, and 35. *J. Med. Virol.* 2010 Jul.;82:1168–1178.

[132] Raiol, T., Wyant, P. S., de Amorim, R. M. S., Cerqueira, D. M., Milanezi N von G., Brígido M de M., et al.: Genetic variability and phylogeny of the high-risk HPV-31, -33, -35, -52, and -58 in central Brazil. *J. Med. Virol.* 2009 Apr.; 81:685–692.

[133] Vrtačnik Bokal, E., Kocjan, B. J., Poljak, M., Bogovac, Ž., Jančar, N.: Genomic variants of human papillomavirus genotypes 16, 18, and 33 in women with cervical cancer in Slovenia. *J. Obstet. Gynaecol. Res.* 2010 Dec. 1;36:1204–1213.

[134] Xin, C. Y., Matsumoto, K., Yoshikawa, H., Yasugi, T., Onda, T., Nakagawa, S., et al.: Analysis of E6 variants of human papillomavirus type 33, 52 and 58 in Japanese women with cervical intraepithelial neoplasia/cervical cancer in relation to their oncogenic potential. *Cancer Lett*. 2001 Setembro;170:19–24.

[135] Nindl, I., Rindfleisch, K., Lotz, B., Schneider, A., Dürst, M.: Uniform distribution of HPV 16 E6 and E7 variants in patients with normal histology, cervical intra-epithelial neoplasia and cervical cancer. *Int. J. Cancer* 1999 Jul. 19;82:203–207.

[136] Gagnon, S., Hankins, C., Tremblay, C., Forest, P., Pourreaux, K., Coutlée, F., et al.: Viral Polymorphism in Human Papillomavirus Types 33 and 35 and Persistent and Transient Infection in the Genital Tract of Women. *J. Infect. Dis.* 2004 Nov. 1;190: 1575–1585.

[137] Chan, P. K. S., Lam, C.-W., Cheung, T.-H., Li, W. W. H., Lo, K. W. K., Chan, M. Y. M., et al.: Association of Human Papillomavirus Type 58 Variant With the Risk of Cervical Cancer. *J. Natl. Cancer Inst.* 2002;94:1249 –1253.

[138] Cerqueira, D. M., Camara, G. N. D. L., Da Cruz, M. R., Silva, E. O., Brígido, M. D. M., Martins, C. R. F.: Variants of human papillomavirus types 53, 58 and 66 identified in Central Brazil. *Virus Genes* 2003;26:83–87.

[139] Wu, E., Zha, X., Yu, X., Zhang, G., Wu, Y., Fan, Y., et al.: Profile of physical status and gene variation of human papillomavirus 58 genome in cervical cancer. *J. Gen. Virol.* 2009 May 1;90:1229–1237.

[140] Ding, T., Wang, X., Ye, F., Cheng, X., Ma, D., Lu, W., et al.: Distribution of human papillomavirus 58 and 52 E6/E7 variants in cervical neoplasia in Chinese women. *Gynecol. Oncol.* 2010 Dec.;119:436–443.

In: Cervical Cancer
Editor: Laurie Elit

ISBN: 978-1-62948-062-6
© 2014 Nova Science Publishers, Inc.

Chapter II

Methods for Cervical Cancer Screening: The Differences Between Developing and Developed Countries

Satoshi Nakagawa, Kiyoshi Yoshino,
Yutaka Ueda and Tadashi Kimura
Department of Obstetrics and Gynecology,
Osaka University, Graduate School of Medicine, Osaka, Japan

Abstract

Cervical cancer is one of the easiest female cancers to prevent, with proper screening for precancerous lesions and adequate follow-up. The Pap screening test, which evaluates exfoliated cervical cells to identify early stage or precancerous cytological abnormalities, has played a central role in this breakthrough in cancer prevention, to the point where some guidelines now recommend a Pap test every 3 years for average-risk women. Although Pap screening was associated with at least a 60% reduction of cancer in developed countries, it has been more difficult to establish similar effective screening program in developing countries. Recently, the HPV (human papillomavirus) test has become an important player in cervical cancer screening. Detection of high-risk HPV infection has revealed a significantly high accuracy rate for diagnosis of cervical intraepithelial neoplasia (CIN). Therefore, guidelines now recommend screening for HPV infection in all women aged 30 or older. Although HPV detection is an effective screening method, the high cost for the test limit its use in developing countries. Another method, known as VIA (visual inspection after acetic acid application), has been widely evaluated as a screening strategy in developing countries. In this review, we will discuss screening methods being used to decrease cervical cancer in both developed and developing countries.

Keywords: Cervical screening, HPV testing, VIA

Pap Test

The Papanicolaou (Pap) test was first introduced in the U.S. in 1941 as a cervical cancer screening method [1]. It has played a central role in screening. The Pap test retrieves exfoliated cells sampled from the 'cervical transformation zone', the junction of the ecto- and endo-cervix, where cervical dysplasia and cancers most often arise. The conventional method is to sample cells from the cervix and vagina with a brush or spatula; the cells are then placed directly on a slide (known as conventional cytology), fixed with an alcohol based solution and then assessed by cytologists.

The Pap screening program greatly facilitates early detection and treatment of precancerous lesions. In a systematic review, Nanda et al. [2] have shown that the sensitivity of the Pap test ranges from 30% to 87% and specificity from 86% to 100%. Both conventional and liquid-based collection (LBC) methods for cervical cytology specimens are found to be acceptable. The cells for LBC are sampled similarly to the conventional method, but are then suspended in a liquid medium, to be subsequently centrifuged or filter concentrated in the laboratory, then set on slides and examined. The sensitivity and specificity of LBC were found to be equivalent to conventional methods [3]. The advantage of LBC is that it allows a single specimen to be used to evaluate multiple parameters, such as cytology and genital infections (with HPV, gonorrhea or Chlamydia) [4].

Criteria for assessing the Pap test is based on the Bethesda System, which is generally accepted in the United States and many other countries. It was first introduced in 1988, and revised in 2001 [5, 6]. One of the major changes made in the Bethesda system involved clear designation of epithelial cell abnormality. This change standardized the results of cytology and improved the clinical usefulness of Pap smear reports.

Some healthcare guidelines for average-risk women recommend starting their Pap-test screening at age 21, regardless of the age of onset of sexual activity, repeat every 3 years thereafter, to be continued until age 65. There is no evidence that annual cervical cytology is superior to every 3 year screening. Annual screening is actually associated with more harms in terms of false positive test results that result in anxiety and require further assessment.

On their webpage, the CDC (Centers for Disease Control and Prevention) has compared the recommendations of three different sets of guidelines, the ACS: American Cancer Society, USPSTF: U.S. Preventive Services Task Force, and ACOG: American College of Obstetricians and Gynecologists [7]. According to this report, although the effectiveness of Pap smear screening for cervical cancer has yet to be demonstrated in a truly randomized trial, it is associated with an at least 60% decrease of cervical cancer incidence and decreasing mortality in developed countries with high population coverage rates. The International Agency for Research on Cancer (IARC), combining data from national programs in eight countries, reported a roughly 90 percent reduction in cervical cancer incidence following periodic screening of the adult female population [8]. There is no doubt about the effectiveness of cytology-based screening programs.

In spite of such great screening programs, cervical cancer statistics show that cervical cancer still ranks as the third most common females cancer and the fourth leading cause of female cancer death worldwide, accounting for 529,800 new cases and 275,100 deaths in 2008 [9]. This poses the question: Why does cervical cancer remain such a common cancer?

In already developed countries, the reason for residual cervical cancer incidence may depend on the sporadic nature of the screening. The participation rates of screening for cervical cancer varies among countries. For example, in Japan the participation rate using the Pap smear for cervical cancer screening is very low, at 23.4% [10]. In the US, more than half of women who develop cervical cancer have either never had cervical cytology, have been seldom screened, or have not been screened within the previous five years [11]. The reasons given for not participating in routine screening programs may be the inconvenience, discomfort, cultural objections or poor socioeconomic status.

On the other hand, more than 85% of the total cervical cancer cases and deaths occur in developing countries [12]. The situation is quite different from that of developed countries and it is a more serious condition. One major factor for the paucity of widespread screening is that cytology-based screening is expensive. It requires extensive modern facilities, staffing of an established laboratory and well-trained cytotechnologists. Moreover, conventional cytology-based screening strategies require multiple patient visits for screening, evaluation and treatment. However, in developing countries, the per capita number of medical institutions and doctors is very low and cytology screening is thus impractical. Therefore, alternative screening tests, for example DNA testing for HPV (human papillomavirus) or direct visual inspection are potentially useful. These methods require fewer clinical visits and they are less dependent on an existing modern laboratory infrastructure [13, 14].

HPV Test

Since the 1970s, the relationship between HPV infection and genital tract neoplasia has been well elucidated. More than 100 different strains of HPV have since been isolated, and the role of an HPV test is increasingly important. About 30 types of HPV infect squamous cells of the anogenital tract. These genotypes can be classified broadly into two groups, high-risk (Types 16, 18, 31, 33, 35, 39, 45, 51, 52, 56, 58, 59 and 68) and low-risk HPV (Types 6, 11, 40, 42, 43, 44, 53, 54, 61, 72, 73 and 81), based on their association with the phenotypic development of cervical cancer [15]. Types 16 and 18 are the most commonly isolated HPV types from invasive cervical cancer. Type 16 is found in approximately 50 percent of cervical cancer patients.

The roles of the high-risk HPV test of can be divided into two, one for primary HPV screening and one for HPV testing as triage. Primary HPV DNA screening with an associated cytology test is more sensitive than conventional screening, especially among women aged 35 or older [16]. Some reports show that HPV testing alone was substantially more sensitive, but also significantly less specific, than the Pap test in detecting CIN2. In an overview of European and North American studies [17], that included results from more than 60,000 women, Cuzick *et al.* compared the sensitivity and specificity of HPV testing with routine cytology, both overall and for a breakdown of ages <35, 35-49 and 50+. HPV testing was substantially more sensitive in detecting CIN2+ than cytology (96.1% vs. 53.0%) but less specific (90.7% vs. 96.3%).

Kitchener *et al.* compared screening by liquid-based cytology with HPV testing to without HPV testing in the ARTISTIC (A Randomised Trial of HPV Testing in Primary Cervical Screening) trial in England. The study population comprised 25,000 women aged

20-64. HPV testing was evaluated over two screening rounds, 3 years apart. Overall rates of CIN 3 or worse stage were equivalent in the two groups over two rounds of screening [18]. HPV sensitivity was uniformly high at all ages. The sensitivity of cytology testing was better in women over 50 than in younger women (79.3% vs. 59.6%). The specificity of both tests increased with age. The ACOG guideline now recommends co-screening with both cytology and HPV testing every 5 years for women aged 30-65 years and screening with cervical cytology alone for women aged 20-29. This is because transient HPV infection is often detected in sexually active women younger than 30 years [19].

One common barrier to participating in screening programs is the need for a pelvic examination with an uncomfortable speculum insertion. As a result, following patient instruction, vaginal self-sampling for oncogenic HPV is being evaluated more broadly as a screening modality [20, 21].

In developing countries, as mentioned before, standard strategies such as cervical cytology are often impractical due to the cost, infrastructure issues and need for more patient visits. Qiao *et al.* reported on the accuracy of the rapid careHPV test (Qiagen, Gaithersburg, MD, USA). The test can detect 14 of the high-risk types of HPV in about 2.5 hours. In their study, the sensitivity and specificity of the screening were 90.0% and 84.2%, respectively, on cervical specimens, and 81.4% and 82.4%, respectively, on vaginal specimens [22]. Moreover, each test cost less than $5 (US). Eduardo *et al.* reported self-HPV-testing was 3-4 times more sensitive than cytology for detecting CIN 2 or worse [23].

A similar study from India [24] compared the efficacy of Pap cytology, visual inspection with acetic acid (VIA) enhancement, and HPV DNA testing for the detection CIN and invasive cancer. HPV testing had a higher sensitivity (100%) and specificity (90.6%) compared to Pap cytology (sensitivity: 78.2%; specificity: 86.0%) and VIA (sensitivity: 31.6%; specificity: 87.5%). However, they concluded that low community participation and high non-compliance were the major impediments for reduction of cervical cancer in India. Therefore, they suggested use of less invasive and more user-friendly primary screening tests, like use of self-collected swabs for HPV DNA testing.

Screening by HPV testing only, without a concurrent Pap smear, is currently under investigation using triaging strategies for HPV positive situation in developed countries, but may be a reasonable option for a once in a life time screening test in rural areas with limited cytology resources. In addition, good education for prevention of cervical cancer and use of less discomfort screening methods are important.

Visual Inspection

Cytology and HPV testing are useful for screening; however, they both need considerable resources and infrastructure. Moreover, these methods are relatively expensive. Therefore, it is difficult to maintain a successful cytology screening system in low-income countries. On the other hand, a visual inspection with acetic acid (VIA) or Lugol's iodine (VILI) enhancement is useful for cervical cancer screening in developing countries where resources are limited [25, 26]. Visual inspection of the cervix for cervical cancer screening was introduced in the 1930s by Schiller. The methods are very simple; require few resources and their results are available immediately. For VIA, dilute (3-5%) acetic acid or vinegar is first applied to the squamous-columnar junction of the uterine cervix with a cotton ball or spray. After one minute, the examiner observes the cervix with the naked eye. CIN and micro-invasive cancers are detected as patches of lasting aceto-whitening. Although aceto-whitening can also be observed transiently in immature squamous metaplasia and in inflamed or regenerating cervical epithelium, it does not persist for long, compared to precancerous and cancerous areas. The test requires ultralow technology and cost. In addition, if the patients need treatment or additional biopsy, they can receive them during the same visit. VIA with magnifying glass assistance is called VIAM. If Lugol's iodine is used instead of acetic acid, it is called VILI (visual inspection with Lugol's iodine). The performance characteristics of these alternative screening tests compared to cytology have been reported by Cuzick *et al.* [27, 28]. According to their report, sensitivity and specificity were VIA (67-79% and 49-86%), VIAM (62-73% and 86-87%) and VILI (78-98% and 73-93%), respectively. They concluded that the most important approach is a 'Screen and Treat' approach. This means that in developing countries, screening and treatment should be done at the same visit. Repeat visits for assessments/treatment may be difficult in developing countries and lead to loss of followup. Changxian *et al.* also reported the sensitivity of VIA, VIAM and VILI in their meta-analysis [29]. In the report, the combined estimates of sensitivity for VIA, VIAM and VILI were77, 64 and 91%, respectively, and the combined values of specificity were 87, 86 and 85%, respectively.

Sue *et al.* found that the country-specific reduction in the lifetime risk of invasive cervical cancer with a single-screening at the age of 35, with either a one-visit or two-visit VIA, ranged from 25 to 31 percent, respectively, and for one-visit or two-visit HPV testing it ranged from 30 to 36 percent. As compared with a single-screening, two-screenings (at 35 and 40 years of age) provided a relative increased reduction in lifetime risk of approximately 40 percent [13].

Treatment following low-specificity testing, such as VIA and HPV testing, results in some women receiving unnecessary treatment. However, 'Screen and Treat' can improve the cost-effectiveness of the program, which is a critical factor in developing countries.

Conclusion

Cervical cancer is easily preventable by application of appropriate screening. However, the best methods for screening may not be the same between different countries and socio-economic regions. The most suitable screening method is dependent on the local economic conditions, infrastructure, care accessibility, religion, sexual activities, etc. Clinical screening decisions can involve more considerations than evidence alone. It is important to choose an appropriate approach for each individual, by considering the patient's social background, hopes, lifestyles and the cost effectiveness of the method to be used. Clinicians have to understand the evidence presented them but they also must still individualize the decision making process to the specific patient or situation.

References

[1] Vilos, GA., et al., The history of the Papanicolaou smear and the odyssey of George and Andromache Papanicolaou. *Obstet Gynecol.* 1998, 91: 479-83

[2] Nanda, K., et al., Accuracy of the Papanicolaou test in screening for and follow-up of cervical cytologic abnormalities: a systematic review. *Ann Intern Med.* 2000, 132: 810-9

[3] Arbyn M., et al., Liquid compared with conventional cervical cytology: a systematic review and meta-analysis. *Obstet Gynecol.* 2008, 111: 167-77

[4] Siebers A., et al., Comparison of liquid-based cytology with conventional cytology for detection of cervical cancer precursors: a randomized controlled trial. *JAMA.* 2009, 302: 1757-64

[5] *ACOG PRACTICE BULLETIN*: Number 131, Nov 2012.

[6] Solomon D., et al., The 2001 Bethesda system: terminology for reporting results of cervical cytology. *JAMA.* 2002, 287: 2114-9

[7] CDC webpage: *http://www.cdc.gov/cancer* Accessed on 19/04/2013.

[8] IARC Working Group on evaluation of cervical cancer screening programs. Screening for squamous cervical cancer: duration of low risk after negative results of cervical cytology and its implication for screening policies. *Br Med J* (Clin Res Ed). 1986, 293: 659-64

[9] Jemal A., et al., Global cancer statistics. *CA Cancer J Clin.* 2011, 61: 69-90

[10] OECD report webpage *(www.oecd.org/els/health)* Accessed on 20/05/2013.

[11] Janerich DT., et al., The screening histories of women with invasive cervical cancer, Connecticut. *Am J Public Health.* 1995, 85: 791-4

[12] Ferlay J., et al., GLOBOCAN 2008 v2.0, Cancer Incidence and Mortality Worldwide: IARC CancerBase No. 10 [Internet].Lyon, France: International Agency for Research on Cancer; 2010. Available from: *http://globocan.iarc.fr.* Accessed on 02/05/2013.

[13] Sue JG., et al., Cost-Effectiveness of Cervical-Cancer Screening in Five Developing Countries. *N Engl J Med.* 2005, 353: 2158-68

[14] Sankaranarayanan R., et al., Effective screening programs for cervical cancer in low and middle-income developing countries. *Bull World Health Organ.* 2001, 79: 954-62

[15] de Sanjose S., et al., Human papillomavirus genotype attribution in invasive cervical cancer: a retrospective cross-sectional worldwide study. *Lancet Oncol.* 2010; 11: 1048-56

[16] Leinonen M., et al., Age-specific evaluation of primary human papillomavirus screening vs conventional cytology in a randomized setting. *J Natl Cancer Inst.* 2009, 101: 1612-23

[17] Cuzick J., et al., Overview of the European and North American studies on HPV testing in primary cervical cancer screening. *Int J Cancer.* 2006, 119: 1095-1101

[18] Kitchener HC.,et al., ARTISTIC Trial Study Group. ARTISTIC: a randomised trial of human papillomavirus (HPV) testing in primary cervical screening. *Health Technol Assess.* 2009, 13: 1-150

[19] Ronco G., et al., New Technologies for Cervical Cancer Working Group.Human Papillomavirus Testing and Liquid-Based Cytology: Results at Recruitment From the

New Technologies for Cervical Cancer Randomized Controlled Trial. *J Natl Cancer Inst*. 2006, 98: 765-74

[20] Harper DM., et al., Randomized clinical trial of PCR-determined human papillomavirus detection methods: self-sampling versus clinician-directed--biologic concordance and women's preferences. *Am J Obstet Gynecol*. 2002, 186: 365-73

[21] Deleré Y., et al., Cervicovaginal self-sampling is a reliable method for determination of prevalence of human papillomavirus genotypes in women aged 20 to 30 years. *J Clin Microbiol*. 2011, 49: 3519-22

[22] Qiao YL., et al., A new HPV-DNA test for cervical-cancer screening in developing regions: a cross-sectional study of clinical accuracy in rural China. *Lancet Oncol*. 2008, 9: 929-36

[23] Lazcano-Ponce E., et al., Self-collection of vaginal specimens for human papillomavirus testing in cervical cancer prevention (MARCH): a community-based randomised controlled trial. *Lancet*. 2011, 378: 1868-73

[24] Gravitt PE., et al., CATCH Study Team. Effectiveness of VIA, Pap, and HPV DNA testing in a cervical cancer screening program in a peri-urban community in Andhra Pradesh, India. *PLoS One*. 2010, 5:e13711. doi: 10.1371/journal. pone. 0013711

[25] Sankaranarayanan R., et al., Effect of visual screening on cervical cancer incidence and mortality in Tamil Nadu, India: a cluster-randomised trial. *Lancet*. 2007, 370: 398-406

[26] Arbyn M., et al., Pooled analysis of the accuracy of five cervical cancer screening tests assessed in eleven studies in Africa and India. *Int J Cancer*. 2008, 123: 153-60

[27] Cuzick J.,et al., Overview of human papillomavirus-based and other novel options for cervical cancer screening in developed and developing countries. *Vaccine*. 2008, 26 (Suppl 10):K29-41. doi: 10.1016/j.vaccine.2008.06.019.

[28] Blumenthal PD., et al., Training for cervical cancer prevention programs in low-resource settings: focus on visual inspection with acetic acid and cryotherapy. *Int J Gynaecol Obstet*. 2005, 89 (Suppl 2): S30-7

[29] Chen C., et al., Accuracy of several cervical screening strategies for early detection of cervical cancer: a meta-analysis. *Int J Gynecol Cancer*. 2012, 22: 908-21

In: Cervical Cancer
Editor: Laurie Elit

ISBN: 978-1-62948-062-6
© 2014 Nova Science Publishers, Inc.

Chapter III

Telemedicine in Cervical Screening

Tsedma Baatar[1] and Laurie Elit[2]

[1]National Center for Maternal and Children's Health Ulaanbaatar, Mongolia
[2]Department of Obstetrics and Gynecology, McMaster University, Hamilton, Canada

Abstract

Introduction: Cervical screening is particularly difficult in geographically isolated regions. Telemedicine offers opportunities for distance consultation, provider education and continuous quality improvement.

Methods and Results: We review the current literature concerning the evaluation of telemedicine in cervical screening at the level of the screening test (ie., VIA, cytology specimen review), and diagnosis (histology and colposcopy). Telemedicine appears feasible and reliable in the static mode. Dynamic telemedicine while feasible and reliable in high resource settings must still be evaluated in low to moderate resource settings. An example where telemedicine was implemented for cytology and colposcopy in Mongolia is provided.

Conclusions: Telemedicine is a new paradigm in the delivery of health care for the patient, continuing education for health care providers and a method of continuous quality improvement. Jurisdictional issues including stable power supply, internet capacity, personal privacy, must still be enhanced to make this a reliable process in low resource countries.

Keywords: Telemedicine, Cervical Screening

Introduction

Access to cervical screening and referral to colposcopy can have several limitations in geographic isolated areas, and low resource settings due to the lack of trained manpower, paucity of financial resources and poor awareness about preventative health. Telemedicine is the practice of transmitting digital images through telecommunication networks to remote viewing locations for the purposes of diagnosis, image storage (for future comparison) and healthcare provider education. Use of telemedicine can fundamentally change the paradigm under which health care is delivered [1,2,3,4]. Telemedicine can have applications with screening for cervical cancer at multiple points in the screening care pathway. For example, telemedicine can be useful at the point of obtaining the screening test. If the screening test is visual inspection with acetic acid (VIA), the cervical image can be transmitted for advice concerning patient disposition. Telemedicine can be useful at the point of evaluating the test. If the screening test is cervical cytology, the stained cytology slide image can be transmitted for advice on the diagnosis. Telemedicine can be useful at the point of diagnosis. Here the magnified colposcopic image of the cervix could be captured and transmitted for advice on patient disposition. There are some principles of telemedicine that can be important in any of the settings described above. For example, a telemedicine diagnosis can be achieved by either use of the image viewed in real time (dynamic systems) or with use of pictures that are first captured in a digital format and then transmitted using a store-and-forward approach to distant observers (static systems). Static systems have the benefit of being lower in cost that dynamic system [4]. In this chapter we will review the feasibility and reliability of telemedicine in cervical screening. Where available we will provide information on comparative research on standard of care versus telemedicine options of static versus dynamic image transfer. We will end this chapter with a pilot study report of the implementation of telemedicine in the cervical cancer screening program in Mongolia.

Methods And Results

Visual Inspection with Acetic Acid (VIA) and Telemedicine

The very earliest inclinings of telemedicine in cervical cancer screening began with a devise known as the cerviscope which was introduced in 1981 by Stafl [4a, 4b]. It was a camera with a fixed telephoto lens that took a photograph of the cervix called a cervigram. The original technology involved capturing a cervical photograph on a 35-mm film using a special camera and light source. Film was sent by ground mail to a certified colposcopists for development and then interpretation. Later renditions of cervicography involved projection of the images on a screen in a dark room. These images could be magnified up to 16 fold as would happen if a physician was examining the cervix through the colposcope. Someone like a nurse could capture the image and an expert later reviewed the image and made a diagnosis and treatment recommendation. More recently this technology was felt to be suitable for developing countries where VIA and digital cervicography improved VIA alone in decision making in low resource settings [6]. Remote cervigram reviewing service are available. The sensitivity of cervicography was generally lower than a Pap test and the specificity was higher [4c].

VIA is the inspection of the cervix with the naked eye after the application of 3-5% acetic acid. VIA is a subjective test with 3 possible diagnoses: negative, positive and suspicious for cancer. In low resource countries, VIA may be performed by trained midwives, nurses or physicians. A strategy for distant preceptorship and supervision of novice health-care staff was evaluated using mobile phone telemedicine to assist non-physician health-care workers in interpreting VIA in Gaborone, Botswana [5]. Of 99 women, all of whom were HIV positive, 93 women had their cervices assessed using VIA and digital image capture and transmission using mobile phones. Thirty-one of the images were not evaluable/insufficient and were excluded by an expert leaving 62 images for comparison. There was concordance with the VIA positive images in 82% of cases and VIA negative cases in 89% of cases for a Kappa of 0.71. A limitation of using mobile phone photographs lay in the lower picture quality compared to conventional digital cameras. Benefits of this strategy were that women could be triaged with immediate treatment where appropriate (using cryotherapy) and reduced referral delays and decreased need for travel from remote sites to regions of greater expertise.

Nurses in Zambia who were trained to perform VIA followed by cryotherapy were aided with digital cervicography (digital camera, laptop computer, television, cell phone and internet) and then distance consultation was sought when needed to help facilitate a screen and treat with cryotherapy program [6]. Digitally obtained images were compressed and tagged with the patient's identification number establishing a standardized file storage system. All images were stored at the University teaching Hospital of Zambia for back up. Communication could be sent by email and no patient identifiers were transmitted. Eventually, an enhanced web-based solution was implemented for remote clinics using open source softward Python (Python Software Foundation, Hampton, NH). All access was password protected. A goal for this system was to respond to distance consultations requests while the patient was still in the clinic so treatment could either be delivered or the patient informed about next steps. Some limitations of this project included image quality (due to obstructed views, inadequate zooming, batteries not being fully charged, improper lighting) and failure of the camera and need to send the camera out of country for repair.

Although these reports suggest using static image relay by cell phone or by a web-based system is potentially feasible, currently there is limited data on reliability. For purpose of patient safety, issues around patient privacy, data storage both the image, recommendation and patient disposition must be worked out.

Cervical Cytology and Telemedicine

Potential uses for telecytology would be for special consultation opportunities to distant laboratories for primary diagnosis or second opinion consultation, archiving interesting cases through slide replication, implement a remote quality assurance program (important method to maintain and improve diagnostic acumen), educational purposes (ie., upgrading laboratory services by producing digital educational material for use in Webbased training systems), proficiency testing programs for assessing the diagnostic expertise of the laboratory medical staff, and board exams [4].

Remote interpretation of digitized images transmitted over the Internet has the potential to provide access to high quality cytology assessment. It has been shown that low-resolution images transmitted over the Internet as e-mail attachments could be adequately interpreted at a distant site without manual microscopy [18]. Telecytology (videomicroscopy) has also been shown to be reliable [19, 20] if the images are of good quality and do not need to be manipulated compared to manual microscopy [21,22]. Accuracy and reproducibility of telecytological diagnosis was evaluated from 404 cervical smears from liquid based collection. The CytoTrainer e-learning telecytology platform developed in the Department of

Cytopathology "ATTIKON" Universty General Hospital Athens Greece was used remotely by 4 board certified cytopathologists. Interobserver agreement was Kappa 0.79-0.97 and intraobserver agreement was Kappa 0.76-1.0 [4]. This study showed that digitized images can be as reliable as those of conventional cytology. Important issues are field selection, sufficient image quality and diagnostic expertise. The role of the person appointed to capture and transmit images is of paramount importance for the success of a static telecytological system.

Reproducibility of 50 cases cervical smears captured as digital images in Georgia and transmitted by electronic mail. Original material and telecytology material was reviewed on two occasions 3 months apart. Interobserver agreement was 0.82 first and 0.68 second time for the glass slide and 0.80 first and 0.66 second for the digital image (Kappa of 0.75-0.84 with the glass slide and 0.7 to 0.8 for digital image). Telecytology requires an experienced cytology at the point of image transfer who is familiar with the technology and trained to recognize and identify highly informative fields for field selection. There is a requirement that the slide be visualized with 100 fold magnification at the point of image transer. High resolution (ie., 2048x1536 pixels) JPEG files this could be interpreted accurately [7].

The Italian NGO Associazione Patologi Oltre Frontiera (APOF) was established in 2000 for the creation or the improvement of histopathology department in low resource countries. APOF is involved in the use of tele-pathology to address lack of pathologists. In 2005, two technicians were trained by Italian volunteers in Chirundu, South Zambia. The technicians could screen Pap smears and could prepare histology sections. Digital photographs were taken of the suspicious or positive cases and sent to one of the 100 volunteers who was on the monthly rotation responsible for diagnosis. For histologic diagnoses, a ditial scanner was used with a satellite connection. The original material was sent to Italy to verify the telemedicine diagnosis [7b].

Feasibility and reliability for telecytology have been clearly reported such that its use is acceptable in cervical cytology assessment given the provisions around image transfer described above.

Colposcopy and Telemedicine

Traditionally the colposcope is a binocular instrument which has the capacity to enlarge the cervix 5 to 15 fold. Digital (video) colposcopy means that the image is projected onto a computer screen and can be easily enlarged. Storage of the image allows opportunity for further digital analyses of the image at another time. With the internet and email, digital colposcopy can take a central role in telemedicine, the electronic transmission of information for the delivery of quality clinical health care from a distance [8,9]. There are 2 types of telecolposcopy – network based versus computer-based. [10,11] Network based telecolposcopy (dynamic) uses an existing infrastructure of technologically advanced hardware, rapid telecommunication lines and trained support personnel. Most provide a real-time or television like video interface at both sites. The computer-based colposcopy (static)– the video images are stored on a computer using customised software and then forwarded. Digital colposcopy has been shown to be as reliable as conventional binocular colposcopy in Europe and North America [2,3,4b 9,13,14,15,16,]. Ferris showed slightly higher rates of unsatisfactory exams with telecolposcopy [8] thus an increase use of biopsies [9]. Studies in patient satisfaction have also shown improved satisfaction as telecolposcopy saves women time and cost related to travel [12]. Because of this women preferred the telecolpscopy [16]. Ferris evaluated both – the sensitivity for detecting CIN 2 or greater is 40.9-43.2% for network based colposcopy and 34.1-40.9% for computer based colposcopy, vs 48% for on site colposcopy. The specificity for CIN2 + is 55.3-58.1% for network and 58.9-59.4% for computer based colposcopy and 59% for on-site colposcopy [8,9,10,11]. In summary telecolposcopy is feasible, reliable, accept to patients and test parameters of sensitivity and specificity have been obtained comparing on site colposcopy to telecolposcopy by both static and dynamic options. All this work has been completed and reported in high resource settings. In the American setting, telemedicine was more costly to the system when compared to a local practitioner conducting colposcopy and biopsy; however, it was less costly compared to referring the patient to a distant centre of excellence [17].

Case study of Implementing Telemedicine for cervical cancer prevention in Mongolia [28-31]

Mongolia is a country of sparse population (2.6 million people) scattered over a vast geographic area. At any point in time, 29.9 women per 100,000 are living with cervical cancer. This disease is the second leading cause of death from cancer for women in Mongolia. In part this is related to the advanced stage of disease at the time of presentation. Currently there is no cervical screening system in the country. Women usually present with symptoms such as bleeding and foul discharge, at this time the opportunity for cure is limited. One of the problems that the Mongolian National Oncology Centre (NOC) faces is the referral of patients from countryside at a point in this disease when cure was no longer possible. Thus patients and families spend a significant percent of limited personal resources to travel the NOC and NCMCH (national center for maternal and children' health) for no benefit to the affected family member. If rural physicians could diagnosis and manage women who had end stage disease, this would free especially human resources from the National Oncology Centre to focus on early stage disease or prevention. The other problems faced by the NOC are a lack of human resources and space to conduct a national cytology based cervical screening program or offer colposcopy for all women with abnormal cytology, should a national program be implemented.

The Mongolian health care system is based on small clinics usually staffed by health care workers (known as feldshers). Patients that need a higher level of care are referred to the district (soum) hospitals. Here the majority of care is provided by family doctors and nurses. If the patient needs yet a higher calibre of care, they are referred to the provincial (aimag) hospital. Some specialty services are available here like general surgery, obstetrics and gynecology, internal medicine. If the patient required focused subspecialty care, she is referred to the capital city, Ulaanbaatar. Here there are numerous specialty based facilities (ie., the National Oncology, Hospital, National center for Maternal and Children health) where care is provided by population (ie., children) or disease (cancer). Health care is funded by a government health insurance system ., the government covers the costs for hospital stays related maternal health, care to children, radiation care. There is a currently small but growing private/commericial (pay be user) health care system.

Telemedicine is an application of modern technology and telecommunications for delivering the health care services, dissemination of knowledge and experience between different parts of the country and a means to provide continuous education for medical personnel. It is most beneficial to the populations living in rural communities and isolated regions. Mongolia had initiated a pilot project with the Telemedicine Network in 2003 focused on cardiovascular disease. Building on this success, this project focused on improving the quality of maternal and newborn health care was birthed. The overall goal of the project was to improve the quality of maternal and newborn services for rural population by establishing and operating a telemedicine communication network and strengthening the capacity of provincial and central service providers to access relevant and necessary information and technical support in a timely manner. One component of this project focused on enhancing cervical cytology capacity and colposcopy image analysis. This later component is the focus of this paper. Thus the 3 objectives were to 1) operationalize internet-based clinical decision-making support for cervical pathology screening based on colposcopy and Pap-smear imaging; 2) strengthen capacity of the MCHRC and provincial hospitals through (a) procurement of diagnostic and medical equipment; (b) training of service providers on new progressive approaches and techniques using updated clinical reference materials; (c) sensitization of the national and provincial governments and health administration; and (d) enhanced professional networking between participating hospitals, national institutions and with professional societies and international partners; and 3) increase access to quality specialized care for the population of 12 provinces of Mongolia with reduction of referrals to the capital city or regional centers that are costly to both health system and patient families.

Project Organization

The technical and operational support for the program was provided by the UNFPA Country Office in Mongolia. The project operated within the National Center for Maternal and Children's Health center of the Ministry of Health, Mongolia. The Joint Steering Committee was defined by a Ministerial Order at MOH. The members of Joint Steering Committee included representatives from MOH, Luxembourg Government, UNFPA, Luxembourg Development Cooperation Agency, implementing hospital directors.

At the level of the policy maker, the UNFPA technical staff worked with the Ministry of Health of achieve a Ministry of Health Order allow implementation of the project. They also supported the development of an eHealth Strategy for Mongolia. This strategy involved many other parties also involved in telemedicine initiatives.

The initial centres for this project in cervical cancer prevention were those provinces most remote from the capital city (Ulaanbaatar): Uvurkhangai, Khovd, Dornogovi, Darkhan, Dornod, Khuvsgul, Selnege,and Orkhon . In 2010, four additional western aimags were added: Bayan-Ulgii, Gobi-Altai, Uvs and Zavkhan.

This project began with a needs assessment addressing the *knowledge* of gynaecologic medical staff concerning cervical cancer prevention, treatment and palliation, *skills* to diagnose and treat pre-invasive disease and *equipment* for conducting cervical assessments and treatment.

In May 2008, the necessary telemedicine equipment (high-speed computer, colour printer with IPod and Iteach capacity) was installed in each rural centre and the National Oncology Hospital and Maternal Children Hospital. The software platform was iPath developed by the Swiss Surgical Team Research Group at Basel University and marketed by Campus Medicus, Gluhammer co. Germany. iPath is a collaborative platform for exchange of medical knowledge, distance consultations, group discussions and distance teaching in medicineiPath is a free and open platform for case based collaboration especially designed for medical applications. The packages included tele-pathology, teaching and hospital. This allowed quality colposcopy, pathology and cytology digital images for consultation, establishment of an electronic database of cases and organize teleconferencing. An information technologist was contracted to develop a database with storage capacity of 8TB to host vital telemedicine servers and Dicom images; secure internet gateway connectivity; method of file sharing; train staff. Digital colposcopes were installed at each site. These allowed not only transfer of colposcopic images but also cytology and histology images (Figure 1).

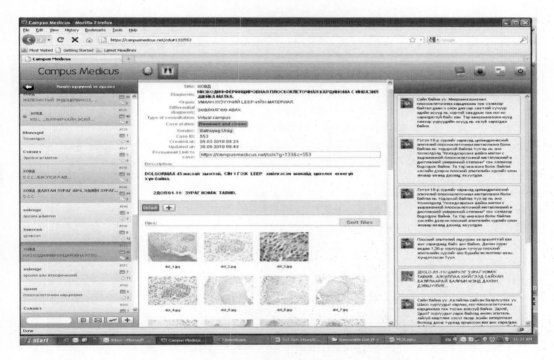

Figure 1. Screen view of a telemedicine interaction concerning cytology and histology assessments.

Training involved both upgrading computer skills, a course in basic colposcopy for gynaecologists and cytology assessment for family doctors with a focused interest in cytology, surgical skills training for the treatment of cervical precancerous lesions using cryotherapy and LEEP, and English language classes to improve professional capacity. These skills were obtained through group workshops and one-on-one training interactions. For example, *colposcopy training* took place for one week on 3 occasions (2008-2010). The training was led by one international expert, 2 members of the division of gynaecologic oncology from the National Cancer Centre and a member of the department of gynecology from the National center for Maternal and Children' Health . The training involved both didactic and practical sessions.

Once the equipment was in place and personnel were trained, patients were seen locally. If there were questions about management, the patient's story and colposcopy pictures were sent to one of two internationally trained colposcopy experts (located at the National

Oncology Hospital and the Maternal Children Hospital); the cytology/histology pictures were sent to the head of cytolopathology at the National Oncology Hospital.

Annual congresses were held for educational purposes and for exchange of experiences among project participants.

Program Assessment

Both qualitative and quantitative research methods were used to evaluate the implementation of the program. Involved were key policy makers, staff from the National Oncology Centre (NOC), National Center for Maternal and Children' Health (NCMCH) and rural staff in the pilot centres (n=82). The overarching goals of this project were: 1. Networking (rural and urban, urban and partners). 2. Capacity Building and 3. Quality and accessibility.

1. Networking

The project was funded by the Government of Luxembourg and implemented by the UNFPA. Relationships were built between the project team and the Ministry of Health, both the leadership and key consultants at the Maternal Children Hospital (MCH) and the National Oncology Centre (NOC), leadership and departments of gynecology and family medicine and Information technology teams and biomedical engineering at the rural hospitals, and international experts. Some of the successes include: partnerships which involved strengthening relationships between organizations including the Swiss Surgical Team, and Department of Obstetrics and Gynecology at McMaster University, Canada; improved leadership, coordination and collaboration of the MOH with this and similar projects has improved.

2. Capacity Building (Figure 2)

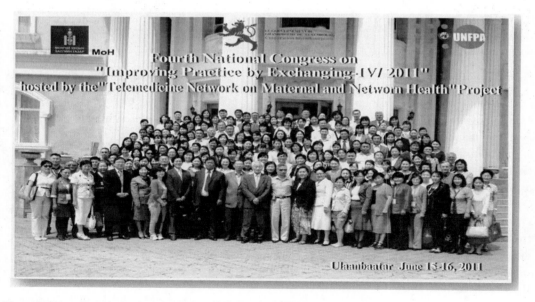

Figure 2. Educational interactions as a result of the project.

A total of 53 gynecologists were trained in *basic colposcopy* assessment and treatment skills (14 in 2008, 12 in 2009, and 27 in 2010). Advanced surgical skills involved training in LEEP. Pre and post knowledge assessment showed that scores improved by 90%. Cryotherapy was not available in Mongolia at the start of the project. Two Mongolian gynecologists were funded to attend further cryotherapy training in Manila, Philippines. Both physicians were certified as a trainer on the single visit approach. They acted as a national resource for skills training sessions.

In the area of *cytology training*, family doctors from each aimag with an interest in extra training in cytology were either self identified or identified by their peers. Eight family doctors received 2 months of full-time training in cervical cytology in the Department of Cytopathology at the National Cancer Centre in 2009. This project funded the publication of coarse material in the Mongolian language.

3. Quality and Accessibility

Prior to this project, colposcopy assessment was not available for patients in rural Mongolia. Now colposcopic assessment is available through the 12 project provincial hospitals. In 121 cases, the rurally located physician had questions and the colposcopy image was assessed by a telemedicine consultant in UB. Cytology is not generally available in the rural areas, thus in 56.7% of cytology cases, the cytology images were assessed centrally. Teleconsultation response-times were as short as 5 minutes and the longest was 9 hours. Over the course of the project, therapeutic questions have become more focused. The numbers of unnecessary referrals from the provinces to the National Cancer Centre have decreased. Prior to the project, cervical cytology assessments were only available in Ulaanbaatar and Dornod aimag. Since the implementation of the project, cytology is available in all the project aimags.

Another benefit of the project was that two annual mini-congresses were held; 79 participants including leadership and/or staff from reference hospitals and other collaborating institutes. Physicians shared their experiences and problem solving took place.

Other successes included: improved capacity of rural specialists to handle medical equipment and information technology applications; timely consultation was provided. An unexpected use of the system was to provide health alerts to the provinces ie., H1N1

Some of the challenges reported from various end users included: equipment issues (ie., electrical fluctuations damaged equipment in 3 provinces so surge protectors were procured, equipment breakdown requires the need for either trained biomedical staff or maintenance service agreements); Internet issues (ie., problems connecting with the internet means the need for trained information technology support; slow internet speed is not sufficient for real time tele-consultation this requires involvement of Ministry of Health and government to improve through policy decisions the eHealth platform; the high cost of internet connection requires involvement of the MOH to address this in their budgets to the hospitals); issues in passing forward knowledge (ie., rurally trained staff needs to be motivated to share their knowledge and skills through a process such as the train the trainer model); on-going learning and problem solving (ie., all staff need to upgrade computer skills and English language skills); need to integrate telemedicine within residency programs and continuing medical education; a system of enumeration is required for time spent by consultants on case reviews.

In Summary

In 2008, there was no organized cervical cancer prevention strategy in Mongolia. We describe the implementation of a project to improve access of women in 8 of 21 geographic isolated regions of Mongolia to cervical screening and assessment of abnormal results. This project involved access to teleconsultation of either/both the abnormal cervical cytology and concerning colposcopic exam. For the women at risk for disease, this technology frees them from the financial burden of travelling to the capital city for screening and/or treatment. As a result of the project, there has been capacity building of the referral centres both in terms of technology, and skill.

We have shown that telemedicine is an excellent resource for providing clinic disposition to women at risk for cervical cancer in geographically remote regions. In addition to now being able to provide cervical cancer screening to women in rural Mongolia, some other benefits of this technology may include opportunities for quality assessment and distance learning opportunities. For Mongolia to move forward at the completion of this project will take problem solving of the issues outlined above, generalization of telemedicine through-out the country, and creating an infrastructure to deal with issues such as updating advanced software programs.

Conclusion

Telemedicine which involves bringing expertise that is physically located at a distance to the bedside for facilitating patient care is clearly a technology that is changing the paradigm of health care delivery across the world. In this chapter we have shown that telemedicine in cervical cancer prevention has best been well evaluated for cytology and colposcopy when delivered in high resource settings. We have shown the issues that exist not just with the technology but also collateral issues related using telemedicine in the system of health care delivery in low resource settings like Botswana, Zambia and Mongolia. When implementing telemedicine in low to middle resource settings, on going evaluation of weaknesses in the process of care delivery is necessary in order to instigate change to continuously improve care for the geographically isolated population.

Acknowledgments

The Mongolian Telemedicine Project was made possible through a grant from the Government of Luxembourg and UNFPA in partnership with the National Center for Maternal and Children' Health (NCMCH), National Cancer Centre (NCC), Ministry of Health, Mongolia and all participating rural hospitals. We wish to specifically acknowledge the following individuals for their involvement in the Mongolian Telemedicine project: Shinetugs B, Baigal G, Munkhbayar Ch, Enkhtuya Sh, Sugar J, Enkhjargalo Kh, Erhembaatar T.

References

[1]   Leong, F.J. Practical applications of Internet resources for cost effective telpathology practice. *Pathology* 2001;33:498-503

[2]   Tan, JHJ; Wrede, CDH. New Technologies and advances in colposcopic assessment. *Best Practice and research Clinical Obstetrics and Gynecology* 2011;25:667-677

[3]   Perisic, Z; Rasic, R; Raznatovic, S. Quality and efficacy of a telecolposcopy programme. *J Telemed Telecare* 2005;11(1):20-2

[4]   Tsilalis, T; Meristoudis, C; Pouliakis, A; Panayiotides, I; Karakitsos P. Assessment of Static telecytological diagnoses' reproducibility in cervical smears prepared by means of liquid-based cytology. *Telemedicine and e-Health.* 2012; 516-520

[5]   Stafl, A. Cervicography: a new method for cervical cancer detection. *Am J Obstet Gynecol* 1981;139:815-25.

[6]   Stafl, A. Cervicography. *Clin Obstet Gynecolo* 1983;26:1007-16

[7]   Parham. GP; Mwanahamuntu, MH; Pfaendler, KS; Sahasrabuddhe, VV; Myung, D; Mkumba, G; Kapambwe, S; Mwanza, B; Chibwesha, C; Hicks, ML; Stringer, JSA. 3C3-A modern telecommunications matrix for cervical cancer prevention in Zambia. *J Low Genit Tr D* 2010;14(3):167-173.

[8]   Louwers, JA; Kocken, M; Harmsel, WA ter; Verheijen, RHM. Digital colposcopy: ready for use? An overview of literature. *RCOG* 2009;116;220-22

[9]   Quinley, KE; Gormley, RH; Ratcliffe, SJ; Shih, T; Szep, Z; Steiner, A; Ramogola-Masire, D; Kovarik, CL. Use of mobile telemedicine for cervical cancer screening. *J Telemed Telecare* 2011;17:203-209.

[10]   Eichhorn, JH; Buckner, L; Buckner, SB; Beech, DP; Harris, KA; McClure, DJ; Crothers, BA; Wilbur, DC. Internet-based gynecologic telecytology with remote automated image selection: results of a first-phase developmental trial. *Am J Clin Pathol* 2008 May;129(5):686-96.

[11]   Eichhorn, JH; Brauns, TA; Gelfand, JA; Crothers, BA; Wilbur, DC. A novel automated screening and interpretation process for cervical cytology using the internet transmission of low-resolution images: a feasibility study. *Cancer.* 2005 Aug 25;105(4):199-206.

[12]   Ziol, M; Vacher-Lavenu, MC; Heudes, D; Ferrand, J; Mayelo, V; Molinié, V; Slama, S; Marsan, C. Expert consultation for cervical carcinoma smears. Reliability of selected-field videomicroscopy. *Anal Quant Cytol Histol* 1999 Feb;21(1):35-41.

[13]   Pinco, J; Goulart, RA; Otis, CN; Garb, J; Pantanowitz, L. Impact of digital image manipulation in cytology. *Arch Pathol Lab Med* 2009 Jan;133(1):57-61.

[14]   Marsan, C; Vacher-Lavenu, MC.Telepathology: a tool to aid in diagnosis and quality assurance in cervicovaginal cytology. *Cytopathology* 1995 Oct;6(5):339-42.

[15]   Kidiashvilli, E; Schrader, T. Reproducibility of telecytology diagnosis of cervical smears in a quality assurance program: the Georgian experience. *Telemedicine and e-Health* 2011;17(7):565-568.

[16]   Micheli, A; Sanz, N; Mwangi-Powell, F; Coleman, MP; Neal, C; Ullrich, A; Travado, L; Santini, LA; et al. International collaborations in cancer control and the Third International Cancer Control Congress. *Tumori* 2009;95:579-596.

[17] Ferris, DG; litaker, MS; Miller, JA; Macfee, MS; Crawley, D; Watson, D. Qualitative assessment of telemedicine network and computer-based telecolposcopy. *J Low Genit Tract Dis* 2002;6:145-9.

[18] Ferris, DG; Bishai, DM; Litaker, MS; Dickman, ED; Miller, JA; Macfee, MS. Telemedicine network telecolposcopy compared with computer-based telecolposcopy. *J Low Genit Tract Dis* 2004;8:94-101.

[19] Ferris, DG; Litaker, MS; Macfee, MS; Miller, JA. Remote diagnosis of cervical neoplasia: 2 types of telecolposcopy compared with cervicography. *J Fam Pract* 2003;152:298-304.

[20] Ferris, DG; Macfee, MS; Miller, JA; Litaker, MS; Crawley, D; Watson, D. The efficacy of telecolposcopy compared with traditional colposcopy. *Obstet Gynecol* 2002;99:248-52.

[21] Etherington, J; Watts, AD; Hughes, E; Lester. The use of telemedicine in primary care for women with cervical cytological abnormalities. *J Telemed Telecare* 2002;8 Suppl 3:S3:17-9.

[22] Etherington, IJ. Telecolposcopy - a feasibility study in primary care. *J Telemed Telecare* 2002;8 Suppl 2:22-4.

[23] Ferris, DG; Macfee, MS; Miller, JA; Litaker, MS; Crawley, D; Watson, D. The efficacy of telecolposcopy compared with traditional colposcopy. *Obstet Gynecol* 2002 Feb;99(2):248-54.

[24] Harper, DM; Moncur, MM; Harper, WH; Burke, GC; Rasmussen, CA; Mumford, MC. The technical performance and clinical feasibility of telecolposcopy. *J Fam Pract* 2000 Jul;49(7):623-7.

[25] Ferris, DG; Litaker, MS; Gilman, PA; Leyva Lopez, AG. Patient acceptance and the psychological effects of women experiencing telecolposcopy and colposcopy. *J Am Board Fam Pract* 2003 Sep-Oct;16(5):405-11.

[26] Bishai, DM; Ferris, DG; Litaker, MS. What is the least costly strategy to evaluate cervical abnormalities in rural women? Comparing telemedicine, local practitioners, and expert physicians. *Med Decis Making* 2003 Nov-Dec;23(6):463-70.

[27] Tsedmaa, B. Telemedicine support on maternal and newborn health to remote provinces of Mongolia 2007-2011. Sydney, Australia 2012

[28] Tsedmaa, B. New Evidence and Strategies for Prevention of Cervical Cancer – Mongolia. *UNFPA*. Dec2010. New York, USA

[29] Tsedmaa, B. Telemedicine support on maternal and newborn health to remote provinces of Mongolia. 2007-2010. *End Evaluation Report*. 30Jul2010

[30] Tsedmaa, B; Shinetugs, B; Genden, P; Baigal, G; Munlhbayar, Ch; Enktuya, Sh; Sugar, J; Navchaa, S; Enkhjargal, Kh; Nizard, J; Elit, L; Erkhembaatar, T. *Telemedicine Model of consultation for Cervical Cancer Prevention. Papillomavirus Conference 7-12July 2010, Montreal, Canada* (poster)

[31] Tsedmaa, B; Shinetugs, B; Genden, P; Baigal, G; Munlhbayar, Ch; Enktuya, Sh; Sugar, J; Navchaa, S; Enkhjargal, Kh; Nizard, J; Elit, L; Erkhembaatar, T. *Telemedicine Model of consultation for Cervical Cancer Prevention. Papillomavirus Conference Montreal, Canada* (presentation 7Jul2010)

In: Cervical Cancer
Editor: Laurie Elit

ISBN: 978-1-62948-062-6
© 2014 Nova Science Publishers, Inc.

Chapter IV

Planning and Implementation of a Cervical Cancer Screening Program

Laurie Elit[1,2], Lars Elffors[3], Baigalimaa Gendendarjaa[4], Erdenjargal Ayush[4], Elena Maximenco[5] and Munkhtaivan Adiya[6]

[1]Ontario Cervical Screening Program, Cancer Care Ontario, Toronto, Ontario, Canada
[2]Dept Obstetrics and Gynecology, McMaster University, Hamilton, Ontario, Canada
[3]EPOS Health Management, Sweden
[4]Division of Gynecologic Oncology, National Cancer Center, Ulaanbaatar, Mongolia
[5] EPOS Health Management, Muldova
[6] Millennium Challenge Account – Mongolia, Health Project, Ulaanbaatar, Mongolia

Abstract

Introduction: Implementing a national cervical cancer screening strategy must meet two conditions. First the incidence of cervical cancer must justify a screening programme and second, the necessary resource must be available and committed for attaining population coverage, and ensuring management of test positive cases. In this chapter, we will discuss the considerations that are important in implementing a cervical screening programme. Using the country of Mongolia, we will provide examples from their recent experience of implementing a national cervical screening program from 2009-2013 to demonstrate these considerations.

Methods: A literature search was conducted using MEDLINE and search terms including "cervical cancer screening", "program planning" and "programme implementation". Various key documents will provide insight into the Mongolian experience including the results of the STEP survey, KAP survey, individual and team reports to EPOS health management and the Millennium Challenge Corporation, and nation and aimag specific program plans.

Results: When introducing a cervical cancer prevention program, policy-level decisions and planning needs to address: 1. Women who are at risk for cervical cancer including their perspectives, socioculture issues, and education; 2. Technology including which screening test is to be implemented, safety, procedures and supplies, costs and acceptability and 3. Services included policies, service availability, health information systems and health care providers. Once resources were secured to implement a national cervical screening program in Mongolia, a planning team (the Project Implementation Unit of the Mongolian Millennium Challenge Corporation) was identified. They were responsible to the Mongolian Ministry of Health. They engaged stake holders, analyzed the situation, developed national policies, guidelines and standards and obtain support for these. The planning phase of the project included engaging local stakeholders to assess local needs, build program capacity, launch and implement the program and then monitor and evaluate the program.

Conclusion: Rates of cervical cancer can be minimized when a cervical cancer screening program is effectively implemented nationally. This process involves engagement at both the policy and at a program management level. The recent implementation of such a program in Mongolia provides examples of options to consider when making program decisions at both levels.

Keywords: Cervical screening program implementation

List of Acronyms

DOH	Department of Health
EPOS	EPOS Health Management
FGP	Family group practice
GAP	Global Assistance Programme
LEEP	Loop electrosurgical excisional procedure
MCA	Millennium Challenge Account Mongolia
MCC	Millennium Challenge Corporation
MOH	Ministry of Health
NCC	National Cancer Centre
NCDI	Non-communicable diseases and injuries
NGO	Non-governmental organization
PIU	Program Implementation Unit
STDs	Sexually Transmitted Diseases
STEPs	WHO STEPwise approach to Surveillance
TMN	Tumor, Metastases, Nodes Classification System
UNFPA	United Nations Population Fund
URC	University Research Co., LLC
VIA	Visual Inspection with Acetic Acid
WHO	World Health Organization
Yo	Years old

May the golden *light in the e*ternal *blue* sky *of Mongolia,*
forever *shine* on the mothers and daughters of the Great Mongol Nation. [1]

Introduction

Cervical cancer is the third most common cancer in women worldwide accounting for 530,000 new cases and 275,000 deaths annually [2]. This is a tragedy as we have had the technology to identify the precancerous stages of the disease for at least 60 years (i.e. the Pap test). Not only do we have screening tests that could help identify women with precancerous changes of the cervix (ie., Pap test, Visual inspection with acetic acid, and careHPV^{TM}), but we also have successful treatments to remove these abnormal cells (ie., cryotherapy, LEEP, laser ablation and cold knife cone biopsy) so as to prevent precancerous cells from becoming cancer. For the last decade, we have also had access to a vaccine which prevents acquisition of the two most common HPV types (16 and 18) that cause 70% of cervical cancers. The principals for implementing a cervical cancer screening program are the same whether you are in a low resource setting or in the developed world, as has been stated for instance by the WHO [3]: "A decision to implement early detection of cancer in health services should be evidence-based, with consideration for the public health importance of the disease, characteristics of early-detection tests, efficacy and cost-effectiveness of early detection, personnel requirements and the level of development of health services in a given setting. Even if the costs of the screening tests are relatively low, the whole process may involve substantial expense and may divert resources from other health care activities".

In this chapter, we will discuss the basic principles for developing or augmenting a cervical cancer screening program. We will liberally provide examples of these principals using our experience in the recently implemented national cervical cancer screening program in Mongolia.

Methods

A literature search was conducted with MEDLINE and GOOGLE using search terms such as 'program planning', 'program implementation' and 'cervical cancer screening'. The examples from the Mongolia cervical screening program were derived from meeting minutes, program reports, research reports from the Mongolian Ministry of Health, Mongolian Millennium Challenge Corporation, and EPOS Health Management.

Results

The Alliance for Cervical Cancer Prevention describes 3 phases in developing a cervical cancer screening program [4]. First there is the initiating or policy phase, then the planning phase and lastly the implementation phase. During the policy phase, there must be a defined need for a screening program based on an analysis of the extent of the problem and a high level of commitment toward developing a screening program. Engaging key stakeholders is critical to drive the process including developing laws, guidelines and standards that will guide the planning and delivery of the program. During the planning phase a program co-ordinator and multidisciplinary team are appointed and they focus on engaging local stakeholders, conducting a situational analysis to understand the training needs, equipment needs, and requirement of collaboration across services, and issues around community engagement. During the implementation phase, there will be a need for ongoing engagement with all stakeholders to ensure availability of the services, access of the services and establishing linkages and referral systems. Monitoring and evaluation will provide information on gaps and successes. In this chapter, we will discuss in more detail, aspects of each of these 3 phases.

A. Policy Phase

When determining that a cervical screening program is needed and then building the components of that program, there are 4 areas that need to be addressed; confirm political commitment, engage stakeholders, conduct a situational analysis, and develop policies to govern services [4].

The first area to address is to confirm political commitment. In other words, there must be an ongoing commitment of high level decision-makers toward developing or strengthening a cervical cancer prevention program. This commitment is reflected by investing the necessary resources and designating a coordinator for cervical cancer prevention who has the mandate, authority and resources to direct the program.

Example:

In 2012, Mongolia was made up of 2.75 million people of which 61.8% lived in urban centres and 38.2% lived in rural areas. 1.071 million (39.2%) lived in the capital city – Ulaanbaatar. Mongolia was divided into 21 aimags (ie., provinces) and each aimag was divided into soums, and each soum was divided into baghs [5]. In 1992, Mongolia moved from a socialist framework in terms of its system of politics, economy, and healthcare. Since that time, their framework has shift to a market economy system with a more democratic political process; however, their healthcare reform has lagged behind.

The funding to develop the Mongolian Cervical Cancer Screening program came through a grant from the Millennium Challenge Corporation. In part the structure to develop the cervical cancer screening program was influenced by the contract of the grant. The Millennium Challenge Account Mongolia was a 5 year health project. It was launched in September 2008 (MCA-Mongolia). This compact made available $284.9 million dollars to reduce poverty in Mongolia through economic growth. The compact covered 6 projects: a property rights project, a peri-urban project, a technical and vocational education and training project, a health project, a north-south road project and an energy and environment project. In the health project the goal was to decrease mortality and disability due to non-communicable diseases and injuries (NCDIs) and thereby increasing the length and quality of life for Mongolians. The long term objective was to increase the productive lives of Mongolians. The short term objective was to increase access to information and services about noncommunicable diseases and injuries which would enable Mongolians to guard their health. The target population covered in the compact was working age Mongolian adults [6]. To this end, the $39 million USD in the health project was directed toward prevention and treatment of hypertension, diabetes, cervical and breast cancer, and road traffic accidents. In this chapter, we will focus on the development of the cervical cancer prevention program.

The second area to address in the Policy Phase involves engaging high-level stakeholders by involving policy makers [4]. Here senior individuals representing key groups will need to be identified. They are usually individuals involved in or affected by the cervical cancer prevention program (ie., decision makers in their own organization, senior MOH officials, heads of medical organizations, university professors, heads of relevant Non-Governmental Organizations (NGOs), high profile community leaders) [4].

Example:

The Mongolian cervical cancer prevention project was managed by the Health Project Implementation Unit (PIU) which was separate from but reported to the Mongolian Ministry of Health and international organizations. The PIU worked within existing structures in Mongolia including specialized organizations, Aimag Department of Health (DoH), training/research institutions (ie.,universities), and legal non-governmental organizations (ie., WHO, UNFPA) [6].

The third area to address is to conduct a situation analysis to determine the burden of disease and relative importance of cervical cancer compared to other health priorities [4]. This could include identifying existing services that could be utilized for a screening program and the technical resources that are available [4].

Example:

A STEPs survey [7] was conducted to understand the prevalence of non-communicable diseases and injuries and risk factors for these among adults. In 2008, the average life expectancy for a Mongolian was 67.2 years. In contrast, healthy life expectancy for Mongolians was 53 years old for men and 58 years old for women. The leading causes of death were cardiovascular disease and cancer [5]. Among cancer deaths, the leading causes of death for women were liver cancer followed by cervical cancer [5,9]. Since the predominant cause of liver cancer was hepatitis, and universal hepatitis B vaccine had been initiated in the country in 1991, interest now shifted to the prevention of cervical cancer [10]. The incidence of cervical cancer had risen from 17.8 per 100,000 in 2000 to 29.9 per 100,000 in 2008 [6]. Mortality had increased from 7 to 7.7 per 100,000 during this time [10]. Seventy-five percent of women presented with Stage 3 and 4 disease resulting in a high case fatality rate. Ninety-one percent of women were diagnosed between 35-55 year old during their reproductive year and economically productive years [10].One major contributor to the high and increasing occurrence rate be the endemically high HPV infection rate reported between 35% and 46% in sexually active women and reaching almost 50% below the age of 25[11,12].

The fourth area to address in the Policy Phase is to develop a policy that will govern the cervical cancer prevention services [4]. This includes identifying the screening test, the target age group for screening, the desired population coverage, the screening frequency, appropriate provider licensing, and whether the program will be a vertical or integrated program within the health services. A vertical program means the health care providers and facilities are devoted to only one health care service (cervical cancer screening). An integrated program means that the client can access more than one health service at the same facility on the same day and from the same health care provider (ie., imbedding cervical screening in to primary care clinics. The strengths and limitations of both approaches will be discussed later in the chapter). The World Health Organization (WHO) recommends that a cervical screening program begin by screening women aged 35-50 years old at least once in a life time before expanding the services and providing repeated screening (ie., once in every 10 years). They also recommend providing a screening test with high sensitivity and treat women with high grade dysplasia and cancer [13].

Example:

A Rapid Needs Assessment was performed in 2009-2010[9] and showed that there was a Mongolian National Cancer Plan but this had not been implemented. There was a National Palliative Care Plan (N37, 2005) which called for 5 palliative care beds in each region according to population [9]. There were palliative care resolutions in the master program of the Ministry of Health 2006-2015 (N72, 2005), the National program on Non-Communicable Diseases (N246, 2005) as well as the Health Law of Mongolia (2006.01.19-paragraph 28 part 1.6)[9]. There was a Document Sub-Programme on Cancer Prevention and Control. 2009 and the Ministry Of Health (MOH) authorized its implementation on 18 Sep 2008 Order of the Minister No 210; however, where cervical cancer prevention was concerned, many of the current technologies, like LEEP, were not available in the country. Thus the Ministry of Health (MOH) gave an order (March 2010) to convene a Cervical Cancer Prevention, Treatment and Palliation Guidelines Working Group. It involved 2 external consultants (Lars Elffors, Laurie Elit), a representative of the National Cancer Centre (G Purevsuren) and several other representatives from local STEs, National Cancer Center (NCC), and other national institutions. The Cervical Cancer Prevention, Diagnosis, Treatment and Palliation Guideline was created in English and back translated into Mongolian. The final guideline document was approved December 1, 2010 as Cervical Cancer Guideline protocol No 020/034 [14,15]. Specific guidelines for pain management in palliative care were also developed, as the first step toward holistic palliative care guidelines, as required by the WHO.

Some of the specific issues that the guideline group grappled with included: the test, the age group to be screened, the frequency of the screening, and management of test positive cases. There was extensive external international assessment-recommendation process. Regarding the test and the age group to be tested, the international recommendations (URC, EPOS Health Management, UNFPA) were for cervical screening of women aged 30-60 year old initially with VIA [9].Three implementation strategies were put forward including: screen all women ages 30 to 59 year old with once in a lifetime VIA which would mean the program needed to reach 485,000 women and 145,000 each subsequent year (assuming 90% coverage). A second strategy involved screening women at age 30 and again at 35 yo. This meant screening 30,000 women initially and 27,000 each year (assuming 90% coverage). A third strategy involved screening women on at age 35 yo which would involve 15,000 women initially and 13,500 each year (assuming 90% coverage). There was a small experience in Mongolia with both Pap test (NCC, private clinics) and VIA [16,17]. Some of the concerns with this approach were the lack of gynaecologists to deal with the high number of expected test positive cases. Using a second test (such as a Pap test or careHPV) was proposed. A proposal at an early stage, to use VIA as a screening instrument, but followed by further assessment, rather than direct treatment was rejected due to the assumed very high rate of false positive results (low specificity), which would bring strain to the very few available pathologists in the country. Concerning the Pap test, the issue was a lack of trained cytologists and cytotechnologists in the country. Concerning careHPV, it was felt to be too expensive. After many meetings, a subcommittee of 12 Mongolian leaders (Specialist in charge of Obstetrics and Gynecology services in the MOH, representative of the Government Implementation agency, vice director of the National Cancer Centre, vice direction of the Ulaanbaatar city Health Department, co-ordinator for UNFPA health reproductive project, Head of cancer research at NCC, head of Gyn-oncology surgery at NCC, head of pathology at NCC, senior chest surgeon at NCC, gynaecologist at NCC, Head of a family practice group No 10, Head of Mongolian Family Clinic Association) recommended the Pap test as the screening test and that cytology capacity be developed throughout the country. They recommended that test positive cases should be evaluated with colposcopy and treated with

Loop Electrosurgical Excisional Procedure (LEEP). Thus, this was the strategy put forward in the national guidelines.

The Mongolian cervical cancer screening policy was planned to be integrated into the public health system of level 1 clinics [5]. Ultimately the Department of Health in each aimag was designated as responsible for the cervical screening program. The Aimag Department of Health would use census lists or lists of populations from the Primary Health Care Centres to identify eligible women. Trained family health workers would visit homes of individual women. Women were invited both verbally and by written invitation to specific family practice clinics based on their address (or job ie., women working on the railroad/army would be seen at the respective railroad/army hospital). The family health workers would issue a screening card to eligible women with her name, age and address filled in. They would also maintain a register of all women invited to participate. Each clinics developed strategies for how screening was delivered (ie., family practice clinics would general offer cervical screening two days a week and Aimag centres would offer screening every day of the week). This information was printed on the invitation card. Women with abnormal results would be referred to the nearest colposcopy clinic usually located at the Aimag hospital or Regional Cancer Diagnostic Centre. All demographic, screening, cytology, and diagnosis information was held within the Aimag Department of Health. A specific call/recall system was designed and developed in order to manage the women as well as the data. This was, however, not yet working properly six months into the full-scale implementation of the policy.

One of the issues encountered involved terminology. Some of the cytology and histology terms in the English document did not have equivalent terms in Mongolian. Thus the Health Sciences University of Mongolia Medical Terminology Committee had to be involved to amend and ultimately approved terminology used in the guidelines protocol No 10/10 from Nov 12, 2010 [14].

Ultimately the following ordinances were passed by the Ministry of Health:

Ordinance #292 (2010) Improve the capacity for prevention of cancer in aimags and district; Ordinance #168 (2011) Cervical cancer guideline(CG-4); Ordinance #76 (2013) Registry statistical guideline (SG-1),Recall system statistical guideline(SG-2), Cancer Palliative Care guidelines (CG-6), Ordinance #96 (2013) Approval of national and local implementation plans, Ordinance #208 (2012) Distribution of equipment like cytology stains, Ordinance #242 (2012) Handling of Drugs [18,19].

A Standards of Practice document in Mongolia describes in detail the tasks various health providers are allowed to perform. Although these existed prior to the development of cervical screening guidelines, this had to be amended to reflect the evolving functions of various disciplines like performing LEEP for gynaecologists (MNS 5855-2:2008)and Cervical Cancer early detection, case management and followup (MNS 5855.2.2011) [14,20,21,22,23]

B. Planning Phase

The second aspect in developing a cervical screening program involves planning the program by engaging local stakeholders, assessing local needs and developing a program action plan. Once these tasks are complete, the management team could aim to build capacity for the program and prepare for implementation [4]. Cervical cancer screening involves many facets: Community information and education increases awareness about cervical cancer and preventative health screening behaviours; screening services including clinics where the test can be completed and cytology laboratory where the test can be analyzed; diagnosis and treatment services for women with a precancer or cancer diagnosis including histopathology laboratory; training for staff in all settings; and monitoring and evaluation [4]. There is interaction of all of these facets for example, the cytology specimen must get from where it was retrieved to the cytology lab. Also the results of the cytology specimen must get back to the health care provider and ultimately the woman who was screening. Planning the program recognizes the there are women in a community who are in the recommended screening cohort, and health care providers who deliver the screening service and follow-up of women with positive tests. Some of the key aspects during this phase involves an assessment of the services currently available including equipment and facilities, training needs for health care provides, and knowledge attitudes and behaviour of the women and their community. Once the assessment is conducted there must be a plan to augment services where needed.

The first aspect in the planning phase involves training. The goal of training is to ensure that there is a sufficient number of competent staff to provide the various aspects of the screening service to eligible women including those identified as having precancer and cancer [4]. Training can involve health care provides like family doctors, gynaecologists and nurses, but it may also include statisticians, clerical staff, cleaning staff, community health workers and biomedical engineers.

Example:

Assessment: The Rapid Needs Assessment [10] done in Mongolia showed that there were deficits in knowledge and understanding about cervical cancer prevention among primary health care providers and their staff, a deficit in number of gynaecologists who could perform colposcopy and treatment of precancers, and a lack of cytologists.

Intervention: Training was undertaken using a train-the-trainer model. Here international and national experts trained an educator and regionally identified peer leaders in their field (Figure 1,2). The educator along with these trained individuals delivered the training in their regions and the surrounding regions using the same material including printed materials, slide decks and videos. The number of individuals to be trained, the length of training and responsible individuals were identified centrally by the PIU. The individuals to be trained were recommended by the regional department of health with input from the local clinics, hospitals ect. Discipline specific training modules were developed (spring 2010), pilot tested (summer-fall 2010) [14] and then implemented with smaller core groups (fall –winter2010) and then eventually across the country (spring- summer 2011). These included both didactic, small group and practical sessions. Although the training emphasized training in the knowledge and skills related to the paradigm of cervical cancer prevention, given results of the community assessment (presented later in this chapter), there was focused training on counselling clients prior to, during and after the medical encounter [24,25]. This counselling involved establishing a respectful rapport with women and addressing their fears and concerns. This was felt to be important in order to encourage women to return for follow-up visits [24,25]. Pre and post tests showed considerable improvement in knowledge (increased by 25%) [10,14,24]. In order to expand the cytology capacity in Mongolia, interested family physicians nominated by their aimag, were brought to the National Cancer Centre (NCC) cytology lab where they underwent an intensive 2 months of didactic and practical training before returning to their Aimag hospital. After this time, case conferencing was possible with the NCC through a telemedicine linkage with the NCC [26]. Separate atlases/training sets (Figure 3,4) were created/translated for colposcopy [27] and cytology [14].

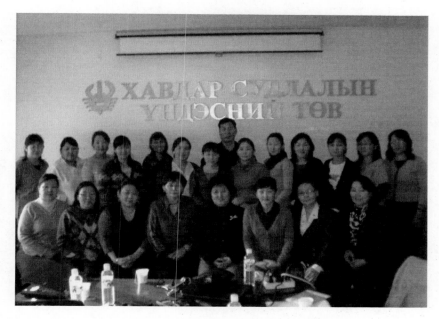

Figure 1. Class picture of physicians attending the January 2011 colposcopy training.

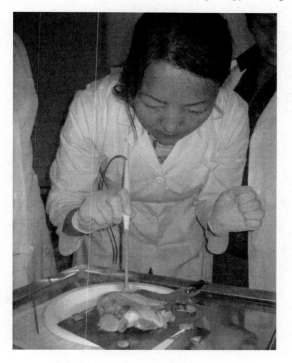

Figure 2. Colposcopy training practicing electrosurgery on a chicken breast.

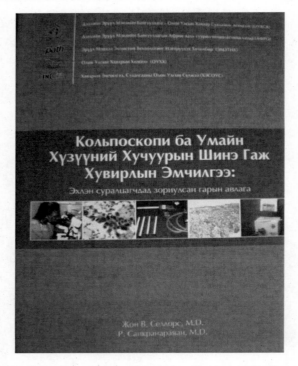

Figure 3. Colposcopy training book developed in conjunction with IARC [27]. The book was translated into Mongolia with permission from IARC.

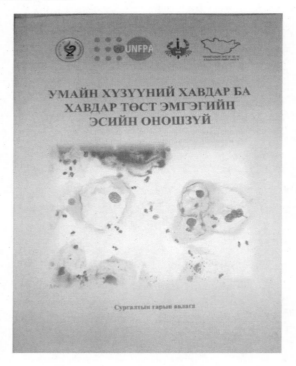

Figure 4. Manual created in Mongolian language for training cytotechnologist.

The second aspect of the planning phase involves facilities and equipment. Preparing and sustaining service facilities means that the screening and treatment services need to have designated space that meets certain requirements (ie., ventilation options for smoke evacuation when a treatment is performed by LEEP). The space also needs to be stocked with appropriate type and volume of supplies and equipment. In addition, strategies must be defined to minimize damage to expensive equipment (ie., surge protectors to prevent power surges). Policies and procedures need to be developed around cleaning the equipment. Procedures are also needed to define individuals who will procure supplies; document receipt of these and problem solve incomplete orders. A strategy of waste management needs to be put into place.

Example:

Background: Health care in Mongolia is organized along a primary, secondary and tertiary system of care [5,21]. Mongolia is made up of 21 aimags (provinces), which are divided into 338 soums (districts) which are further divided into baghs (villages).Primary care is offered by bagh feldshers (ie., health care workers and midwives), family group practice (FGP) clinics or family health centre of which there are 228 across the country and soum health centres and inter soum hospitals (35 in the country). Secondary care is offered at District General Hospitals and Aimag General Hospitals. Tertiary level care is available in UlaanBaatar where there are major hospitals and specialized professional centres like the National Cancer Centre (NCC) and Regional Diagnostic and Treatment Centres (3 in the country) [5].

In the 1990s, the only cancer treatment (ie., radiation, curative surgery and chemotherapy) was available at the NCC. In the last decade, 3 regional Cancer Diagnostic and Treatment Centres were developed as a place closer to home where patients could be assessed and if they have a potentially curative cancer referred to the NCC [29]. If the cancer was considered palliative, then the pain and symptom management, if offered via oncologists, could be administered at these regional centres, closer to home.

Assessment: A Facilities Based Impact assessment [10] showed that all centres were lacking in the equipment necessary for screening (ie., speculums, preservatives). The labs were lacking in Pap test stains. The Hospitals and Regional Diagnostic and Treatment Centres did not have operable colposcopes, biopsy forceps, or LEEP/cryotherapy units [10]. The units that were present had been procured originally from international donors [10].

Intervention: One of the priorities of the project was to define the type and amount of equipment needed at each service level. Unfortunately delivery of procured equipment which was planned for early 2011, was delayed until the spring of 2012.

Part of one's care is paid for by the national insurance but people must contribute to the cost of their care. Prior to the MCC project, Pap tests were designated to be paid for by the individual. During the conduct of the project, one Pap test per woman age 30-60 years old was free.

There are two aspects of the Planning Phase that are related to the education of women and the community. First involves the broader scope of educating the community about cervical cancer and the opportunity to prevent this disease through vaccination and screening. Second involves the one on one counselling with a woman at the time when she is considering or presents for the screening test.

Educating the community: It is important to have an information and education plan that informs women in the target age group and their partners about the benefits and availability of cervical cancer prevention services. This plan focuses communication at different levels such as the community, facilities and media. Although the media can reach a large proportion of the community at one period in time, its impact is different than that of direct contact with health workers and peer educators. Group awareness followed by individual counselling can address a client's specific informational and emotional needs, motivate her to follow treatment recommendations and establish a satisfied client who will encourage other women to attend screening. Printed material is helpful to reinforce messages but should not replace direct provider contact.

Educating individual women: Since the women at highest risk for cervical cancer usually have completed childbearing and so are unlikely to access family planning or maternal health services – special approaches for screening are required [30]. Creating culturally relevant methods are needed (ie., through input from local women's or community groups); by linking screening to an important event in an older woman's life (ie., becoming a grandmother) or linking screening to other mid-life events (ie contraceptive sterilization). Use of multiple communication strategies is most successful [30]. The most valued education comes from the physician to the woman and this interaction strongly influences whether the woman returns for her follow-up or rescreening appointments. The interaction with a physician should take place in a private and safe place for the woman.

Example:

Assessment: In Mongolia there were several types of assessments used to understand the knowledge, attitudes, beliefs, and behaviour of women and their partners concerning cervical cancer and cervical cancer screening

A cross-sectional survey was conducted in 2009 using the WHO STEPS survey methodology [8]. A total of 3,221 women were randomly selected from ages 15-64 years old. Mongolians participated from 36 soums of 20 aimags and 6 Ulaanbaatar city districts. The demographics of the women were that 6.9% (5.2-8.5%) currently smoke usually starting at 23.2 (21.3-25.1) years. The population included 496 aged 15-24yo, 992 aged 25-34 yo, 876 age 35-44yo, 626 age 45-54 yo, and 301 age 55-64yo. The mean number of years of education was 10.8 year. Women were more likely than men to have post-secondary school education. The average annual income was 1,282 USD. Cervical cancer screening coverage was reported to be very low; 5.2% (95%CI 4.2-6.1%) of females surveyed reported having had a VIA test and 11.4% (95%CI 9.9-13%) a Pap test. The highest cervical screening rate was in women 35-54 years old. Cervical screening coverage was the same in urban and rural settings.

A qualitative study was conducted through Mongolia involving women ages 30-60 years old and their husbands [6,7]. The women in the study either presented for cervical screening or were diagnosed with cancer. They either had a one on one interview or they were interviewed in focus groups. The first theme involved female knowledge, attitudes, behaviour and perceptions of risk factors related to cervical cancer screening. Women appeared to know about cervical cancer if a family member or acquaintance was affected. Rural women appeared to present in the late stages of the disease. Women reported higher satisfaction with treatment at the NCC with a lower complication rate than women treated at private clinics. Women reported a lack of information about cervical cancer and its cure rates. There was a considerable difference in knowledge levels between urban and rural women; for example, rural women thought the causes of cervical cancer were smoking, heavy drinking, complicated delivery, stress and chronic illness. Urban women thought the causes were not being faithful to husband, multiple sex partners, early age of sex, abortions, STD, husband's education level. The second theme involved the perceptions, misconceptions and knowledge of signs and symptoms of cervical cancer as pain, bleeding, and discharge. Women found it hard to tell their husbands this was going on, but when they did tell their husbands they were encouraged to get medical care. The third theme was perceptions, knowledge, and attitudes related to screening. Urban women found it easier to seek health care from private clinic even though its more expensive. Rural women went to local hospitals for treatment. Most women did not know anything about cervical cancer screening. Women claimed that health providers do not give information about screening. The fourth theme was the experience with screening and referral. Women found the waiting rooms of screening service locations crowded, inconvenient and they lack information about cervical cancer. In urban centres, the husbands came with the women and helped in decision making. In rural settings women came to the hospital alone. MDs do not explain things, too busy.

A cross-sectional survey of knowledge, attitudes and practices related to non-communicable diseases among Mongolian general population was conducted in 2010 [31]. This survey included 2,037 randomly selected women ages 15-64 yo from 24 soums of 20 Aimags and 18 Khoroos of 7 districts of Ulaanbaatar. Data was collected in 2010. 594 were ages 15-24yo, 441 wee 25-34 yo, 396 were 35-44 yo, 311 were 45-54 yo, and 295 were 55-64 yo. 11.9% of women complete college and 25.7 completed university. 22.2% of women were employed in the public organizations, 6.7% in NGOS, 18.1% in private sector and 1.2% irregular employment, with 16.1% unemployed. More than half of the women 30 yr and older (57.6%) did not know about cervical cancer. The 4-point scale showed that 22.1% (18.1-26.6%) had no understanding, 35.5% (30.7-40.7%) had heard the term, 31.5% (28.1-35.1%) know a little, and 10.9% (8.2-14.3%) knew it well.21.4% did not know how often to have a Pap test and 71.6% (66.6-76.1%) thought it should occur annually, 6% (4.1-8.8) every 3years, 1% (0.5-1.9) every 5 years. Reasons for not having a Pap test were that 63.1% (58.1-67.9) did not know that they needed a Pap test and 14.5% (11.4-18.2) said they did not have time while 13.2% (10-17.4) did not know where to go to get a Pap test, 2.5% (1.4-4.4) said it was expensive and 2.1% (0.8-5.5%) said it was embarrassing. In terms of prevention: 15.3% (said it was preventable by vaccine and 84.7% said it was not preventable. Responses were similar in rural and urban women. 45.7% (39.9-51.7%) said they never worry that cervical cancer could affect them or their families, and 48.4% (43.4-53.5) said they seldom worry about this while 5.8% (3.9-8.6) were very worried. Women have a lack of knowledge about cervical cancer and thus have a low risk perception. They have lack of a risk perception leading to a lack of preventive behaviour. This study showed a need to develop a nation wide education and health promotion.

The School of Public Health in Mongolia did a health seeking behaviour study involving six hundred and thirty four teachers from 60 schools in 2010 [32]. These teachers were predominantly female (90.2%) and represented urban (49%) and rural schools (51%). Mean age was 37.2 year. 93.7% considered cervical cancer preventable. 40.5% named the Pap test as a method for early detection while 3.6% named colposcopy as a method for early detection. Knowledge about cervical cancer and screening appeared to be better in educated women.

Intervention: A multipronged approach was planned around education of Mongolians concerning cervical cancer and preventative health care.

Opportunistic Media opportunities: The media coverage concerning the success of receiving the Millennium Challenge project in Mongolia in and of itself raised awareness about health issues in Mongolia. During the time frame of the Millennium Challenge project, the first lady of Mongolia who was also involved in the Hope Foundation, was instrumental in procuring the HPV vaccine through GAP for Mongolian girls aged 14yo. This also resulted in media attention which further educated the public on primary prevention and cervical cancer.

Planned educational events: The project planned for time on national television to provide in depth education on the need for screening to prevent cervical cancer. In addition, at each health clinic offering cervical screening there were large posters hung either outside the clinic or on the clinic walls in the waiting area (Figure 5). These serve to reinforce the message about the importance of cervical screening. Family health workers were trained concerning cervical cancer risks and prevention strategies. Family health workers were instrumental in handing out the invitations for cervical cancer screening and were often the first level of trained personnel that the Mongolia general public interacted with one on one concerning information needs or specific questions related to cervical cancer prevention (Figure 6,7,8). Nurses and doctors were trained in counselling concerning the Pap test and giving results. This model of educating and counselling patients was novel for many health care providers.

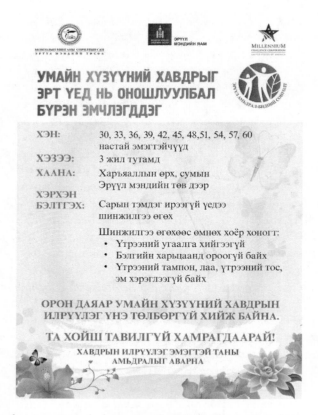

Figure 5. An example of posters on cervical screening found in family practice clinics.

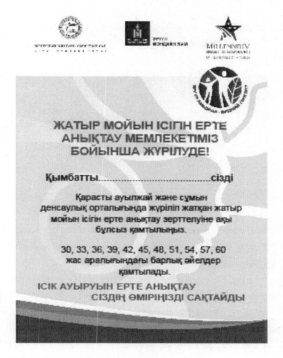

Figure 6. An example of an invitation card for the Kazak region.

The fourth aspect of the Planning Phase related to information systems. In order to understand how well the cervical screening program is functioning, the program requires good records whether paper based or electronic. Ideally the system should be able to identify who needs to be invited to be screened and track their results, including the test positive cases that required further investigations and treatment. Indicators like screening coverage can be determined with access to such information and allows the program management team to focus on specific issues that are identified.

Example:

Assessment: Prior to developing the Mongolian Cervical Screening Program, every Mongolian had a 6"x 8" paper based medical record that they were personally responsible for. This record and any ancillary pieces of paper with test results or XRay films were carried by the patient from health care provider to health care provider. During the time frame of this project, cell phone use was possible throughout most of the country. Although internet was available throughout the country, it was exceedingly slow and costly especially in more rural locations.

Plan: National standardized screening invitation logs and screening participation logs were developed. National data collection forms were developed for lab results (ie., cytology and histology), and clinical assessment (Pap test completed, colposcopy record, treatment record). One copy would follow the patient but one copy would go to the Aimag Department of Health either in paper or by electronic data capture. When data capture did not occur directly at the clinic/lab, these results would be transferred from paper based forms into an electronic system specifically created for cervical screening program by the statistics department at the Aimag Department of Health [14,15].

During the creation of a strategy for data collection for the cervical screening program, it became clear that the National Cancer Registry which is a part of the National Cancer Centre and is regulated by a HM Order no 203 2005 [33] was not operating optimally. In part this was due to multiple issues including incompatibility of the CANREG 5 system to the in country hardware and the lack of a Mongolian translation of morphology coding and TMN classification. Thus, Mongolian cancer statistics only reflected data from patients who were seen and registered at the National Cancer Centre and not about cancers occurring throughout the country. This cervical screening project created an opportunity to improve upon the status of the national cancer registry.

C. Implementation Phase

The third phase of developing a cervical cancer prevention program involves a plan for implementing, monitoring and evaluation [4]. All the work of the policy and the planning phase comes to fruition during the launch of the program. As discussed above, the components of the program include providing the community with information and education to address both the community and client's needs; delivery of the clinical services and the linkages between services; and ensuring trained providers are performing to standard [4]. Once the program is operational, ongoing monitoring is focused on ensuring that quality services are provided and taking time to collect and analyze data related to the program's goals and taking timely corrective action to optimize quality of care. This may be at the local level, the regional level or the national level. Evaluation is a formal process of measuring indicators to determine if the program is meeting its goals including the reduction of advanced stage cervical cancer (an outcome variable). As part of implementation, the management team works toward ensuring the availability of service, ensuring access to services, and maintaining linkages and referral systems.

Example:

In Mongolia, each aimag Department of Health received a Cervical Cancer Screening Manual. This manual included: 1.The cervical cancer screening guideline, 2.Procedures, 3. Standards (ie., how to label Pap test slides with the patient identifiers), 4. Instructions related to equipment like cleaning and maintenance, 5 Waste management protocols, 6. Standards for the size of the room and equipment requirements, 7. Human resources in terms of number and type of personnel required with their job description, 8. Equipment lists, 9. Quality assurance plan, and 10. The monitoring and evaluation plan.

There were implementation plans for both the national and locoregional level. These outlined in detail the 1.Human resources issues; 2. Guidelines, standards and procedure protocols, 3. Supplies and Equipment, 4. Facilities, 5. Data registry and call back, 6. Community Education, and 7. Monitoring and Evaluation. Each item had a list of activities to be accomplished, time frame, agency responsible, a list of cooperating agencies, expected outcomes, and indicator(s). By and large the national plan was under the direction of the MOH and PIU. The locoregional plan was under the direction of the Department of Health.

The first aspect of implementation involves ensuring availability of services for all women in the target age. Within this section all components for cervical cancer prevention must be in place and functioning including all components of the clinical service (counselling, screening, laboratory services (cytology and histology), diagnosis (colposcopy) and treatment of precancer (LEEP), post treatment followup, a referral system for treatment of cancer or end stage disease (palliative care)). This task also involves focusing on making sure appropriate staff is available and trained at every level of care. It also means preparing and sustaining facilities for the task that they have been designated to conduct.

Example:

Each family practice/public health clinic needed to define how the Pap test specimens would go to the lab. In one centre this meant the nurse would walk the specimen to the lab when she walked home from work. In rural settings, there was discussion that a multi-use driver would pick up and deliver the specimens on a weekly schedule. Each jurisdiction problem solved the portion of the program that was under their control.

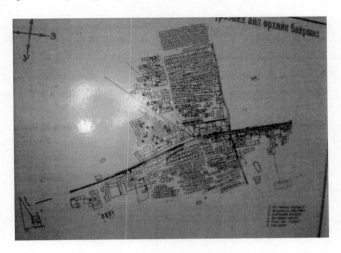

Figure 7. In one clinic, this is a survey of the households served by that clinic. The green dots represent who has been invited to participate.

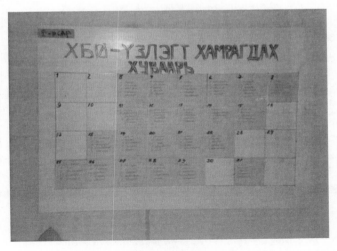

Figure 8. To handle the increase of patient volume, this clinic created a list of women who would be invited to attend screening each day of the month.

The second aspect involved in implementation involves ensuring access to cervical cancer prevention services. There are several strategies to optimize the chance a woman gets the care she needs which involves decreasing barriers [4]. A strategy of single visit versus multi-visit approach can minimize the number of health care visits for the woman screened. For example, a "see and treat" approach where screening and treatment take place at the same visit is a beneficial strategy for rural women and minimizes loss to follow-up due to geographic barriers to care. The multi-visit approach is associated with additional recalls and revisits for diagnostic evaluation and treatment and may pose added logistic difficulties. These may act as barriers to participation in the program [13]. Another consideration with respect to implementing the service involves a vertical versus integrated service. A *vertical service* means that clinics are run with the sole purpose of offering cervical cancer screening means that the staff roles and responsibilities are clearly defined but is more costly to implement and more difficult for the client to access. *Integrating* cervical cancer prevention services with other health programs that offer related services and/or reach women in their 30-40s [4,30] has the benefits of dealing with several health problems during one visit, using existing referral networks, and access to a wider range of onsite staff. A disadvantage of the integrated service is that there are competing priorities and prevention always seems less important than treating illness. An integrated service requires a higher level of planning and organization. It has the potential to excessively increase the providers' workload. The clinic staff's roles and responsibilities may be less well defined. Another strategy for implementing the service involves *static services* such as going clinics compared to high coverage onetime event outreach clinics like the Pap test bus.

Example:

The Mongolia MOH ultimately agreed to the choice of a multiple visit cervical screening approach. It was well known that this approach has many opportunities for loss to follow-up (ie., patient needs to return to get her results, patient needs to travel to a colposcopy clinic for diagnosis, patient needs to attend the colposcopy clinic for her results, the patient needs to attend the colposcopy clinic for treatment). In part loss to follow-up is related to geography (ie., distance from home to clinic), and other pressing priorities for the woman (ie., child care or work). The recently completed Healthy Mongolian project [9,17] showed some of the difficulties of carrying out a multiple visit cervical screening approach. In the Healthy Mongolian project, women were screened for cervical cancer using a questionnaire and/or VIA. 2,919 women were recommended to have further assessment. Only 332 (1 in 9) were confirmed while the rest (8 of 9) never attended follow up [9]. Mongolia did choose an integrated approach of including cervical cancer screening within the family practice model currently accessible throughout the country. This was augmented by the work being done by one of the NGOs known as the Daffodil project. Here the rotary club has volunteers who provide Pap test screening services to geographically isolated women [34].

As part of ensuring access to the cervical cancer screening program, there is a need to identify and address bottlenecks to effective service delivery [30].

Example:

Given that screening was an entirely new concept for most Mongolians and because the first Pap test would be free of charge, it was anticipated that many women would want the service. In order not to overwhelm health care providers including family practice/public health offices and cytology services, several implementation strategies were discussed. For example, there could be a once in a life time invitation of all women aged 30-60 years old to attend screening when the service was ready to start. Alternatively, women could be invited during the month of their birthday to attend the service which would spread out the demand over 12 months. Alternatively, the first year of the program women 30-39 yo could be invited and the next year 40-49 yo, and the final year women 50-59 yo could be invited. Alternatively since screening was to take place every three years, women aged 30, 33, 36, 39, 42, 45,48, 51, 54,57,60 yo could be invited to attend screening during the month of their birthday and this would smooth out attendance for a new service over the 3 year initiation. The last strategy was chosen in Mongolia [35].

The third aspect of implementation involves establishing and maintaining linkages and referral systems. A well-functioning referral network facilitates issues such as where the Pap test is analyzed, where the regional colposcopy clinic is located and its days and times of operation, how data flows between providers and how the system interacts with the community. Referral systems for patients with a newly diagnosed early stage cancer and end stage cancer are important. Within this system there needs to be methods of two-way communication, protocols for referral, tools like standardized referral letters and counter-referral letters.

Monitoring and evaluation helps determine whether the program is meeting its goals and objectives. Monitoring is about ensuring high quality processes of care. Monitoring determines whether the program is delivering appropriate services, reaching the women at risk (coverage) and allows for correction of problems in the operation of the program [4,30]. The outputs of monitoring include creating a quality service with available screening and treatment services run by competent staff and a community that is knowledgeable about cervical cancer. Evaluation is about being effective. Here questions are answered including: what is the screening coverage, what is the treatment rate of women with precancers. The ultimate goal is a decrease rate in late stage cervical cancer and eventually a decrease rate in all cervical cancers. Positive results in monitoring and evaluation can mobilize continued financial and political support for the program [30].

Example:

An example of monitoring in Mongolia involved the initial program launched in Tuv aimag. This was planned as a pilot study to identify key issues and rectify them so that later in the winter of 2012, the launch of the national cervical screening program would be more smooth. Another example of monitoring took place in the summer and fall of 2012. Here several individuals representing, health care providers, trainers, equipment, and health services planners conducted monitoring visits throughout the country. One focus was to verify that the equipment had arrived, was accounted for and operational. Another focus was to evaluate whether the health care staff understood how to complete forms and patient logs, and that the DOH statisticians understood the importance of timely data entry. Processes were reviewed at every level of the screening chain of events to ensure that each level had a plan and that those involved understood the plan.

The cervical screening program began in August 2012. The first 5 months of the program was evaluated and results discussed at the Second International Conference of Prevention and Control of Major non-communicable diseases and Injuries in May 2013.

1. *Knowledge Attitudes and Practice study from 2010 was compared to 2013. Here women of mean age 15-64 years old were surveyed and one of the questions involved awareness of cervical cancer. 54.2% of women had attended cervical screening. The*

awareness of the need for a Pap test had increased from 6% in 2010 to 34.2% in 2013, p<0.01. Awareness of the ability of a vaccine to prevent cervical cancer improved from 15.3% in 2010 to 45.3% in 2013, p<0.01.

2. *The Facilities Based Impact Study from 2010 was repeated in 2013. 88 urban facilities and 98 rural facilities were involved. There were 10 questionnaires completes by primary care practitioners, feldshers and nurses and managers or coordinators. On a 4 point score ranging from sufficient, middle, low, and insufficient, the overall score was sufficient. In terms of trained staff 78.7% scored sufficient; screening activity 85.1% scored sufficient; availability of guidelines 81.4% scored sufficient; available health education material 37.2% scored sufficient; and access to equipment 68.8% scored sufficient.*

3. *Knowledge, Attitudes and Practice study in school teachers involved urban regions (9 districts of Ulaanbaatar and 2 major cities), and rural areas (16 aimags and 9 soums). In 2010, 40.5% of teachers knew about Pap test and this rose to 71.60% in 2013.*

4. *Using the electronic data capture system, the coverage of invited women 30-60 year old for the first 5 months of the national program was 29.9%.*

It must be high-lighted, that there myst be clear ownership and management of a public health policy during the implementation phase, to ensure sustainability. A high-level Committee, provided with professional, political and financial authority must govern the implementation, monitoring and evaluating it, assuring quality and rapidly responding to any malfunctioning. This has been stressed as a necessary prerequisite for cancer screening programmes, particularly in low- and middle-resource health systems, by the WHO [3].

Example:
The recall system was developed for three purposes:

1. *To manage flows of patients and data through the screening process, according to the screening algorithms and Guidelines on cervical cancer*
2. *To deliver health data and data on the health system's performance for statistical analyses*
3. *To monitor the process and identify malfunctioning, bottle-necks and misunder-standings, in order to correct them*

It was early requested, and several times repeated, by the Project implementer, that a standing "Monitoring Committee" should be formed, already before the start of the implementation phase, with the tasks to actively monitor and evaluate the policy implementation, to collect and analyze data, and to promptly take any necessary actions of correction, whenever needed.

Almost one year into the implementation, such a Committee had yet not been formed, and it was not clear whether the Mongolian health system had understood the importance. As a result, data from the recall system had yet not been processed, and there was no clear understanding on how the policy was running. During a mission from the international cancer screening expert, data were processed and analyzed, together with the Mongolian counterpart, in a hands-on demonstration.

When this Chapter is written, there is finally a decision taken to follow the recommendations to harbour the policy on the MOH level (ownership),and to nominate a management for Monitoring and Evaluation, and Quality Assurance.

Conclusion

Creating or changing a cervical cancer program is not a unidirectional path of activity. It involves empowering a manager who sets into action the project plan which has clear objectives and timelines. This manager is ultimately responsible for the daily operations of the program. There is an interdisciplinary management team which is involved in raising concerns and problem solving issues. A clearly defined ownership and a staged management is a must in the implementation and maintenance of any public health policy. This clear ownership and firm management can minimize flaws in the systems that go undetected. In a national cervical screening program, there are also many stakeholders and partnerships. A change in one area has predictable and unpredictable ramifications. Thus communication is a key skill set in the leadership of the cervical cancer screening program. The plan and ongoing communication and problem solving will allow all the players to move forward there part of the cervical screening program plan. Monitory and evaluation will be critical to inform the successes and identify problems to information areas where adjustments are needed so that the ultimate goal (decreasing the rate of cervical cancer) is reached.

Next Steps

It is early days in the Mongolian cervical cancer screening program. The Mongolian Ministry of Health will need to continue to invest financially in the cervical screening program when the Millennium Challenge project comes to a close in September 2013. Identification of a responsible agency within the MOH has yet to occur. Monitoring will be needed to understand local issues and help problem solve these. Evaluation will be needed on an ongoing basis to determine if the rates of cervical cancer actually decrease with the screening strategy that was implemented. Location and responsibility for the electronic health record and recall system has yet to be defined. Mongolian office the WHO has indicated strong support for navigating this transition process.

Afterward

My Mongolian counterparts in the healthcare sector recently asked me, "Do you remember when you first came to Mongolia in 1999? You gave a lecture on cervical cancer prevention and most of us had never heard about a Pap test." It has been an amazing journey to participate, however, small in the implementation of a National Mongolian Cervical Cancer screening strategy. How well this program meets the needs of the Mongolian women at risk for cervical cancer is a story that will be written using the creativity, ingenuity and perseverance that the Mongolians have been known for since the time of their ancestors like Ghenghis Khan.

Acknowledgments

The Mongolian project was financed by the Millennium Challenge Corporation, USA, implemented by MCA-Mongolia and the institutional contractor was EPOS Health Management, Germany.

References

[1]   Edited from Weatherford J. *The Secret History of the Mongol Queens. How the daughters of Genghis Khan Rescued his empire.* Ney York;Crown Publishing Group c2010.

[2]   Sankaranarayanan R, Ferlay J. Burden of Breast and Gynecological cancers in low-resource countries. In Shetty ME (eds). *Breast and Gynecological Cancers: An integrated approach for screening and early diagnosis in developing countries.* Springer Science and Business Media, New York 2013.

[3]   WHO: National Cancer Control Programmes. Policies and Managerial Guidelines. *WHO, Geneva,* 2002 (2nd edition).

[4]   Alliance for Cervical Cancer Prevention (ACCP). Planning and Implementing cervical cancer prevention and control programs. *A manual for managers. Seattle: ACCP;* 2004.

[5]   Tsilaajav T, Ser-od E, Baasai B, Byambaa B, Shagdarsuren O. Mongolia Health System Review. Health Systems in Transition. Editors Kwon S, Tichardson E. Asia Pacitic Observatory on Health Systems and Policies, Vol 3 Issue 2 *WHO Press*:Geneva, Switzerland c 2013.

[6]   Report on Health Seeking Behaviour with regard to cervical cancer screening in Ulaanbaatar. Millennium Challenge Account – Mongolia Health Project, School of Public Health, Health Sciences of Mongolia. *Ulaanbaatar:EPOS;* 2010.

[7]   Erdenechimeg E, Tholmon Ch, Naransukh D, Myagmarchuluun S, Khishgtogtokh D, Tsevegdorj Ts et al. *Study Report on Health Seeking behaviour with regard to cervical cancer screening. MCA-Mongolia Health Project and School of Public Health, Health Science University of Mongolia. Ulaanbaatar,* 2011.

[8]   WHO. Mongolian STEPS Survey on the Prevalence of Noncommunicable Disease and Injury Risk Factors – 2009. *Ulaanbaatar:WHO;*2010.

[9]   Cervical Cancer: Programmatic Strategies Mongolia. *CC Mongolia – Cervical Cancer Screening and Treatment and HPV Pilot Program: Draft Report.* 7Jan2009.

[10]   Mongolia MCA-Millennium Challenge Account Mongolia, The Government of Mongolia. Institutional Technical Assistance contractor for the prevention and control of major non-communicable diseases and injuries. Rapid needs assessment report – main Body. *Ulaanbaatar:MMCA;* Feb 2010.

[11]   Dondog, B; Clifford, GM; Vaccarella, S; Waterboer, T; Unurjargal, D; Avirmed, D; Enkhtuya, S; Kommoss, F; Wentzensen, N; Snijders, PJ; Meijer, CJ; Franceschi, S; Pawlita, M. *Human papillomavirus infection* Cancer Epidemiol Biomarkers Prev 2008:17(7);1731-8. doi: 10.1158/1055-9965.EPI-07-2796.

[12] *Possible difference in the protective (to cervical cancer) efficacy between the two HPV vaccines Gardasil ® and Cervarix ®. Elffors L, letter to the MCA PIU*, November 12, 2010.

[13] Sankaranarayanan, R; Budukh, AM; Rajkumar. Effective screening programmes for cervical cancer in low- and middle-income developing countries. *Bulletin of the WHO* 2001;79(10);954-962.

[14] Mongolia MCA-Millennium Challenge Account Mongolia, The Government of Mongolia. Institutional Technical Assistance for the Prevention and Control of Major Non-communicable diseases and injuries. Phase 2 Report. *Ulaanbaatar:MMCA*; Dec 2010.

[15] EPOS, MCC. Institutional Technical: Assistance for the prevention and control of major noncommunicable diseases and injuries. First midterm report Phase 3. Ulaanbaatar: *EPOS Health Management;*June 2011.

[16] Elit, L; Baigal, G; Tan, J; Munkhtaivan, A. Assessment of two cervical screening methods in Mongolia: Cervical cytology and visual inspection with acetic acid. *Journal of LGTD* 2006; 10(2):83-88.

[17] Healthy Mongolian Project (Survey) 2007-2008 in MCC Mongolia. *Cervical Cancer Screening and treatment and HPV Pilot Program. Ulaanbaatar: MMCA.* Dec7, 2009.

[18] *http://www.moh.mn* Accessed 31May2013.

[19] *http://www.ncdi.mn* Accessed 31May2013.

[20] *http://www.estandard.mn* Accessed 31May2013.

[21] *http://www.estandard.gov.mn* Accessed 31May2013.

[22] *http://www.estandard.mn* Accessed 31May2013.

[23] *http://www.masm.gov.mn* Accessed 31May2013.

[24] Training Program for the MCA---Mongolia Non---Communicable Diseases and Injuries (NCDI) Health Project submitted by Onum Foundation and Eurasian Medical Education Program (EMEP) Partnership and . 2011 first quarterly report. *Ulaanbaatar:EPOS Health Management*;2011.

[25] Training Program for the MCA---Mongolia Non---Communicable Diseases and Injuries (NCDI) Health Project submitted by Onum Foundation and Eurasian Medical Education Program (EMEP) Partnership and . 2011 second quarterly report Jun 25, 2011. *Ulaanbaatar:EPOS Health Management*;2011.

[26] Tseedma B, Elit L. Telemedicine in cervical screening. In: Cervix cancer: screening methods, risk factors and treatment options. *Elit L* (Ed) Nova Press.

[27] Sellors J, Sankaranarayananan R (eds). Colposcopy and treatment of cervical intraepithelial neoplasia: A beginners' manual. *IARC Press;*France c2003.

[28] Mongolia MCA-Millennium Challenge Account Mongolia, The Government of Mongolia. Institutional Technical: Assistance for the prevention and control of major non-commuicable diseases and injuries. *Design of the facility based impact study. Ulaanbaatar:MMCA*; Mar2010.

[29] Elffors, L. Activities in the cancer area under the MCC funded health project on non-communicable diseases and injuries in Mongolia. Technical Report. *Ulaanbaatar; EPOS Health Management*;December 12-21,2009.

[30] Sherris JD, HerdmanC. Preventing cervical cancer in low resource settings. *Outlook.* 2000;18(1):6,7.

[31] *http://www.path.org/publications/detail.php?i=326* Accessed 5Apr2013

[32] Lkhagva, L; Tsetsegdary, G. Knowledge, Attitudes and Practices related to Non-Communicable Diseases among Mongolian General Population. Survey Report 2010. *Ulaanbaatar:EPOS Health Management*; 2011.

[33] School of Public Health HSUM. Report of Knowledge, *Attitudes and practices on non communicable diseases and injuries among school teachers in Mongolia.* Ulaanbaatar:HSUM; 2010.

[34] Esteban, DB. *Cancer registration in Mongolia. Mission Report to the MCA NCDI Project*, November 2010.

[35] *Daffodil   Project.   http://www.rotary.org/en/MediaAndNews/TheRotarian/Pages/ Health0910.aspx (Accessed 5April2013).*

[36] Elffors, L. *Assumptions on approaches to cervical cancer screening in Mongolia.* Technical Report. 30Apr2010.

In: Cervical Cancer
Editor: Laurie Elit

ISBN: 978-1-62948-062-6
© 2014 Nova Science Publishers, Inc.

Chapter V

Risk Factors for Recurrence or Progression in Women Treated for Cervical Intraepithelial Neoplasia

Begoña Martínez Montoro, Mónica González Macatangga,
Ignacio Zapardiel, Margarita Sanchez-Pastor, María
Serrano Velasco and Javier de Santiago
Gynecology Department, La Paz University Hospital, Madrid, Spain

Abstract

Cervical cancer ranks second for incidence and mortality associated with cancer in developing countries. In developed countries, thanks to the implementation of screening programs we have achieved a decrease of a 75% in incidence and mortality caused by this cancer. The purpose of the screening is to diagnose this serious disease in early stages and treat precursor lesions, also called cervical intraepithelial neoplasia (CIN), in an attempt to stop the carcinogenic evolution. Despite performing cervical conization to remove these premalignant lesions and appropriate cytologic and colposcopic following up, some of these treated patients develop cervical cancer. The risk of progression to invasive carcinoma in treated women remains higher compared to the general population for 20-25 years. Even women undergoing hysterectomy with removal of the cervix should be followed more closely than the general population because of the possibility of recurrence, although scarce, in vaginal vault or other locations. Hence the importance of finding predictors of recurrence of lesions in women already treated for precancerous lesions, despite attempts has not reached clear conclusions. We find conflicting results in the literature and few studies with long term follow-up.

With the main objective to determine what factors are associated with recurrent disease in women treated for precancerous lesions we conducted a retrospective study of 871 women diagnosed with HSIL or persistent LSIL treated in the service of Cervical Pathology of La Paz Hospital in Madrid from 1998 to 2008 and followed by cytology, colposcopy and histology for at least a year (mean follow-up time 33.35 months). The sample was divided according to the appearance of recurrent lesions, and studied the possible differences in age, type of lesion, treatment received, status of the margins of the surgical specimen, type of HPV infection found and by HIV presence.

As a result we found 13.5% of recurrence between patients under cone biopsy. (46% LSIL, 45% high-grade (5% CIN II, 6% CIN II-III, 16% CIN III y un 25% unspecified degree.) A 43.7% of patients with affected surgical margins recurred; this was statistically significant compared with the rest.

Besides HIV-positive women had a 50% of recurrent or persistent lesions, statistically significant comparing with 12.2% of recurrence in HIV-negative patients. Variables such as age, lesion type, treatment and subtype of HPV implicated no statistically significant differences. We conclude that the status of the surgical margins and the inmunosuppression caused by HIV infection were significant factors for predicting recurrence, and earlier development. Research for new predictors of recurrence is necessary for a better follow-up of the high-risk patients and to avoid overtreating low-risk ones.

Keywords: Intraepithelial lesion; HPV; Risk factors; Cervical cancer; Recurrence

Introduction

1.1. Objectives

The main objective of this study is to determine what factors are associated with the appearance of both persistent and recurrent disease in women treated for high grade intraepithelial cervical lesions (HSIL) or persistent low-grade squamous intraepithelial lesions (LSIL) in the service of Cervical Pathology in "La Paz" Hospital in Madrid, from 1998 to 2008. First we will describe the types of premalignant lesions and its carcinogenic evolution, different classifications, epidemiological data, the relationship with the human papillomavirus (HPV), methods of diagnosis and treatment and monitoring protocols. We attempt to provide an overview, though briefly, to help understand the importance and complexity of the issue at hand.

1.2. Epidemiology, Definition and Classification

In 2005 according to WHO, 500,000 new cases of cervical cancer were diagnosed. In 2008, the United States reported 11,070 new invasive cervical cancer; among them 3870 women are expected to die from this, which means 1% of all cancer deaths in women [1]. Although there has been a 75% of decline in incidence and mortality from cervical cancer in developed countries (due to the implementation of screening programs), it should be noted that this represents the second leading cause of morbidity and cancer associated mortality in developing countries.

Cervical cancer has been exceeded by breast cancer since the 1990s [2]. The descrepancy in morality between high and low resource countries is due to the lack of screening programs in countries with fewer health resources.

Throughout the last century and as the knowledge about the process of cervical carcinogenesis progressed, different nomenclatures have been appearing over time. At first we used the term 'dysplasia' to define premalignant cytological changes produced in the squamous epithelium classified into three grades from lowest to highest severity.

A few years later the term `Cervical Intraepithelial Neoplasia´ (CIN) was coined to describe the histological alterations observed and it was divided into three grades, depending on the thickness of the epithelium affected (Richart classification):

- CIN 1 is considered a low-grade lesion. They is mild atypia that only affect the lower third of the epithelium.
- CIN 2 is considered a high-grade lesion. There is moderate atypia bounded to the basal two-thirds of the epithelium remaining the upper third with preserved cell maturity.
- CIN 3 is also a high grade lesion. The atypia is severe and occupies more than two thirds of the thickness, invading even the entire epithelium but without actually breaching the basement membrane, which is what differentiates carcinoma from CIN.

The annual incidence of CIN in women undergoing screening in the US is estimated at 4% for CIN 1 and 5% for high grade lesions (CIN 2 and CIN3) [3]. At the conference in Bethesda in 2001 another classification was created which introduced new cytological terms like:

- LSIL: low grade squamous intraepithelial lesion
- HSIL: high grade squamous intraepithelial lesion.
- Other terms were ASC-US (Atypical Squamous Cells of Undetermined Significance) and AGUS (Atypical Glandular Cells of Undetermined Significance).

1.3. Etiology

Studies have been showing consistently that sexual activity is the most important risk factor for developing cervical cancer; in fact, both the cancer and its precursor lesions are virtually nonexistent in people without sexual activity [4].

Through epidemiological and molecular biology studies it has been seen the causal relationship between infection by the Human Papilloma Virus (HPV) and cervical cancer as well as other types of genitals cancer such as most of anal cancer, vagina, vulva, penis and from a third to a half of oropharyngeal cancers.

Table 1. Terminology

BETHESDA (2001)	Negative for malignancy	Reparative changes	ASC-US	LSIL	HSIL				AGUS AIS AC
RICHART (1993)	Normal	inflamation		CIN 1	CIN 2		CIN 3		
OMS (1979)	Normal	inflamation		Mild dysplasia	Moderate dysplasia	Severe dysplasia	Carcinoma in situ		

HPV is a double stranded DNA virus belonging to the family of Papilomaviridae and affects only humans because papillomaviruses are very species-specifics. There are over hundred types of HPV, more than 40 of them have tropism for mucous membrane and can infect the lower female genital tract. They have a very clear geographical distribution and are classified according to their carcinogenic potential in low or high risk. Common types are:

- High-risk (oncogenic or cancer-associated) types: 16, 18, 31, 33, 35, 39, 45, 51, 52, 56, 58, 59, 68, 69, 82.
- Low-risk (non-oncogenic) types: 6, 11, 40, 42, 43, 44, 54, 61, 72, 81

The most common high-risk types are 16, 18, 31, 33, 35, 45, 52 and 58 jointly causing 95% of cervical cancers [5]. It is noteworthy that only between 16 and 18 HPV types cause approximately 70% of cervical cancers (HPV16 in 60% of cases, and HPV18 in 10%)[6 and 8)]. The non-oncogenic types 6 and 11 cause about 90% of condyloma acuminatum and genital warts. Thus, it is estimated that the vaccines developed against HPV (the bivalent against HPV 16 and 18, and the quadrivalent againt HPV 6, 11, 16 and 18) will prevent about half of the high-grade precancerous lesions and 70% of cancers of the cervix, as well as most of genital warts [6].

Transmission usually occurs through genital contact during sex. Penetration is not required for the acquisition of infection [7], HPV infection has been identified in homosexual women who have never had sexual contact with men. HPV can be transmitted only by close personal contact in the case of cutaneous warts. It has been also described papillomatosis in respiratory tract of newborn due to the passage through the infected birth canal.

HPV is the most common sexually transmitted infection in the world. A meta-analysis performed in 157,897 women with normal cytology has shown that HPV prevalence is approximately 10% [8].

In the US, the estimated prevalence of anogenital tract infections by HPV is twenty million and the annual incidence of 5.5 million. It is also estimated that between 75-80% of sexually active adults will acquire this infection before the age of fifty. In view of all these data, it is curious that both the uterine cervical carcinoma and its precursor lesions are not much more frequent than they are already, generating a true pandemic. This is because over 50% of infections are removed between six and eighteen months from the acquisition and up to 80-90% are resolved in the first two years [6, 9, 10, 11].

We must know the mechanism of action of HPV in the cell to understand why the majority of HPV infections are transient and asymptomatic. HPV infects basal cells through small epithelial erosions produced during intercourse and uses the cellular machinery to generate new viral particles. The low-risk HPV are not inserted into cellular DNA and only use the cell to replicate, thus generating low-grade lesions. In contrast, the high-risk types, although they can also produce low-grade lesions, are closely related to high-grade lesions, persistence and progression of the lesions, as they are able to integrate into the host DNA.

HPV 16 and 18 generate 25% of LSIL, 50-60% of HSIL and 70% of cervix carcinomas [12]. Normal cells activate their defense mechanisms against viral presence and check their DNA sequence before splitting. If viral DNA is found, the cell enters apoptosis to prevent the infection from spreading. However, high-risk oncogenic HPV have evolved a mechanism capable of blocking this cellular defense system.

They block the apoptosis mechanism and the ability of the cell to check his DNA sequence, thus generating immortal cell clones that will be the basis of all the neoplastic process. So the neoplastic transformation capacity will depend on whether the virus is or not integrated in the cell genome and the host immunocompetence. We can find different situations after infection:

– Latent infection: is the most common (occurring in greater than 90% of infected women)
– Active infection: the virus replicates using the cellular machinery but is not integrated into the genome. It produces typical cytological changes.
– Resolution of infection: previously seen cellular changes disappear. It is resolved by the action of macrophages and by activated lymphocytes T CD4 antibody production. [13, 14, 70]
– Neoplastic transformation: with integration of HPV into the genome and therefore possibility of progression to high-grade lesions or cancer.

So we understand why HPV is considered a necessary but not sufficient cause for the development of cervical neoplasia, since the vast majority of infected women do not develop high-grade lesions or cancer [15, 16]. That is, the clearance of the virus is much more common than its persistence.

Several factors can influence the persistence of the virus such as:

1 The type of virus and its ability to produce a genomic integration (as previously explained)
2 Viral load
3 Cofactors such as those detailed below

The association between this virus and cervical neoplasia is so intense that the following socio-economic, sexual or life habits factors have been found as dependent variables for the presence of HPV and not like independent risk factors.

Risk factors for developing cervical cancer and its precursor lesions are (see section 3 for further expansion on each risk factor) [17-27]:

3.1. Early onset of sexual intercourse (before age 18 and more than three years of active sex life)
3.2. Multiple sexual partners
3.3. Sexual partner with high-risk factors: promiscuity, previous partners with HPV infection, not circumcised
3.4. STDs such as herpes simplex or chlamydia.
3.5. Smoking (direct carcinogenic effect and on local immunity)
3.6. Multiparity (> 3 children)
3.7. Immunosuppression (HIV, other diseases, iatrogenic factor)
3.8. Prolonged use of oral contraceptives (> 5 years)
3.9. Previous history of VIN, VAIN or condylomata
3.10.Age

It is known that in women over 55 years the virus persists by 50% while it is 20% in women under 25 years. Age is closely related to the development of cervical cancer. The high-grade precursor lesions are usually diagnosed between 25-35 years, with a mean of diagnosis of invasive cancer usually greater than 40 years (47 years in the US), between eight and thirteen after the diagnosis of high grade lesion [28].

1.4. Prevention

1.4.1. Primary Prevention

Previously, primary prevention consisted only in protection against the risk factors discussed above. Nowadays a new form of prevention is possible with vaccines. To avoid the risky sexual behaviors is the best preventive measure but other factors should be avoided as far as possible: continued use of hormonal contraceptives, nutritional status, to correct immunosuppressive states and avoid smoking are other important measures to prevent the occurrence of preinvasive lesions of female genital tract and subsequent progression to carcinoma.

Currently there are two different vaccines: one of them is a bivalent vaccine against 16 and 18 serotypes (Cervarix); and another is the quadrivalent against 6, 11, 16 and 18 serotypes (Gardasil). There are already many studies supporting the safety of the two formulations. It is not ethical or feasible to assess as an efficacy´s variable the changes in the incidence of cervical neoplasia, therefore intermediate variables are used for this purpose. In this way, studies have shown effectiveness achieving a lower incidence of HPV infection, a less persistence of viral infection and a lower detection of precursor lesions CIN II-III. Thus, the evidence shows that both formulations provide a high efficacy in preventing both transient and persistent infection and also in the development of cytological lesions.

Therefore the bivalent and quadrivalent vaccines generate immunogenicity with a seroconversion rate (generation of antibodies against HPV) very close to 100%. The level of these antibodies is maximum on seventh month (80 times greater than the produced by natural infection) and after it decreases gradually and remains stable at a level that is 14 times higher than the natural immune response generated (which is usually able to clear the virus). In animal studies a persistent protection has been seen despite low levels of antibody.

Although both vaccines contain only two types of high-risk oncogenic HPV, as previously mentioned, they are the two most frequent, so the immunization of 100% of the population could prevent 70% of cervical neoplasia. Furthermore it is noteworthy that due to the phylogenetic and antigenic similarities between the different types of HPV, it has been found a cross-protection against other HPV serotypes such as 45 and 31.

The vaccine should be inoculated before the first sexual intercourse. Even women who have had sex relations could also benefit from the vaccine because it is unlikely to have been infected with all HPV types included in it, in addition to the aforementioned cross-protection. Currently it is even recommended in women who have been treated for a premalignant lesion, for the same reasons.

It is anticipated that with the new vaccines in countries where there is a screening system, a significant reduction will be observed in the rates of CIN 2 and 3 (to 50%) and CIN 1 and ASCUS (by 20-30%) [29] This would reduce the number of abnormal Pap smears and therefore, a considerable decrease in the associated healthcare costs.

It has been speculated that a substitution can be occurred in the most frequently viral genotypes, yielding the space now occupied by subtypes included in the vaccine. More long-term studies are needed to demonstrate the certainty of this assumption. This also will help in the future to review the screening strategies, which may allow in this way, for example, to delay the age of onset of screening or to space out the subsequent controls. However it is necessary to continue with screening programs until there is a polyvalent vaccine that generates protection against all subtypes of HPV.

1.4.2. Secondary Prevention

There are only three types of cancer for those there are secondary prevention methods or screening: cervix, breast and colon. The first for which a screening method was introduced was the cervix in US in 1941 and was called Pap test. It consist in collecting, using a small brush or spatula, the cervix and vagina cells, and place them directly on a slide and fixed with chemicals.

Since its implementation the cervix cancer screening is in continuous reassessment and the technique has evolved. So, years later, a new technology called liquid-based cytology appeared and began to replace the old method. It involves extracting the sample similarly and then suspends the cells obtained in liquid transport medium; the cells are then filtered in the laboratory to be placed on a slide so it can be analyzed by cytologists or pathologists. It has failed to demonstrate a higher reliability compared to the other technique.

The main objective of this test is to detect in asymptomatic patients, cellular changes that occur by action of HPV in cervical epithelium. Specifically in the transformation zone (the junction between the ectocervix and endocervix) which is where cervical dysplasias and neoplasias settle, allowing to diagnose the process of carcinogenesis in early or preneoplastic stages. Adenocarcinoma is originated from endocervical tissue while if the neoplastic process begins in the ectocervical epithelial, the result will be a squamous carcinoma.

In the US between 50 and 60 million Pap test are performed every year. Approximately 3.5 million have any abnormalities on cytology, so about 2.5 million should undergo colposcopic study. Despite the implementation of population screening policies in UUEE, half of cervical cancers diagnosed between 2004 and 2006 were in advanced stages because they have not undergone screening (the most were elderly women and Hispanic race) [30]. In fact, more than half of women who had cervical cancer, had never been subjected to cytology, had done it very sporadically, or had not been seen in the last five years [31].

The Pap test gives cytological results, thereby allowing only to examine cells but not the tissue or the structure. It can diagnose LSIL or HSIL but not CIN, since this is a histological concept that requires obtaining a tissue sample by biopsy. Although the cytological abnormalities predict histological changes, there is not an absolute correspondence between the findings thus always histological diagnosis is required for the diagnosis of carcinoma of the cervix. Cervical cytology has many steps that could lead to errors in sampling or analysis. It has a quite important interobserver variability but it decreases with increasing severity of the abnormalities present in the sample. The test has a sensitivity and specificity that varies widely among studies. In fact it has never been evaluated in a randomized controlled trial. All the evidence of their effectiveness in reducing the incidence and mortality from cervical cancer (around 75%) is very consistent, although it comes exclusively from observational studies, it has been adopted as a screening method in all developed countries and many developing ones.

In UK, for example, the cervical cancer screening based on perform the cytology in its population since 1988 has prevented the death of 1 in 65 British women born since 1950 and about 6000 deaths per year in that country [32]. The average cervical cytology coverage in Spain is 76%, with differences between regions [33].

Cervical cytology has a low sensitivity for CIN 2-3, so it needs to be supplemented. Thus, it will be jointly used with the colposcopy or with the HPV detection test. Using cytology and colposcopy with or with HPV testing results in a negative predictive value of 100% for CIN 3 or higher. We will briefly describe the complementary techniques mentioned.

The HPV DNA´s determination can be accomplished by Hybrid Capture, in situ hybridization (FISH), or by polymerase chain reaction (PCR). They are designed to detect the presence of any of the 13 or 14 high-risk HPV subtypes. The sensitivity of the viral DNA´s detection by any technique is greater than cytology, so making a combined use of both techniques; it shows an improvement of the sensitivity of the screening. If both are negative the HPV´s infection is virtually impossible so the screening interval could be lengthened if this technique is added to the Pap test [34]. However, the DNA detection cannot be used as independent primary screening due to its low specificity, although it might be interesting as a strategy for screening in resource-poor areas for the cytology.

The indications for high risk HPV DNA´s detection include:

- Women with ASCUS in the cytology to know if it is necessary the colposcopy
- Postmenopausal women with LSIL in their cytology
- To follow-up women with CIN 1 after colposcopy and biopsy
- Control after treatment of intraepithelial neoplasia
- As a single screening test in conjunction with cytology

There is scientific evidence that the HPV DNA test becomes negative in the lesions have been extirpated completely, while if it continues detectable, the lesion will persist or recur. So, a positive DNA test at 6-12 months after therapy, even in the presence of normal cytology, allows us to recognize early treatment failure [35].

Colposcopy is a complementary technique enabling the exploration of the entire lower genital tract and to locate and describe the lesions, used especially for cervical study. It forms part of the diagnostic protocol of intraepithelial lesions and invasive cancer in these locations. This technique involves exploring the entire of lower genital tract with different optical magnification. It is performed with and without acetic acid and with and without iodine (Schiller's test).

A colposcopy is considered satisfactory when the entire transformation zone (T.Z.) can be seen, and unsatisfactory if displayed incompletely. So we can distinguish:

- T.Z. type 1: in ectocervix completely visible
- T.Z. type 2: the endocervical component is present although fully visible
- T.Z. type 3: the endocervical component is present but not totally visible.

The findings obtained with this technique are classified like major or minor changes according to the severity. Biopsy should be performed in all colposcopies with major changes and also in minor if it presents LSIL cytology or higher.

Not every abnormal finding corresponds to a cancer precursor lesion. Most of minor changes correspond to metaplasia or low grade lesion; the major changes usually correspond to high grade lesion or to an invasive lesion. Colposcopy has a high sensitivity and united to cytology allows to diagnose the most of the lesions. Despite all this, the screening of adenocarcinoma is less effective than squamous lesions because adenocarcinomas can settle in the channel and be more difficult to detect.

The recommended age for the end of the screening for cervical cancer is between 65 and 70 years, provided that they have had 3 or more consecutive normal Pap tests and without any abnormal in the last 10 years. However, it is always needed to individualize based on the patient's personal situation: life expectancy, sexual activity and other risk factors.

The introduction of vaccines will probably make obsolete this screening system. It will lead to an adaptation to the new situation and the rethinking of the protocol. There are certain exceptions to the usual protocols, as some risk groups that require more frequent screening than the general population: HIV positive women, other immunodeficiency as an organ transplant or SLE and women with intrauterine exposure to diethylstilbestrol.

We take into special consideration women undergoing hysterectomy. It is important to know which type of hysterectomy was performed because, although there are few studies about the cytological screening in women with hysterectomy, it is known that if the treatment was subtotal hysterectomy (preserving the cervix); they share practically the same risk as women who keep their entire uterus. So their screening should be equal to population general. However, it is known that those who underwent total hysterectomy (including removal of the cervix (95% of hysterectomies performed in the US currently) [36]) maintain virtually nonexistent risk of cervical cancer. Among women undergoing total hysterectomy it is important to differentiate two groups depending on the intervention's purpose. For women whose surgery indication was not related to any gynecologic malignancy, such as cervical cancer or precursor lesions, it is not recommended the screening for malignancy due to the low incidence discussed above in this subgroup. However, if the reason for the hysterectomy was associated with uterine cervical neoplasia, screening should be performed to rule out local recurrence at the site of the anastomosis, VAIN or vaginal carcinoma, despite its low frequency (The probability of cervical cancer after hysterectomy performed for CIN 3 is 1 in 5037 cases in a study) [37]. And the likelihood of developing VAIN after being treated with hysterectomy for CIN 3 is 1.7 compared to 0.12 for women without previous CIN. Vaginal cancer is even more rare [38]. So screening in these women can be spaced after three consecutive negative screening.

1.5. Treatment of Lesions Found by Screening

In the management of women with CIN, the aim is to prevent the progression to invasive cancer and also to avoid overtreating the lesions that are more likely to disappear. In the handling of CIN we can choose to keep waiting or treat immediately. Decision-making of one of the two options requires taking into account the correlation between cytological and colposcopic findings, the histological results of the biopsy, the patient characteristics such as age, pregnancy and the probability of adherence to monitoring, and the desire of future offspring.

The decision depends on several factors because pre-invasive lesions of the cervix usually appear in women's reproductive period and any excessive treatment may compromise their reproductive capacity.

There are two large groups of different therapeutic methods among which no significant differences were observed in terms of results (the average is 90% of cure) [39] so that the success of the treatment depends on the correct selection of the method as well as the surgeon's experience, because regardless of the method the complete elimination of the transformation zone is required:

- Ablative methods: it is only useful for treatment, not for diagnosis. Due to tissue destruction, there is no sample for analysis by the pathologist. This can be done using diathermocoagulation, thermocoagulation, cold coagulation or laser vaporization. It has a low incidence of adverse effects and complications (1-2%).

- Excisional method: This method results in a tissue sample for histopathological study. It should be used if the patient will not be able to attend follow-up, if invasive disease is suspected or if there was an unsatisfactory colposcopy. There are basically two techniques, hysterectomy or conization. Hysterectomy should not be done as a first choice for initial treatment of CIN II or III as it has higher morbidity than other techniques described. The cone can be made by scalpel, CO2 laser or loop diathermy. Comparative studies between different types of cone found no significant differences in the rate of recurrence of CIN or in terms of postoperative bleeding.

Although heat artifact is produced with laser and LEEP, is nonexistent when the cone is done with a scalpel. The length of the cone should be the minimum necessary in women of reproductive age. Conization´s technique involves cleavage (cone-shaped) of the portion of cervix around the endocervical canal including the transformation zone.

Conducting a cone biopsy versus observation depends on the diagnosis. Observation criteria are as follows: age <35years, the cytology and biopsy are consistent, if there are minor changes in colposcopy, the extension is small, if the lesion is peripheral, the endocervix is not affected, monitoring is possible or if it does not persist for long time. In contrast, the recommended criteria for an excisional biopsy would be: age > 35 years, if there are discrepancies between cytology and biopsy, if there are major colposcopic changes, the extension is large, the lesion is located in the center, if the endocervix is affected, the monitoring is not feasible or if the lesion persisted for over two years.

CIN I Lesions

Generally, CIN 1 does not required aggressive intervention. Not excisional treatment is needed if the histological diagnosis has been preceded by cytology findings of low-grade lesion as ASCUS, ASC-H or LSIL. This is so because a great number of them regress while very few progress to CIN II-III or carcinoma. However, if the lesion that was observed on cytology performed prior to biopsy showed a high-grade lesions, this could imply a serious lesion exists, and it has not been diagnosed by colposcopy and biopsy. HSIL on cytology implies more than 70% of prevalence of CIN II, III or higher on biopsy. For this reason, an excisional procedure is recommended. If CIN I on biopsy persists for more than two years, treatment is an option.

In adolescent females there is a high rate of spontaneous regression of the CIN 1. In pregnant women, there is a high rate of regression of these lesions after delivery and also a high risk of complications related to these therapeutic techniques during pregnancy (ie., bleeding, pregnancy loss). For this reason, treatment is not recommended during pregnancy for lesions unless there is a suspicion of invasion. Women with CIN 1, 2,or 3 should be reassessed with colposcopy at six weeks postpartum.

CIN 2 and CIN 3 Lesion

Both CIN 2 and 3 lesions are managed in the same way because histological distinction is complicated and difficult to reproduce. Due to the high risk of progression it is recommended immediate treatment with except in adolescents and pregnant (many high-grade lesions diagnosed during pregnancy tend to return in the postpartum period, although colposcopic monitoring is recommended).

CIN 2 lesions regress spontaneously in 40-58%, while 22% progress to CIN 3 and 5% to invasive carcinoma.

CIN 3 lesion regression rate without treatment is between 32%-47% and progression occurs in 12%-40%. So there is a lower rate of progression to CIN 2 as compared to CIN 3 and this could be explained because the CIN 2 is more frequently associated with HPV subtypes that are less prone to carcinogenesis.

1.6. Follow Up After Treatment

The goal of treatment after follow up is detecting both persistence (residual disease) and recurrence (disease of new onset after a year of close monitoring in which no residual disease was detected). Although it must be mentioned that there is no consensus about the time limits to differentiate between persistence and recurrence, so in the literature many classifications are found, and in our study we will refer to both of them as recurrence.

Despite treatment and long term follow up, the risk of invasive cancer in women treated stays higher than among women in the general population, even for 20 or 25 years later (56 per 100,000 women per year compared to 5.6 per 100,000 women per year). Furthermore, the rate of recurrence is by any of the methods discussed, between 5-17%. The influencing factors in a greater recurrence: the size of the excised lesion, endocervical gland involvement, positive surgical margins and maintenance of detectable viral DNA (especially if it is HPV 16). In this study one of the goals is to see what kind of factors affect the recurrence or persistence in our population.

Regarding surgical margins it has been demonstrated in a metaanalysis with more than 35,000 women undergoing excisional procedures with any degree of CIN, comparing those with positive margins against presenting free margins or uncertain edges, the first one has an increased risk for 5.47 times to present CIN post-treatment of any grade [40]. It shows that there is a higher cure rate when the lesion. Positive margins imply an increased risk of persistent disease and thus greater chance of having to be subjected to re-excision or hysterectomy. There is an even increased risk if both margins, endocervical and ectocervical, are affected. Although there are still few studies with long term follow up.

It is also noted that, although the involvement of the cone margins is consistently related with residual disease, both concepts are not synonymous, as there may be impairment of the surgical margins and no detectable residual disease and vice versa. Some use different protocols for monitoring after treatment depending on whether the margin is involved.

1.7. Special Considerations for HIV Positive Women

The greatest evidence of the importance of the immune response in the natural history of HPV has been obtained from studies that correlated the incidence of cervical cancer in women with HIV. A meta-analysis has shown that there is an increased risk of cancer attributable to papillomavirus among HIV positive patients. In 1988 it began to corroborate the evident relationship between cervical neoplasia and Human Immunodeficiency Virus. It was observed the high proportion of HIV positive women requiring colposcopy, younger age at diagnosis of cervical cancer and its greater severity.

It is now known that the cervical neoplasia is one of the malignant diseases more related with AIDS [41]. The incidence of CIN is 4-5 times higher among HIV-infected women than among HIV-negative women [42, 43] and cervical cancer risk is multiplied from 5-8 times in the seropositive women [44, 45]. This is because the prevalence of HPV infection in women with HIV is 64% compared to 27% in HIV negative women. Those affected by HIV have a higher risk of HPV infection (RR 17). It is also known that in these patients, cancer develops in a shorter time of period than in those women who are immunocompetent (The interval between the diagnosis of carcinoma in situ (CIS) and invasive carcinoma is 3.2 years according to studies in HIV positive compared to 15.7years in HIV negatives) [46].

There are differences depending on the severity of the immunodeficiency that occurs within all HIV-infected women. Women with lower CD4 counts and higher viral load (viral RNA detected) have a higher prevalence of HPV infection [47]. It is believed that HIV infection may, directly at the molecular level promote oncogenesis associated with HPV. It is recommended that the assessment of these women is by cytology and colposcopy and they require more frequent monitoring. Given this it is more common to see abnormal Pap smears among HIV positive women, colposcopy should be performed to evaluate all abnormalities found by cytology except for ASC-US [48]. The appropriate management of CIN in these patients is with excision followed by topical agents. How to follow patient in terms of frequency and method requires more research. It is clear that it must be performed by qualified personnel experienced in these pathologies.

Some recommendations include:

- After a diagnosis of HIV, cervical cancer screening should be performed twice during the first year and annually thereafter as long as the results are normal. A colposcopic exam should also be done as a routine, and will not be repeated unless abnormal cytology is found. After two normal Pap smears it is recommended to perform a complete inspection of the rest of the lower genital tract (vagina and vulva) and anus. There is no consensus on whether HPV typing in these women should be done routinely. The knowledge of HPV positivity should increase the surveillance to every six months.
- There are few studies concerning low-grade lesions there and there is allot of discrepancy between the results published, so there are no recommendations

specially designed for HIV patients. Expectant management is recommended for a diagnosis of CIN I if colposcopy is satisfactory. If the lesion persists for 2 years or progresses, it should be treated.

− In the case of persistent CIN 1 or with CIN 2 or CIN 3, these can be treated by local destructive or excisional techniques as long as colposcopy is satisfactory. Otherwise, destructive techniques would be contraindicated. It is important to obtain tissue and rule out an occult carcinoma.

As mentioned, the success rate after treatment is very high (90%) in HIV negative women. In contrast, in HIV-positive patients the success rate is much lower and therefore the persistence or recurrence of lesions is more common in this group. Recurrence rates are up to 56% and even 87% in severely immunocompromised patients [49, 50]. One of the factors that may influence in worse outcome after treatment is the highest rate of incomplete ablation of CIN that tends to occur in these patients, although the reason is not known. Comparing women whose surgical margins were free among HIV (+) and HIV (-) there is a greater risk of recurrence and persistence in the first group, which leads to the conclusion that, besides the margin status, other factors are important for recurrence of the disease.

The high persistence rate after excisional treatments in HIV + women has led to assessment of adjuvant therapeutic modalities. Adjuvant therapies as treatment with beta-carotene, isotretinoin or interferon have not shown consistently good results. In contrast, when 5-fluorouracil is applied topically, it is recommended as adjuvant destructive or excisional treatment for CIN 2 or 3. Although the therapy that produces greater differences in results is undoubtedly the Highly Active Antiretroviral Therapy (HAART). It has been an important improvement in the prognosis of HIV patients and it has reduced the incidence of many AIDS-related neoplastic complications, including the cervical neoplasia. HAART is associated with higher rate of regression and thus lower rate of recurrence in HIV-infected women. In fact it is believed that HIV-infected women treated with HAART with low viral load and stable CD4 levels, could be considered in terms of handling similarly to HIV-uninfected women [51, 52].

There is much to discover in relation to patients with HIV and precursor lesions of cervical cancer. In the general population, the new vaccines represent the future of prevention of these diseases. However, the vaccinated women are likely to have a different distribution of HPV subtypes presented compared with seronegative women. In addition, the most common route of transmission of human immunodeficiency virus is sexually, making it very likely that before vaccination, the majority of them are already infected with HPV. Not yet known how is the immune response to the vaccine in HIV positive women. Further research is needed in this field.

Material and Methods

For this retrospective study we used our patient records from the Cervical Pathology service of La Paz Hospital. From the group of patients who underwent surgery from 1998 to 2008, we included those who have been followed successfully for at least 12 months after the surgery.

We excluded also patients with carcinomas already diagnosed by cytology who were treated to confirm the diagnosis and extension. Using these criteria our sample was reduced to 873 patients.

We used our archived records of the patients in the Cervical Pathology service and their pathology reports, we extracted the data needed to complete the study variables which are:

i.   Age of the woman (at the treatment date)
ii.   Cytologic or histologic diagnosis, maintaining the highest degree found (either in the previous biopsy or in surgical specimen removed by conization or hysterectomy.)
iii.   Type of treatment
iv.   If any HPV DNA test was done, and the type found.
v.   The surgical margins status, classifying the findings into four groups:
       -    Free edges: if no lesion was found contacting any of the surgical margins
       -    Affected edges: if at least one of the margins was not free of lesion
       -    Edges not assessable: the sample does not allow an assessment of the edges because of artifacts of different origin such as thermal damage from LEEP or laser.
       -    Proximity: if the edges are free but the lesion is located in the immediate proximity of the surgical margins.
vi.   The time (in months) the patient was followed until discharge or until the last revision performed if she was lost to follow up, or months until recurrence is diagnosed.
vii.   We searched for the appearance of residual disease (recurrence or persistence) understanding this as the diagnosis of any lesion severity from LSIL (without therefore consider the appearance of ASCUS) by cytological or histologic control. Twenty-four recurrences (21%) were observed only by cytology. All of them were LSIL.
viii. The type of treatment realized in case of recurrent lesions.
ix.   Immunosuppression of the patient, especially if the patient was HIV carrier to see if we found more recurrence in this group, as we explained in the introduction.

After collecting the data mentioned, all were analyzed, with help from our Biostatistics Service with the program SPSS version 9.0.

Results

We included 873 women treated because of diagnosis of HSIL or persistent LSIL. The mean and median age of the sample were both 36 years with a standard deviation of 9.5 years. The minimum age was 17 years and the oldest patient treated was 87 years old. As shown in the graph below, the majority of the sample was treated because of HSIL 805 women (92%) and persistent LSIL were only 47 (5%). In 7 (less than 1%) women, we could not find the grade of the SIL for which they were treated; we include them in the unspecified SIL group. 14 carcinomas (1.6%) were discovered in the conization or hysterectomy sample that had not been diagnosed on previous biopsy.

The literature indicates that about 0.5% of the samples obtained by excision present as AIS or microinvasive squamous cell carcinoma that had not been suspected by cytology or colposcopy [53]. All of the cancer and AIS lesions were eliminated from the study because we were interested only in premalignant lesions. Our final sample was 859 women.

The chart below tries to clarify the pathological diagnoses included in the sample, dividing into different subtypes this 92% of high-grade lesions (805 women).

Treatment varied based on the characteristics of the patient and the grade of the lesion observed. The vast majority of patients underwent cone biopsy (93%) and hysterectomy was performed as first choice only to a 7% of the total. Below there is a graphic trying to outline the distribution of the different types of conization used.

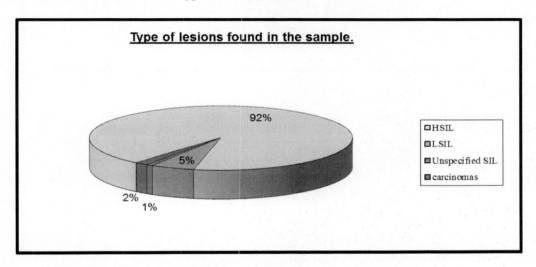

Figure 1. Type of lesion in the population (n=873).

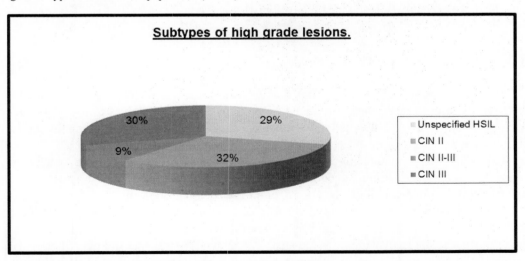

Figure 2. Types of high grade lesions (n=805).

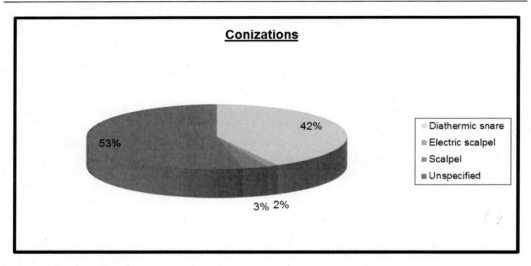

Figure 3. Treatement types.

Table 2. Rate of recurrence in women treated by conization

Conizations	Frequency	Proportion
Recurrence	688	86.5%
No recurrence	107	13.5%

It should be noted that in 54%, the type of cone was not reported; nevertheless the use of diathermy loop was the most commonly encountered. It is worth highlighting that, due to the low risk of recurrence in patients with total hysterectomy and the small percentage of women who underwent hysterectomy (64 patients), for analysis of the relapse and risk factors they were studied separately (a group for hysterectomy and a group for conization).

3.1. Recurrence or Persistence

We studied separately the recurrences found in the 64 patients with hysterectomy, among them only 5 cases of recurrence were found (7.81%): two were LSIL, one was a VAIN I, and two HSIL although one was only a cytological finding and was not or could not be corroborated by histology.

Excluding this hysterectomy group, we have 795 cases of women who underwent conization. Subsequent lesions occurring in 107 women there were found at least in the cytology, LSIL or higher risk lesions (13.5% of the conization group).

If we represent this data in a survival curve, understanding survival as the time until the studied event occurs, namely the diagnosis of cervical cancer precursor lesions. It is placed on the ordinate axis the percentage (in value respect to the unit) of patients and in the horizontal axis the following time (in months.) The crosses indicate patients who reach their maximum follow-up time.

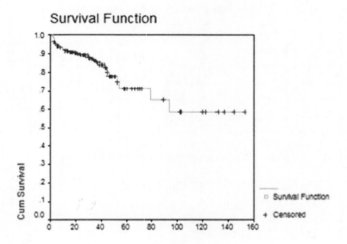

Figure 4. Recurrence free survival of women treated by conization.

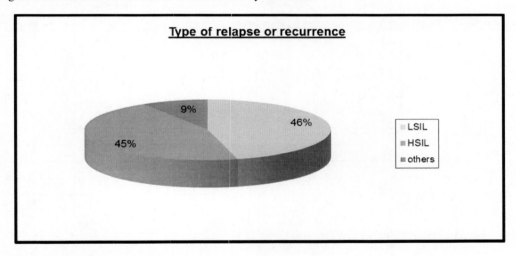

Figure 5. Type of the lesions at recurrence.

We can see, for example, that within two years approximately 90% of the patients remained healthy (without detection of any premalignant or malignant cervical lesion). Within 5 years (60 months), this percentage remains still higher than 70%.

3.2. Type of Lesions Found As Recurrence

After reviewing the rate of relapse, we will describe the type of recurrence based on histological classification.

The following table classifies by subtypes the 45% of high-grade lesions.

Table 3. Subclassification of high grade lesions

HIGH GRADE LESIONS	Frequency	Proportion of all the recurrences	Proportion of the total of patients
CIN 2	5	4.46%	0.6%
CIN 3	16	14.28%	1.8%
CIN 23	6	5.35%	0.7%
Unspecified HSIL	25	22.32%	2.9%

Table 4. Subclassification of other lesions

Others	Frequency	Proportion of all the recurrences	Proportion of the total of patients
Carcinomas	3	2.67%	0.3%
VIN 2	1	0.89%	0.1%
VIN 3	1	0.89%	0.1%
VAIN 1	2	1.78%	0.1%
Unspecified SIL	3	2.67%	0.3%

Table 5. Treatment for recurrent disease

Treatment	Frequency	Proportion of all the recurrences	Proportion of the total of patients
Conization	13	11.6%	1.5%
Hysterectomy	28	25.0%	3.3%
Control	63	56.3%	7.3%
Others	8	7.1%	0.9%
TOTAL	112		

3.3. Treatment of Relapses

The following table summarizes the different types of treatments performed after the diagnosis of recurrent disease. Expectant management (realizing only a closer surveillance) was the most frequently performed. Among the active treatments the most common was hysterectomy. Among those classified as "others", we did 2 cervical amputations, one subsequently had to undergo a hysterectomy because of yet another relapse, 1 brachytherapy, 3 conizations that subsequently underwent a hysterectomy, a vulvectomy and a colpectomy.

3.4. Possible Prognostic Factors for Recurrence

3.4.1. Age

The average age in the sample was 36.76 years (among the women who had a hystectomy, the mean age was higher). Among patients who underwent a cone biopsy, we divide the sample depending on whether or not they recurred and considered their age.

Table 6. Age of those who recurred

	Number of patients	Mean age (years)	Standard deviation of the age (years)
No recurrence	688	35.67	8.39
Recurrence	107	36.21	10.16

Table 7. Decade during which recurrence is identified

AGE	No recurrence	Recurrence	Total	Proportion of recurrence
< or = 19	5	0	5	0%
20-29	152	27	179	15.0%
30-39	345	51	396	12.9%
40-49	189	19	208	9.1%
50-59	37	11	48	22.9%
60-69	12	3	15	20.0%
> or = 70	6	1	7	14.3%
TOTAL	746	112	858	

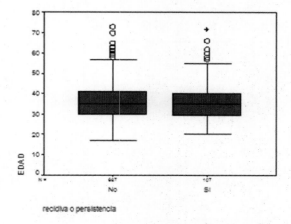

Figure 6. Age of those who recurred compared to those who did not recur.

Performing a Student T test we prove that there are no statistically significant differences between the two groups. P value is 0.602 two-tailed with a 95% confidence interval of -2.58 to 1.50. If we assess the sample by age (in decades), we obtain the following results in function of the probability of relapse.

3.4.2. Type of Lesion Diagnosed and Treated at the Beginning

To see if there are differences between the various types of SIL in the frequency of recurrence we have built the following table.

When comparing by the Fisher test we can say that there are no statistically significant differences between groups (p = 1). Moreover, this following Kaplan-Meier table shows the cumulative survival functions.

Table 8. Original Lesion and rate of recurrence

	No recurrence	Recurrence	Total
HIGH GRADE SIL	645 (86.7%)	99 (13.3%)	744 (100%)
LOW GRADE SIL	38 (86.4%)	6 (13.6%)	44 (100%)
Total	683 (86.7%)	105 (13.3%)	788 (100%)

Table 9. Recurrence based on degree of abnormality in the original lesion

Cytology/Histology result	No recurrence	Recurrence	Total
No specified SIL	5 (71.4%)	2 (28.6%)	8 (100%)
HSIL. No histology	196 (89.9%)	22 (10.1%)	218 (100%)
HSIL. CIN 2-3	55 (77.5%)	16 (22.5%)	71 (100%)
HSIL. CIN 2	215 (89.2%)	26 (10.8%)	241 (100%)
HSIL. CIN 3	178 (83.6%)	35 (16.4%)	213 (100%)
LSIL. No histology	38 (86.5%)	6 (13.6%)	44 (100%)
TOTAL	688 (86.5%)	107 (13.5%)	795 (100%)

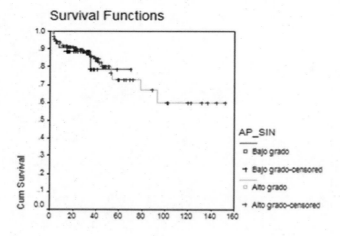

Figure 7. Recurrence free survival.

From the curves shown we obtain a p-value of 0.84 so it is concluded that there is no statistically significant difference in terms of the rate of recurrence.

We divided the sample into different subcategories based on high and low grade lesions.

The table shows that CIN 2 recur or persist in a 10.8% while there is a higher rate of recurrence in CIN3 (13.6%). There are differences between the two types in terms of the type of lesion appeared if they recur.

Among CIN 2 there are only 7 cases of high-grade lesions recurrence (2.9%), while among CIN 3 we found 23 high-grade lesions (a recurrence rate of high-grade lesion of 10.8%). This means that higher grade lesions more likely present relapse to high-grade lesions.

3.4.3. Type of HPV

One of the objectives of the study was to know what HPV subtypes are the most frequent in patients treated in our hospital and if some of them recur more likely than the others. In order to do so we collected all subtypes of HPV found in patients who underwent determination of viral DNA. 468 women had HPV assessment and in some, more than one subtype of the virus was detected. A total of 579 times, a type of HPV was detected. In Table 10, one can see the different subtypes found and the rate of recurrence or persistence within each one.

Table 10. HPV type associated with recurrent disease

HPV TYPE	WITHOUT RECURRENCE	RECUR	TOTAL	PROPORTION OF THE TOTAL	CUMULATIVE PROPORTION	RECURRENCE PROPORTION
16	282	50	332	57.34	57.34	15.06
31	45	5	50	8.63	65.97	10.00
51	40	7	47	8.11	74.08	14.89
58	28	6	34	5.87	79.95	17.65
33	24	7	31	5.35	85.30	22.58
18	26	0	26	4.49	89.79	0.00
6	7	3	10	1.72	91.51	30.00
52	5	4	9	1.55	93.06	44.44
35	4	2	6	1.03	94.09	33.33
11	2	2	4	0.69	94.78	50.00
56	1	2	3	0.51	95.29	66.67
54	2	1	3	0.51	95.80	33.33
53	1	2	3	0.51	96.31	66.67
27	2	0	2	0.34	96.65	0.00
39	2	0	2	0.34	96.99	0.00
45	1	1	2	0.34	97.33	50.00
70	2	0	2	0.34	97.67	0.00
42	1	0	1	0.17	97.84	0.00
66	1	0	1	0.17	98.01	0.00
13	1	0	1	0.17	98.18	0.00
83	1	0	1	0.17	98.35	0.00
72	1	0	1	0.17	98.52	0.00
82	1	0	1	0.17	98.69	0.00
76	1	0	1	0.17	98.86	0.00
64	1	0	1	0.17	99.03	0.00
62	1	0	1	0.17	99.20	0.00
2	1	0	1	0.17	99.37	0.00
13	1	0	1	0.17	99.54	0.00
59	1	0	1	0.17	99.71	0.00
40	1	0	1	0.17	99.88	0.00

It is important to clarify that such high proportions of relapse in viral genotypes without a very high oncogenic risk may result because in most cases they appeared as a co-infection with a high-risk type such as HPV 16. It is very interesting to see that we only found the most common 6 subtypes HPV 16, 31, 51, 58, 33 and 18 in almost 90%. This is also shown in the following chart.

Several studies have found that HPV 16 has a higher association with precancerous lesions and cancer compared to the other oncogenic types. (It is said that the risk of developing a CIN 3 or a more severe lesion was significantly higher among women with HPV 16 infection (30-40%) than in women infected with other high risk subtypes (8-10%) [54].) Therefore, we compared the relapse among patients infected by HPV 16 (as a single infection or in co-infection with other genotypes) with all those patients who were infected by other serotypes.

When we compare relapse rates of the patients who underwent cone biopsy, using Fisher's exact test, we realize that there are no statistically significant differences. (p = 0.574) in the percentage of relapses according the HPV subtype they present.

We also wanted to compare the survival functions by type of HPV, to see if there was significant difference in the rate of recurrences or relapses between both groups. By log-rank test on the Kaplan-Meier tables we found no statistically significant differences (p = 0.7338).

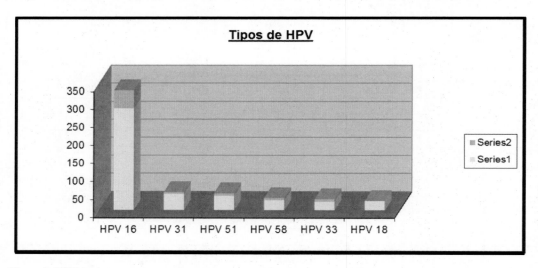

Figure 8. HPV types seen.

Table 11. Rates of HPV type in the original cervix

	Frequency	Proportion of the total sample	Proportion among patients with a HPV detected
HPV 16	325	37.8%	69.4%
Other HPV types	143	16.6%	30.6%
TOTAL	468	54.5%	100

Table 12. Relapse rate based on HPV type

	No recurrence	Recurrence	Total
HPV 16	267 (85.3%)	46 (14.7%)	313
Other HPV type	115 (83.3%)	23 (16.7%)	138
TOTAL	382 (84.7%)	69 (15.3%)	451

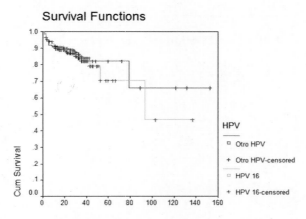

Figure 9. Relapse free recurrence based on HPV type.

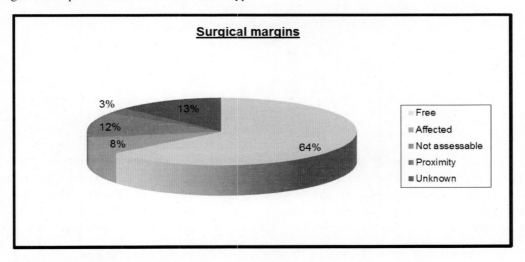

Figure 10. Margin status of the specimen.

3.4.4. Surgical Margins

The graph below shows the proportion of the four subgroups of the surgical margins classification presented in the materials and methods section.

To compare the proportion of relapse among the four groups we have created this chart.

Using "Chi Square" test we obtain a value of p <0.001, so that the higher percentage of recurrence or persistence found between patients with affected surgical margins is statistically significant.

Table 13. Margin status and risk of recurrence

Margin status	No recurrence	Recurrence	Total
Involved	40 (56.3%)	31 (43.7%)	71 (100%)
Free	480 (91.3%)	46 (8.7%)	526 (100%)
Not assessable	85 (82.5%)	18(17.5%)	103 (100%)
Proximity	21 (91.3%)	2 (8.7%)	23 (100%)
TOTAL	626 (86.6%)	97 (13.4%)	723 (100%)

Table 14. HIV status impact on recurrence

	No recurrence	Recurrence	TOTAL
HIV NEGATIVES	675 (87.8%)	94 (12.2%)	769 (100%)
HIV POSITIVES	13 (50.0.%)	13 (50.0%)	26 (100%)
TOTAL	688 (86.5%)	107 (13.5%)	795 (100%)

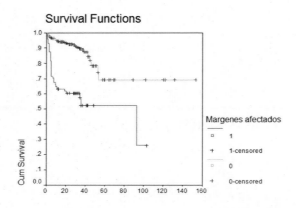

Figure 11. Relapse free survival based on margin status.

Despite having already demonstrated the importance of the surgical margins in the appearance of lesions after treatment, the sample was divided into two groups: one with affected edges patients and another group including the other three subcategories. By making the graphical representation of recurrence in the two groups we objective a greater recurrence-free interval in the second group. Cases with affected margins recur more and do so early. These are statistically significant differences (p <0.001).

3.4.5. HIV Status

The sample in the study included 26 HIV seropositive patients (3.1%). In the table below we see the proportion of relapses or recurrences depending on whether they are infected or not by the Human Immunodeficiency Virus.

There is a clearly higher recurrence rate among HIV patients, and these differences are statistically significant because using Fisher's exact test we obtain a value of p <0.001. It also shows statistical significance (p <0.001) the observed differences comparing the two survival functions of HIV negative patients and HIV positive ones.

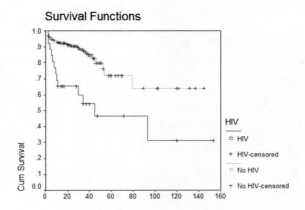

Figure 12. Relapse free survival based on HIV status.

The following chart shows very intuitively that the time to new diagnosis of lesion is longer in seronegative women, which means that persistent or recurrent lesions appear earlier in HIV positive patients.

Conclusion

In order to clarify this section we will organize the most relevant data in ten different interesting aspects:

Natural Evolution of the Lesions

The changes produced in the tissue by the action of HPV, namely preneoplastic lesions, are common (4% of women who undergo screening in US present CIN I while there is a 5% of high-grade CIN lesions (CIN II and III).

This is relevant because as it has been explained they can develop through the process of carcinogenesis an invasive carcinoma if not treated. (22% of CIN II lesions progress to CIN III and 5% to invasive cancer if left untreated. 12-40% untreated CIN III lesions progress to cervical cancer) [55]

As seen in the results section, even treating these premalignant lesions and following them cytologically and with colposcopy, some of the treated patients also develop cervical cancer.

It is known that the risk of invasive carcinoma in treated women remains higher compared to the general population even for 20 or 25 years. In our sample three invasive carcinomas were diagnosed in patients who had previously have a cone biopsy, representing 2.7% of total relapsing or recurrent lesions found and 0.3% of the total of treated patients.

CONCLUSION: The treatment greatly reduces the proportion of women that evolve to cancer from precursor lesions but this still remains higher than women in general population.

Screening

The use of population-based screening methods in developed countries has achieved a reduce of approximately 75% of both the incidence and mortality of cervical cancer and this enormous clinical relevance makes the decision about what type of screening method to implement a continual revision. Numerous types of protocols of screening and follow-up have been proposed combining the use of HPV DNA test, cytology, endocervical curettage and colposcopy at very different intervals. None of them have been compared by randomized clinical studies and comparisons between available studies are limited because of the mentioned design differences.

Further review of the screening protocol will be required because of the introduction of new vaccines against HPV (it is expected a decrease of the incidence of cervical cancer precursor lesions found in the vaccinated population), although screening probably cannot be eliminated completely.

CONCLUSION: We have to keep searching for the most appropriate and efficient screening and follow-up model so more studies are needed comparing the results of the different methods to find the optimal combination.

HPV Type

It is known that the most common oncogenic subtypes of HPV are 16 and 18 and that vaccines create immunization against these two viral subtypes. It is curious to note that while HPV 16 is the most frequently detected in our sample (57.34% of total detected HPV), type 18 is the sixth in frequency, exceeded by the types: 31,51,58 and 33 (in descending order). The six mentioned subtypes represent together a total of nearly 90% of the HPV detected whereas the other 24 different subtypes found represent the remaining 10%. It is also worth noting that none of the 18 subtypes was detected in women with persistent or recurrent lesions, which is not consistent with the high oncogenic potential of this virus. It may be explained by the low percentage of type 18 detected in the sample and/or because we do not have data about what HPV was infecting most of the patients.

As a result of the lower prevalence of HPV 18 subtype observed, the vaccination against HPV in the sample would not be as useful as in the general population. Although a certain degree of crossreactivity has been demonstrated due to antigenic similarities and common phylogenetic origin with subtypes 45 and 31(the second in frequency detected).

It may also be worth noting that, although it has been shown by several studies that HPV 16 infection poses a greater risk of recurrence or persistence of HSIL [56] and also tend to appear earlier, our sample did not find statistically significant differences in this respect, which may be due to the same reason as for HPV type 18. One of the main problems of our study is precisely the reason discussed above, the lack of information in most patients about HPV type that infected each one.

It has been consistently shown that the HPV test carried out between 6 and 12 months post-treatment has a sensitivity of 90% to predict recurrence [57, 73]. In our sample this is what we have been realizing in these recent years, but in most patients especially those in the first years, it was not done due to lack of resources or because there was no scientific evidence yet.

CONCLUSION: It can be very useful to analyze the genotype of HPV for the clinic because it could predict the evolution of disease in the woman and it is helpful in order to make treatment decision. The problem is that such tests are not currently available in many jurisdictions [58, 71].

Recurrence or Relapse

The treatment success rate in our study (86.5%) is similar to those reported by most authors, between 81% and 98% [59]. The published rate of recurrence for treated premalignant lesions varies between 5 and 17%. In our sample, the percentage was 13.5% which is consistent with the literature studied.

CONCLUSION: Our study shows a relapse rate and treatment success similar to most published studies on the subject.

Time to Recurrence or Persistence and Follow-Up Time

According to the literature, the *average time from diagnosis and treatment* of high-grade cervical lesions until the development of carcinoma is between 8 and 13 years. In our sample, the mean time to diagnosis carcinoma after treatment was 33 months (less than 3 years). The average follow up time of women who showed no recurrence was 33.35 months. This is consistent with the current recommendation that after three annual consecutive negative cytologies the patient returns to the screening of the general population. The mean time until detection of persistent or recurrent disease in our sample was 15.53 months. As the survival curves show that after two years 10% of the sample has already relapsed. (The vast majority of the recurrences found have appeared in that period.)

CONCLUSION: The majority of women who relapse after treatment do so in the first two years post-treatment so the follow up must be maximized during this period and it can be subsequently less frequent.

Type of Found Lesions

In our study, persistent LSIL and HSIL have a very similar ratio of recurrence or persistence (13.6% vs. 13.3%). Our finding does not agree with what is seen in most studies [60]. Usually high-grade lesions are more aggressive. This could be explained because of the small number of treated LSIL and their persistent nature, involving a greater aggressiveness than LSIL that disappear. However, we observed a higher percentage of recurrence in CIN 3 (16.4%) than CIN 2 (10.8%). This is because less oncogenic viral types are usually involved in CIN 2. Although this percentage could have been modified if we had known the exact histology (CIN 2 or CIN 3) in the group classified as HSIL. Also as seen in the attached tables when CIN 2 recur it does so as lesser degree lesions than those present in patients with CIN 3. Most recurrences found were LSIL (46%) that is the reason why the most common treatment of new lesions is simply the strict control of the patient. The next most common lesion among recurrence or persistence was CIN 3 (14.28% of them all).

Notably, 21% of relapses were diagnosed only by cytological techniques and did not or could not have histological verification; this can be a problem in the sample, because although cytological abnormalities usually predict histological changes there is no absolute correspondence between the findings.

Another indication that there is not an absolute correspondence between the cytological and histological findings is that it is estimated that a 0.5% of the samples obtained by excisional techniques show a CIS or microinvasive carcinomas that have not been previously detected by cytology or colposcopy [53].

In our sample this percentage was 1.6%. (14 cases). This high proportion can be in part explained by possible bias in which classified by cytology patients without evidence of neoplasia could undergo excision because of suspicion not reflected in the report.

CONCLUSION: A higher degree lesion predicts a larger percentage of recurrence and it also tends to be higher grade. Cytological and colposcopic findings are not always predictive of the histology

Age

We find contradictions in the literature regarding age as a prognostic factor of recurrence or persistence [61]. In our study we found no statistical significance comparing the ratio of recurrence with the age of the patient.

In the general population screening usually finishes at the age of 65 years. If we had treated the patients in our study as general population, we would not have diagnosed two cases of HSIL with possible progression to carcinoma and the corresponding need for treatment. (In our sample, 16.6% of women recurred over 65 years.) So this argues for the need of a special monitoring protocol for women who have been treated for premalignant lesions different than the general population.

CONCLUSION: It is still unclear if age is a predictor of recurrence in women treated for cervical cancer precursors. These patients need to be followed with different protocols from the general population and that includes changes in the recommended age of completion.

Patients with Hysterectomy

Women who undergo total hysterectomy for reasons unrelated to cervical cancer do not present risk of lower genital tract premalignant or malignant lesions. By contrast those who undergo total hysterectomy because of cervical precancerous lesions have more risk of recurrence, although still low.

In our sample, five patients with hysterectomy relapsed but it is important to note that two were LSIL, another one was a VAIN I. Two HSIL appeared although these may be false positives because they were cytological findings and do not have a histological corroboration.

CONCLUSION: Women undergoing hysterectomy for reasons related to cervical cancer precursor lesions, must maintain a more intense followup than the general population because of the possibility of recurrence.

Surgical Margins

Although there are few long-term studies, it is known that there is a 5.47 times higher risk of presenting any type of CIN after treatment of precursor lesions if surgical specimen margins were affected [62]. In our study, it is statistically very significant the increased risk of relapse or recurrence in the group of patients without complete removal of the lesion. Furthermore, we have observed that patients with affected surgical margins not only recurred more but they do so much earlier.

As already explained, affected margins and residual lesion are not synonymous since in the literature and in our study, we found that women with affected margins who did not relapse and women presenting residual lesion whose surgical edges were free of lesion. This could be explained by the existence of multifocal lesions, by an inadequate classification by the pathologist or because of the existence of places with epithelial dysplasia hidden under normal epithelium because of reepithelialization produced by traumas from biopsy or cytology.

Although in our work, the women with questionable margins had a recurrence rate is similar to the uninvolved margins group, according to the literature these patients should be followed more intensely because they present a higher risk of recurrence [63].

CONCLUSION: The surgical margin status is a prognostic factor for recurrence or persistence.

HIV

HIV positive women have a higher risk of persistent or recurrent CIN after treatment. Recurrence rates are up to 56% (even 87% if they are in a phase of severe immune-suppression.) In our study, we did not take into account the severity of the inmmuno-suppression since we had no available data of viral load, CD4 count or if the patient was treated with HAART. (As explained if these three factors are favorable the patient can be treated as a seronegative.) In our work we found a rate of relapses or recurrences of 50% among HIV infected women and this was statistically significant compared with HIV-uninfected women. Recurrences also occurred quicker in the HIV infected women. The best way to follow-up these women, is still unclear. There is no consensus about the need of a routine test for detection of HPV DNA. In contrast, it is clear viewing the results of our study supported by the available literature that seropositive patients treated for precursor lesions of cervical cancer, require a closer monitoring than HIV negative ones [64]. Managing the HIV positive woman, involves not focusing on cure rather focusing on prevention of cervix cancer [72].

References

[1]   Comino, R., Cararach, M., Prevención del Cáncer de cérvix uterino. *Documento de Consenso SEGO* 2005; 126-178.

[2]   Parkin, D. M., Bray, F., Ferlay, J., Pisani, P. Global cancer statistics, 2002. *CA Cancer J. Clin.* 2005;55:74-108.

[3]   Insinga, R. P., Glass, A. G., Rush, B. B. Diagnoses and outcomes in cervical cancer screening: a population-based study. *Am. J. Obstet. Gynecol.* 2004; 191:105.

[4]   Shepherd, J., Weston, R., Peersman, G., Napuli, I. Z. Interventions for encouraging sexual lifestyles and behaviours intended to prevent cervical cancer. *Cochrane Database Syst. Rev.* 2000; :CD001035.

[5]   Kahn, J. A. HPV vaccination for the prevention of cervical intraepithelial neoplasia. *N Engl. J. Med.* 2009; 361:271.

[6]   Greer, C. E., Wheeler, C. M., Ladner, M. B., et al. Human papillomavirus (HPV) type distribution and serological response to HPV type 6 virus-like particles in patients with genital warts. *J. Clin. Microbiol.* 1995; 33:2058.

[7]   Winer, R. L., Lee, S. K., Hughes, J. P., et al. Genital human papillomavirus infection: incidence and risk factors in a cohort of female university students. *Am. J. Epidemiol.* 2003; 157:218.

[8]   De Sanjosé, S., Diaz, M., Castellsagué, X., et al. Worldwide prevalence and genotype distribution of cervical human papillomavirus DNA in women with normal cytology: a meta-analysis. *Lancet Infect. Dis.* 2007; 7:453.

[9]   Centers for Disease Control and Prevention, Workowski, K. A., Berman, S. M. Sexually transmitted diseases treatment guidelines, 2006. *MMWR Recomm. Rep.* 2006; 55:1.

[10]   Rodríguez, A. C., Schiffman, M., Herrero, R., et al. Rapid clearance of human papillomavirus and implications for clinical focus on persistent infections. *J. Natl. Cancer Inst.* 2008; 100:513.

[11]   Castle, P. E., Solomon, D., Schiffman, M., Wheeler, C. M. Human papillomavirus type 16 infections and 2-year absolute risk of cervical precancer in women with equivocal or mild cytologic abnormalities. *J. Natl. Cancer Inst.* 2005; 97:1066.

[12]   Bosch, X., Harper, D. Prevention strategies of cervical cancer in the HPV vaccine era. *Gynecol. Oncol.* 2006; 103:21.

[13]   Carter, J. J., Koutsky, L. A., Hughes, J. P., et al. Comparison of human papillomavirus types 16, 18, and 6 capsid antibody responses following incident infection. *J. Infect. Dis.* 2000; 181:1911.

[14]   Arany, I., Tyring, S. K. Activation of local cell-mediated immunity in interferon-responsive patients with human papillomavirus-associated lesions. *J. Interferon. Cytokine Res.* 1996; 16:453.

[15]   Walboomers, J. M., Jacobs, M. V., Manos, M. M., et al. Human papillomavirus is a necessary cause of invasive cervical cancer worldwide. *J. Pathol.* 1999; 189:12.

[16]   Moscicki, A. B., Hills, N., Shiboski, S., et al. Risks for incident human papillomavirus infection and low-grade squamous intraepithelial lesion development in young females. *JAMA* 2001; 285:2995.

[17]   Berrington de González, A., Green, J., International Collaboration of Epidemiological Studies of Cervical Cancer. Comparison of risk factors for invasive squamous cell carcinoma and adenocarcinoma of the cervix: collaborative reanalysis of individual data on 8,097 women with squamous cell carcinoma and 1,374 women with adenocarcinoma from 12 epidemiological studies. *Int. J. Cancer* 2007; 120:885.

[18]   Castellsagué, X., Bosch, F. X., Muñoz, N., et al. Male circumcision, penile human papillomavirus infection, and cervical cancer in female partners. *N Engl. J. Med.* 2002; 346:1105.

[19] Anttila, T., Saikku, P., Koskela, P., et al. Serotypes of Chlamydia trachomatis and risk for development of cervical squamous cell carcinoma. *JAMA* 2001; 285:47.

[20] Wallin, K. L., Wiklund, F., Luostarinen, T., et al. A population-based prospective study of Chlamydia trachomatis infection and cervical carcinoma. *Int. J. Cancer* 2002; 101: 371.

[21] Hawes, S. E., Kiviat, N. B. Are genital infections and inflammation cofactors in the pathogenesis of invasive cervical cancer? *J. Natl. Cancer Inst.* 2002; 94:1592.

[22] Castle, P. E., Wacholder, S., Lorincz, A. T., et al. A prospective study of high-grade cervical neoplasia risk among human papillomavirus-infected women. *J. Natl. Cancer Inst.* 2002; 94:1406.

[23] International Collaboration of Epidemiological Studies of Cervical Cancer, Appleby, P., Beral, V., et al. Carcinoma of the cervix and tobacco smoking: collaborative reanalysis of individual data on 13,541 women with carcinoma of the cervix and 23,017 women without carcinoma of the cervix from 23 epidemiological studies. *Int. J. Cancer* 2006; 118:1481.

[24] Muñoz, N., Franceschi, S., Bosetti, C., et al. Role of parity and human papillomavirus in cervical cancer: the IARC multicentric case-control study. *Lancet* 2002; 359:1093.

[25] International Collaboration of Epidemiological Studies of Cervical Cancer. Cervical carcinoma and reproductive factors: collaborative reanalysis of individual data on 16,563 women with cervical carcinoma and 33,542 women without cervical carcinoma from 25 epidemiological studies. *Int. J. Cancer* 2006; 119:1108.

[26] International Collaboration of Epidemiological Studies of Cervical Cancer, Appleby, P., Beral, V., et al. Cervical cancer and hormonal contraceptives: collaborative reanalysis of individual data for 16,573 women with cervical cancer and 35,509 women without cervical cancer from 24 epidemiological studies. *Lancet* 2007; 370:1609.

[27] Waggoner, S. E., Darcy, K. M., Tian, C., Lanciano, R. Smoking behavior in women with locally advanced cervical carcinoma: a Gynecologic Oncology Group study. *Am. J. Obstet. Gynecol.* 2010; 202:283.e1.

[28] American Cancer Society - Cancer Facts and Figures 2008. At: http://www.cancer.org/downloads/STT/2008CAFFfinalsecured.pdf (Accessed May 21, 2008).

[29] Clifford, G. M., Smith, J. S., Plummer, M., Munoz, N., Franceschi, S. Human papillomavirus types in invasive cervical cancer worldwide: a meta-analysis. *Br. J. Cancer* 2003;88:63-73.

[30] Henley, S. J., King, J. B., German, R. R., et al. Surveillance of screening-detected cancers (colon and rectum, breast, and cervix) - United States, 2004-2006. *MMWR Surveill Summ.* 2010; 59:1.

[31] Janerich, D. T., Hadjimichael, O., Schwartz, P. E., et al. The screening histories of women with invasive cervical cancer, Connecticut. *Am. J. Public Health* 1995; 85:791.

[32] Peto, J. The cervical cancer epidemic that screening has prevented in the UK. *Lancet* 2004; 364: 249-56.

[33] Puig Tintoré, L. M. Cobertura del cribado del Cáncer de Cérvix en España y factores relacionados (Estudio Afrodita). *Comunicación a la XVIII Reunión de la AEPCC.* Bilbao, Noviembre 2006.

[34] Wrigth, T. C. Jr, Schiffman, M., Solomon, D., Cox, T., Garcia, F., Goldie, S., Hatch, K., Soller, K. L., Roach, N., Runowicz, C., Saslow, D. Interim Guidance for the Use of

Human Papillomavirus DNA Testing as an Adjunct to Cervical Cytology for Screening. *Obstet. Gynecol.* 2004;103:304-9.

[35] Puig-Tintoré, L. M., Cortés, X., Castellsague, X., Torne, A., Ordi, J., de Sanjose, S., Alonso, I., Cararach, M., Vidart, J. A., Alba, A., Martínez-Escoriza, J. C., Coll, C., Vilaplana, E., Hardisson, D., Bosch, X. Prevención del cáncer de cuello uterino, ante la vacunación frente al virus del papiloma humano. *Prog. Obstet. Ginecol.* 2006; 49 Supl. 2:5-62.

[36] Sirovich, B. E., Welch, H. G. Cervical cancer screening among women without a cervix. *JAMA* 2004; 291:2990.

[37] Stokes-Lampard, H., Wilson, S., Waddell, C., et al. Vaginal vault smears after hysterectomy for reasons other than malignancy: a systematic review of the literature. *BJOG* 2006; 113:1354.

[38] Stokes-Lampard, H., Wilson, S., Waddell, C., et al. Vaginal vault smears after hysterectomy for reasons other than malignancy: a systematic review of the literature. *BJOG* 2006; 113:1354.

[39] Martin-Hirsch, P. L., Paraskevaidis, E., Kitchener, H. Surgery for cervical intraepithelial neoplasia. *Cochrane Database Syst. Rev.* 2000; CD001318.

[40] Ghaem-Maghami, S., Sagi, S., Majeed, G., Soutter, W. P. Incomplete excision of cervical intraepithelial neoplasia and risk of treatment failure: a meta-analysis. *Lancet Oncol.* 2007; 8:985.

[41] Maiman, M., Fruchter, R. G., Clark, M., et al. Cervical cancer as an AIDS-defining illness. *Obstet. Gynecol.* 1997; 89:76.

[42] Wright, T. C. Jr, Ellerbrock, T. V., Chiasson, M. A., et al. Cervical intraepithelial neoplasia in women infected with human immunodeficiency virus: prevalence, risk factors, and validity of Papanicolaou smears. New York Cervical Disease Study. *Obstet. Gynecol.* 1994; 84:591.

[43] Ellerbrock, T. V., Chiasson, M. A., Bush, T. J., et al. Incidence of cervical squamous intraepithelial lesions in HIV-infected women. *JAMA* 2000; 283:1031.

[44] Frisch, M., Biggar, R. J., Goedert, J. J. Human papillomavirus-associated cancers in patients with human immunodeficiency virus infection and acquired immunodeficiency syndrome. *J. Natl. Cancer Inst.* 2000; 92:1500.

[45] Serraino, D., Carrieri, P., Pradier, C., et al. Risk of invasive cervical cancer among women with, or at risk for, HIV infection. *Int. J. Cancer* 1999; 82:334.

[46] Frisch, M., Biggar, R. J., Goedert, J. J. Human papillomavirus-associated cancers in patients with human immunodeficiency virus infection and acquired immunodeficiency syndrome. *J. Natl. Cancer Inst.* 2000; 92:1500.

[47] Palefsky, J. M., Minkoff, H., Kalish, L. A., et al. Cervicovaginal human papillomavirus infection in human immunodeficiency virus-1 (HIV)-positive and high-risk HIV-negative women. *J. Natl. Cancer Inst.* 1999; 91:226.

[48] Wright, T. C. Jr, Massad, L. S., Dunton, C. J., et al. 2006 consensus guidelines for the management of women with abnormal cervical cancer screening tests. *Am. J. Obstet. Gynecol.* 2007; 197:346.

[49] Fruchter, R. G., Maiman, M., Sedlis, A., et al. Multiple recurrences of cervical intraepithelial neoplasia in women with the human immunodeficiency virus. *Obstet. Gynecol.* 1996; 87:338.

[50] Heard, I., Potard, V., Foulot, H., et al. High rate of recurrence of cervical intraepithelial neoplasia after surgery in HIV-positive women. *J. Acquir. Immune. Defic. Syndr.* 2005; 39:412.

[51] Frisch, M., Biggar, R. J., Goedert, J. J. Human papillomavirus-associated cancers in patients with human immunodeficiency virus infection and acquired immunodeficiency syndrome. *J. Natl. Cancer Inst.* 2000; 92:1500.

[52] Ahdieh-Grant, L., Li, R., Levine, A. M., et al. Highly active antiretroviral therapy and cervical squamous intraepithelial lesions in human immunodeficiency virus-positive women. *J. Natl. Cancer Inst.* 2004; 96:1070.

[53] Bigrigg, M. A., Codling, B. W., Pearson, P., et al. Colposcopic diagnosis and treatment of cervical dysplasia at a single clinic visit. Experience of low-voltage diathermy loop in 1000 patients. *Lancet* 1990; 336-229.

[54] Castle, P. E., Solomon, D., Schiffman, M., Wheeeler, C. M. Human papillomavirus type 16 infections and 2-year absolute risk of cervical precancer in women with equivocal or mild cytologic abnormalities. *J. Natl. Cancer Inst.* 2005; 97:1066.

[55] McCredie, M. R., Sharples, K. J., Paul, C., et al. Natural history of cervical neoplasia and risk of invasive cancer in women with cervical intraepithelial neoplasia 3: a retrospective cohort study. *Lancet Oncol.* 2008;9:425

[56] Gok, Coupe, Berkhof HPV 16 and increased risk of recurrrence after treatment for CIN. *Gynecologic Oncology* 104 (2007) 273-275.

[57] Paraskevaidis, E., Arbyn, M., Sotiriadis, A., et al. The role of HPV DNA testing in the follow-up period after treatment for CIN: a systematic review of the literature. *Cancer Treat. Rev.* 2004;30:205.

[58] Khan, M. J., Castle, P. E., Lorincz, A. T., et al. The elevated 10-year risk of cervical precancer and cancer in women with human papillomavirus (HPV) type 16 or 18 and the possible utility of type-specific HPV testing in clinical practice. *J. Natl. Cancer Inst.* 2005; 97:1072.

[59] Baldauf, Dreyfus Ritter. Cytology and Colposcopy After Loop Electrosurgical Excision: Implications for follow-up. *Obs. and Gyn.* 92 no.1, july 1998.

[60] Geoffery Hulman, Clive J. Pickles, Clive A. Gie, Frecuency of cervical intraepithelial neoplasia following large loop excision of the transformation zone. *J. Clin. Pathol.* 1998; 51:375-377

[61] Orbo, A., Arnesen, T., Arnes, M. Resection margins in conization as prognostic marker for relapse in high-grade dysplasia of the uterine cervix in northern Norway: a retrospective long-term follow-up material. *Gin. Onc.* 93(2004)479-483

[62] Sadaf Ghaem-Maghami, Slomi Sagi. Incomplete excision of cervical intraepithelial neoplasia and risk of treatment failure: a meta-analysis.

[63] Hulman, G., Pickles, C. J., Frecuency of cervical intraepithelial neoplasia following large loop excision of the transformation zone. *J. Clin. Pathol.* 1998;51:375-377

[64] Instituto Fernandes Figueira, Fundacao Oswaldo Cruz. Recurrence of cervical intraepithelial neoplasia grades 2 or 3 in HIV-infected women treated by large loop excision of the transformation zone. (LLETZ) *Sao Paulo Med. J.* 2008;126(1):17-22.

[65] Parkin, D. M., Bray, F., Ferlay, J., Pisani, P. Global cancer statistics, 2002. *CA Cancer J. Clin.* 2005; 55:74.

[66] D'Souza, G., Kreimer, A. R., Viscidi, R., et al. Case-control study of human papillomavirus and oropharyngeal cancer. *N Engl. J. Med.* 2007; 356:1944.

[67]   Kreimer, A. R., Clifford, G. M., Boyle, P., Franceschi, S. Human papillomavirus types in head and neck squamous cell carcinomas worldwide: a systematic review. *Cancer Epidemiol. Biomarkers Prev.* 2005; 14:467.

[68]   De Sanjose, S., Quint, W. G., Alemany, L., et al. Human papillomavirus genotype attribution in invasive cervical cancer: a retrospective cross-sectional worldwide study. *Lancet Oncol.* 2010; 11:1048.

[69]   Moore, E. E., Danielewski, J. A., Garland, S. M., et al. Clearance of human papillomavirus in women treated for cervical dysplasia. *Obstet. Gynecol.* 2011; 117: 101.

[70]   Bontkes, H. J., de Gruijl, T. D., Walboomers, J. M., et al. Immune responses against human papillomavirus (HPV) type 16 virus-like particles in a cohort study of women with cervical intraepithelial neoplasia. II. Systemic but not local IgA responses correlate with clearance of HPV-16. *J. Gen. Virol.* 1999; 80 (Pt 2):409.

[71]   Meijer, C. J., Snijders, P. J., Castle, P. E. Clinical utility of HPV genotyping. *Gynecol. Oncol.* 2006; 103:12.

[72]   Laura, L. Reimers, Susan Sotardi. Outcomes after an excisional procedure for cervical intraepithelial neoplasia in HIV-infected women. *Ginecologic oncology* 119(2010)92-97.

[73]   Marielle Kocken, Theo, J. M. Helmerhorst. Risk of recurrent high-grada cervical intraepithelial neoplasia after successfurl treatmente: a long-term multi-cohort study.

In: Cervical Cancer
Editor: Laurie Elit

ISBN: 978-1-62948-062-6
© 2014 Nova Science Publishers, Inc.

Chapter VI

Quality Indicators for the Practice of Colposcopy in the Screening and Prevention of Cervical Cancer

Lua R. Eiriksson[*1], Clare J. Reade[2] and Laurie Elit[1]

[1]Department of Obstetrics & Gynecology, Division of Gynecologic Oncology,
McMaster University and Juravinski Hospital and Cancer Centre, Hamilton, Canada
[2]Department of Obstetrics & Gynecology, Division of Gynecologic Oncology,
University of Toronto, Toronto, Canada

Abstract

Cervical cancer screening has been a significant public health success in primary prevention. Since the development of the "Pap test" in the 1940's by Georgios Papanikolaou, the incidence and mortality from cervical cancer have dramatically decreased in countries where programs of cervical screening exist.

The objective of the delivery of health care services is to improve patient outcomes and quality of life. The quality of health care is a measurement of the degree to which health care services increase the likelihood of improved health outcomes. Quality of care is a multidimensional concept which requires a broad range of performance measures. Performance is often measured using indicators or standards of care, and determining whether programs of health care delivery and outcomes are consistent with the established standards. Indicators may measure program structure, the process of health care delivery, or outcomes. The selection of indicators to be used in the evaluation of a program should ideally be based on evidence that the indicator is a valid measurement of program quality, is reflective of the scope of care, and is feasible to implement. The indicator should be sensitive to differences in quality of care, easily interpreted, and inform efforts aimed at quality improvement.

* Correspondence concerning this article should be addressed to Lua Eiriksson, Dept of Obstetrics and Gynecology, Division of Gynecologic Oncology, Hamilton, Canada. Email: lua.eiriksson@jcc.hhsc.ca.

Program indicators for cervical cancer screening are in use, including coverage, cytology performance, system capacity, follow-up and outcome indicators. However, indicators specifically focused on the performance of colposcopy have not undergone the same rigor of identification and evaluation. Colposcopy is the procedure whereby suspicious lesions, identified through cervical screening techniques, are identified, followed, and/or treated in order to prevent progression to invasive cancer. While the Pap test is a screening procedure, colposcopy is a diagnostic procedure with the potential to treat pre-invasive disease. The success of cervical cancer prevention as a whole depends not only on screening, but also on diagnosis and treatment. As such, quality indicators for the practice of colposcopy are also needed.

The objective of this chapter is to review the available literature related to colposcopy quality indicators, and to propose colposcopy quality indicators for use in program evaluation in the screening and prevention of cervical cancer.

Introduction

Globally, cervical cancer is the third leading cause of cancer in women [1]. The low rate of cervical cancer in high resource countries is directly related to the presence of cervical cancer screening strategies using the Papanikolaou test (i.e. Pap test) [2]. Canada was one of the early adopters of cervical screening in sexually active women and a clear reduction in cervical cancer incidence over time has been described [3].

The objective of the delivery of health care services is to improve patient outcomes and quality of life. The quality of health care is a measurement of the degree to which health care services increase the likelihood of improved health outcomes [4]. Quality of care is a multidimensional concept that requires a broad range of performance measures [5]. Performance is often measured using indicators or standards of care, and determining whether programs of health care delivery and outcomes are consistent with the established standards [5]. Indicators may measure program structure, the process of health care delivery, or outcomes [6]. Ultimately, the application of quality indicators in the assessment of health care delivery is to improve the quality of health care and thereby improve patient outcomes.

The selection of indicators to be used in the evaluation of a program should ideally be based on evidence that the indicator is a valid measurement of program quality, is reflective of the scope of care, and is feasible to implement [7]. The indicator should be sensitive to differences in quality of care, easily interpreted, and inform efforts aimed at quality improvement [5].

The Delphi method is an evidence-based collaborative approach to the development of quality indicators (Figure 1) [8]. It uses questionnaires and a consensus conference to systematically translate available evidence into objective performance measures. Indicators are first identified through a comprehensive literature search. An expert review panel is then nominated. Indicators are compiled in a questionnaire, which is completed by the expert panel, followed by a group discussion of the results. The process continues with a second questionnaire to assess indicators requiring further assessment, followed by prioritization of indicators selected from the first and second rounds. Feasibility assessment involves refining indicator definitions and identifying data sources to be used for indicator measurement. Data analysis using the chosen indicators is then applied to programs, reviewed for accuracy, and then presented as evaluations of program performance [5].

Cervical cancer screening has been a significant public health success in primary prevention. Since the development of the Pap test in the 1940's by Georgios Papanikolaou, the incidence and mortality from cervical cancer have dramatically decreased in countries where programs of cervical screening exist. In Ontario, Canada, roughly 1.5 million Pap tests are performed annually. In those 5% of women who have an abnormal Pap test, further assessment is recommended using high-powered magnification of the cervix via colposcopy. Colposcopy allows identification of an abnormal area on the cervix, which if biopsied and proven to be a high-grade abnormality (otherwise known as cervical intra-epithelial neoplasia (CIN) 2 or 3), can be removed by freezing (cryotherapy), or excision (cold knife cone, Laser or Loop Electrosurgical Excision Procedure (LEEP)). Such treatments are intended to prevent the development of invasive disease. While the Pap test is a screening procedure, colposcopy is a diagnostic procedure with the potential to treat pre-invasive disease.

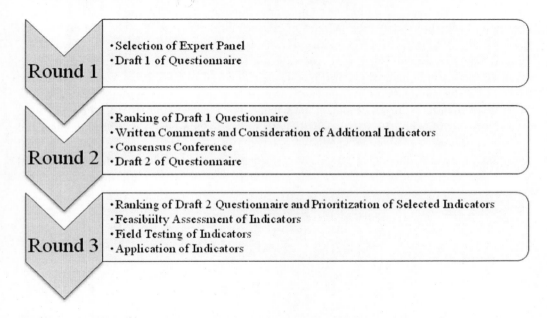

Figure 1. The Modified Delphi Process.

Program indicators for cervical cancer screening have been identified and evaluated. They include screening coverage, cytology performance, system capacity, follow-up and outcome indicators. Indicators specifically focused on the performance of colposcopy have not undergone the same rigor of identification and evaluation. The success of cervical cancer screening as a whole depends not only on screening, but also on diagnosis and treatment. As such, widely accepted quality indicators for the practice of colposcopy are also needed.

The objective of this chapter is to review the available literature related to colposcopy quality indicators and to make the argument that the Delphi process should be used to define colposcopy quality indicators for widespread use in cervical cancer prevention program evaluation.

Methods

A literature review was performed using the search terms 'colposcopy', 'uterine cervical neoplasms', 'uterine cervical dysplasia', 'delivery of health care', 'health services accessibility', 'physicians' practice patterns', 'quality of health care', 'clinical competence', 'outcome and process assessment (health care)', 'outcome assessment (health care)', 'treatment outcome', 'process assessment (health care)', 'program evaluation', 'quality assurance, health care or benchmarking', 'quality indicators, health care', 'nursing audit', 'nursing care', 'medical audit', 'utilization review', 'indicator', 'quality', 'report card', 'scorecard', and 'performance measurement'.

Fifty-six articles were found in the peer-reviewed literature to be relevant. These were reviewed, and potential quality indicators were abstracted. Relevant grey literature was also retrieved and examined, including the Guidelines for the National Health Service Cervical Screening Programme [9], the Canadian Partnership Against Cancer Guidelines on Performance Measurement for Organized Cancer Screening Programs [10], the CPAC Cervical Cancer Screening in Canada: Monitoring Program Performance 2006 – 2008 [11], and the Cancer Care Ontario: Ontario Cervical Screening Program 2003 – 2008 Evaluation Report [12]. The candidate quality indicators were then condensed into the main categories of "Program Structure" (the environment in which health care is provided), "Process" (the method by which health care is provided) and "Outcome" (consequences of health care) and relevant subcategories, with associated references [7]. The target population of cervical cancer screening is women aged 20 – 69 years. For the purpose of this chapter, women aged 20 – 69 years who qualify for colposcopic examination according to referral guidelines are the target population of interest.

Quality Indicators

Program Structure

One of the first potential quality indicators for the practice of colposcopy is whether a formal colposcopy program is in effect [13-16]. Such a program should be integrated into the regional cervical screening initiatives. Formalized systems of patient referral and recall are as necessary for colposcopy as they are for cervical screening. Mechanisms to ensure that follow-up is received may further increase the likelihood that pre-invasive cervical lesions are diagnosed and treated, with expected declines in rates of invasive cervical neoplasia.

The use of an established registry or database to compile clinical details and colposcopic results would allow for linkage of cytologic, colposcopic and histologic findings [9,12,13,16-18]. Furthermore, linkage of cervical screening data with cancer registry data would allow for direct assessment of screening, colposcopy and cancer outcomes. This may be used to produce national statistics. Databases of cytology, colposcopy, and histology results (or linked databases) might also be linked to patients' electronic medical records [15,19-21]. This would allow previous cytology results to be made available to the colposcopist, and cytology results and the colposcopic impression to be made available to the interpreting pathologist. This additional information may assist with establishing a diagnosis and formulating a treatment plan for individual patients.

The practice of colposcopy requires knowledge not only of the pathogenesis of invasive cervical neoplasia, but also an understanding of the risk-benefit ratio of diagnosis and treatment of pre-invasive cervical lesions. A program of formal training and (re-)certification for the qualification of colposcopists has been highlighted as a pre-requisite for proficiency in the practice of colposcopy [9,13-15,17,19,22-27]. A recognized training program under the supervision of qualified colposcopy preceptors, with a formal evaluation process to ensure proficiency would be ideal, providing both a theoretical as well as a practical knowledge base. Case logs may be employed, with the use of Objective Structured Clinical Examinations (OSCE's), a valid method of assessment of training [26]. Formal procedure-specific courses or programs, such as LASER certification, should also be offered. Once competency is achieved, continuing medical education workshops should be available to maintain competence [13,15,19]. The minimum number of new cases seen per year to maintain competence has been debated, with some authors suggesting a minimum of 100 new patients per year [13,15,28].

Objective measures of quality would allow for the monitoring of individual colposcopists' performance and practice. Regular audits of practice to maintain ongoing quality would serve such a purpose [9,13-15,18,19,23,25,28-34]. Indicators of quality within such audits might include whether biopsies taken during colposcopic evaluation are suitable for histologic interpretation, and complication rates for both diagnostic and therapeutic procedures. When deficiencies are identified, standardized programs of upgrading skills or remediation programs for suboptimal colposcopic practice may serve to improve the quality of care provided [19,23].

Process

As an initial measure of the quality of colposcopy in terms of process, it should be determined whether referrals to colposcopy are appropriate; i.e. in accordance with guideline recommendations [9,10,13,35,36]. The referral rate, defined as the number of screened women referred to colposcopy in a given time period divided by the number of women screened during that same time period should be calculated and compared, while taking into consideration population demographics and risk factors. Whether patients are managed in an appropriate centre is a question of interest, particularly when specialized expertise is required for selected sub-populations, such as those with immunosuppression. The time from cytology to colposcopy must be acceptable based on the degree of severity of the cytology prompting colposcopy referral [9,10,12,13,15,16,28,37,38]. According to cytology, the time to colposcopy should be measured (3 months/6 months/9 months/12 months/>12 months) to determine the adequacy of colposcopy services and the appropriateness of patient triaging.

A satisfactory practice setting has been identified as a necessity for the provision of high quality colposcopy services [9,13,39]. Measures of the adequacy or appropriateness of a facility might include whether there is privacy for patients to change and adequate toilet facilities. A permanently sited room specific for colposcopy, with a permanent examination table/chair and colposcope has been identified as a pre-requisite, in addition to appropriate sterilizing facilities, resuscitation equipment, and the availability of refreshments if needed.

Safety guidelines should be put into effect for treatment equipment (e.g. LASER and electrosurgical units), with at least two nurses trained in colposcopy in each clinic. Separate waiting and recovery areas prior to and following assessment and/or treatment, respectively, would be expected to improve patient comfort and safety. In cases of diagnostic services only, automatic referral to treatment units should be available. Dedicated clerical support should facilitate the flow of patients through the clinic.

An assessment of patient perspectives regarding the colposcopic experience might serve to further increase patient satisfaction with the cervical cancer prevention continuum [13,15,25]. Assessments of patient comfort, a patient's impression of the degree of emotional support provided, and anxiety levels prior to and following clinic encounters may be instructive. Surveys may determine whether the clinic is culturally appropriate, including the availability of translation services for ethnic minorities. The clinic should be accessible, both in proximity to the population of interest, as well as by the availability of clinic hours.

Patient counseling and education should be integrated into the colposcopic assessment process [9,13,15,25,40]. Written or verbal information explaining the procedure prior to the appointment should be provided, in addition to personalized counseling with explanation of colposcopic examination procedures, findings, and expected outcomes. The pathogenesis of disease should be reviewed, with the opportunity for patients to ask questions, since there are often numerous misconceptions surrounding the Human Papillomavirus (HPV), its acquisition and persistence, the timeline from infection to development of cervical dysplasia, and the role of preventive versus treatment efforts. Video-colposcopy may be of benefit to patients to improve understanding of the diagnostic and treatment process. Formal letters of invitation and reminder letters should be sent to patients, with additional information provided to explain the rationale for continued follow-up [15,16].

To facilitate a formalized program of colposcopy, standardized reporting forms incorporating standardized terminology should be used [9,13,18,19,25,31,33,41]. Minimum data to be collected could include personal identification, and reason for referral. Forms should also include grade of cytologic abnormality, whether the transformation zone could be adequately visualized, reasons for not performing a biopsy (e.g. pregnancy), diagnosis, documented consent for treatment, biopsy with histologic diagnosis prior to destructive treatment, details of treatment and follow-up. Comprehensive reports should be generated from patient encounters and sent to both referring and family physicians, with follow-up of referrals to gynecologic or gynecologic oncology services to optimize compliance [13]. The proportion of patients who can be safely managed as outpatients, under local analgesia, should be recorded as an additional quality measure [28,33].

A multi-disciplinary colposcopy team may serve to improve quality in the practice of colposcopy [9,13,22]. To evaluate the multi-disciplinary team itself, attendance should be recorded, identifying the proportion of meetings attended by each member and the frequency of meetings. Decisions made by the multi-disciplinary team should be recorded, with letters sent to the managing colposcopist from the multi-disciplinary team reviewing the case. Clinical-pathologic correlation meetings should be a component of an organized program of colposcopy [13,37,42]. Analysis of all cases of invasive cervical cancer should also take place, to evaluate the potential for colposcopic or systems/process errors [9,15,18,43,44]. This would include complete reviews of the screening histories of women diagnosed with invasive or micro-invasive cervical cancer as well as determination of the ratio of "observed:expected" cases of invasive carcinoma. A gynecologic cancer centre multi-disciplinary team should also review all cases of cervical cancer.

Outcomes

In the assessment of outcomes, several authors describe the correlation between colposcopic impression and cytology/histology, or the agreement between cytology and histology as a measure of quality [12,13,20,23,25,28,31-33,41,43,45-49]. Typically the percentage agreement between examinations should be within 1 degree of severity. An additional measure would be the percentage of high-grade Pap test results (e.g. ASC-H/HSIL+) with CIN 2+ or CIN3+ biopsy results within 12 months of the Pap test.

Women presenting to colposcopy with high-grade Pap test results would be expected to undergo a biopsy at the time of clinical examination [9,11,12,13,25,28,31-33,37,44,50-52]. The biopsy rate in these circumstances would be determined as the proportion of women with a high-grade Pap test result who underwent a biopsy within 12 months of a Pap test with the denominator set as all women with a high-grade Pap test result within the defined 12 month time period. This measure would assess adherence to referral guidelines as well as the quality of colposcopy itself. Included in this measure could be the number of biopsies performed per encounter and the manner in which they are taken, as improved sensitivity has been demonstrated when more than 1 biopsy is taken [50] and colposcopically directed biopsies demonstrate greater sensitivity than a 4-quadrant approach [51].

The practice of colposcopy is successful when pre-invasive lesions are detected. Useful measures of outcome quality are understood in the context of disease incidence as well as test sensitivity, specificity, positive and negative predictive value. One useful measure is the colposcopic detection rate of CIN 2 or greater lesions [9-12,28,36,44]. This rate would be calculated as the number of pre-cancerous lesions (CIN2, CIN3) detected per 1000 women screened in a 12-month period. The number of micro-invasive carcinomas detected, as well as the invasive cancer detection rate could be similarly calculated and compared.

The sensitivity of colposcopy in correctly identifying the presence of disease using clinical examination and directed biopsies is a measure of the quality of the testing procedure [10,19,25,50,53-55]. This would be calculated as the number of test-positive subjects per number of diseased subjects. The sensitivity of initial colposcopic examination in the detection of CIN 2+ could be compared to follow-up assessments. A test with high sensitivity is considered a reliable indicator when the result is negative, since it rarely misses cases with disease. The specificity of colposcopy (i.e. the rate of colposcopy correctly identifying the absence of disease) is calculated as the number of test-negative subjects by the number of non-diseased subjects [19,25,54,55]. Highly specific tests rarely miss cases without disease. Therefore, when a highly specific test suggests the presence of disease, there is a high probability that disease is present.

A biopsy of CIN 2+ is typically the threshold that would trigger excisional therapy. Therefore, of the women with a colposcopically guided biopsy of CIN 2+ at enrollment, the proportion of women with a cumulative CIN 2+ diagnostic excision would allow for the calculation of the positive predictive value of an initial CIN 2+ biopsy. The positive predictive value of a test, the proportion of positive test results that make the correct diagnosis (i.e. the proportion of disease-positive and test-positive women compared to all test-positive women) is an important measure of the performance of a diagnostic test, since it reflects the probability that a positive test reflects the underlying condition being tested for. This is particularly important if excisional treatment is to be offered, especially in young women with fertility desires, given the increase in preterm rupture of membranes and preterm delivery following LEEP and cone biopsy procedures [56-64]. Similarly, the negative predictive value of a test, the proportion of non-diseased and test-negative women compared to all test-negative women, evaluates the ability of a negative test to reassure patients and practitioners of the absence of disease. Both positive and negative predictive values are influenced by the prevalence of disease, and therefore can differ for a particular test based on the population of interest.

The association between high-grade dysplasia (CIN 2+) and treatment should be determined (the number of patients with CIN 2+ who are treated compared to the number of patients with CIN 2+ disease) to see whether there has been adherence to treatment guidelines [13,22,37]. The rate of over-treatment should also be determined [13,15,19,28,37,65]. The number of patients with less than CIN 2 on excisional biopsy compared to the number of patients undergoing excisional biopsy procedures is one potential measure of over-treatment. High-grade dysplasia should be identified on histology in >90% of patients who are treated at the first visit if colposcopic impression of high-grade dysplasia is to be relied upon as a sufficient diagnostic tool. Adherence to treatment guidelines should be evaluated, as treatment guidelines may differ by region and population served. The adequacy of treatment may require several indicators, such as measures of the wait time between biopsy report and treatment, the completeness of lesion excision, and clearance of disease as reflected by negative follow-up [9,15,18,28,48,49]. Treatment may be considered inadequate if a lesion is incompletely excised or dysplasia is documented on subsequent follow-up cytology, as it has been suggested there should be no dysplasia at 6 months follow-up in over 90% of patients treated.

The incidence of cervical cancer may be a reflection of the performance of colposcopy where rates of cervical screening are optimized [11,18]. Calculated as the number of new cases of invasive cervical cancer per 100 000 women, it is expected that this incidence should decrease with the increased effectiveness of cervical screening, diagnosis of pre-invasive lesions, and treatment. It is acknowledged that programs of cervical screening must be considered in the context of a population, with issues of access, culture, education, and poverty presenting barriers to cervical cancer prevention strategies. However, many of these barriers can be overcome with organized systems that take into consideration the unique needs of the population served. The stage of cancer at the time of diagnosis is one of the best known prognostic indicators. The primary purpose of screening programs is to diagnose disease at the earliest stage in order to improve overall outcomes and reduce treatment-related morbidity. The proportion of cancers diagnosed at stage I, calculated over a 12-month period, may thus be considered an indicator of the success of a cervical cancer screening and prevention program [10,11,18]. While in some instances disease may not be prevented in the pre-invasive phase, the identification and treatment of cervical cancer when confined to the cervix allows for more conservative treatments and is associated with significantly improved survival outcomes compared to more advanced stage disease.

Finally, compliance with the recommendation for colposcopy and colposcopy follow-up assesses the ability of a system to engage and retain participants [9-11,13, 15,19,22, 25,28,38,44]. The participation rate is the number of patients referred who attend colposcopy compared to the total number of patients referred. The retention or follow-up rate is the number of patients who return for colposcopy follow-up compared to the number seen in colposcopy and advised to return for follow-up. The participation and retention rates can be analyzed by subgroup according to the grade of cervical dysplasia. Women may have special circumstances that contribute to delayed diagnosis or treatment, such as those with cytology or biopsy-proven CIN diagnosed during pregnancy. These cases should be assessed separately, with unique measures such as the number of women assessed post-partum per women diagnosed with CIN during pregnancy. The rate of missed appointments (i.e. defaults) should be known, with written protocols for management of non-attendees. The duration of follow-up should be appropriate, with patient retention within the system only for as long as is necessary.

The indicators identified in this chapter are based on results from the peer-reviewed literature, systems of cervical cancer prevention in effect, and expert opinion. In order to determine which indicators are of most usefulness in the assessment of the practice of colposcopy within programs of cervical cancer prevention, a consensus is required.

The Delphi Process

The Delphi Process is a commonly used consensus method used in medical, nursing and health resources research. Consensus methods allow for a wider range of study types to be considered compared to standard statistical reviews, with the added component of qualitative assessment of evidence. Features of consensus methods include anonymity, several iterations allowing participants to modify their opinions, controlled feedback demonstrating the group's responses, and statistical group responses expressing judgment using summary measures of the entire group's responses. Consensus methods are typically employed when unanimity of opinion is lacking due to either insufficient evidence, or contradictory evidence [8].

The Delphi process involves a series of rounds. During Round 1 an expert panel is selected. Based on knowledge, experience, and relevant literature, a questionnaire is drafted under a limited number of subheadings and statements to circulate to all participants. Round 2 requires Delphi participants to rank their agreement with statements posed on the questionnaire. These rankings are summarized and included in a second questionnaire, which is circulated in Round 3. Participants re-rank their agreement with each statement of the questionnaire with the opportunity to change one's previous scoring based on the group's response. If an acceptable degree of consensus is achieved, the final results are provided to the participants. Otherwise, Round 3 is repeated. In certain situations, a face-to-face meeting may be organized to discuss the process and modify the questionnaire. One of the benefits of the Delphi process is the ability to achieve consensus between a large number of experts with limited time commitment and expense [8].

Expert panels of participants should be selected by nomination from physicians, administrators, and managers of ambulatory care with the aid of hospital CEOs. The panels should include colposcopy clinic administrator(s), colposcopy clinic nurse(s), colposcopy clinic physicians (including gynecologists, family physicians and gynecologic oncologists), and pathology and laboratory medicine specialists. Representatives from both hospital-based and non hospital-based colposcopy clinics should be included. The indicators identified and discussed in this chapter may be used as the basis for the first questionnaire in a modified Delphi process to be presented to an expert panel of participants (Figure 1). The first questionnaire should list all of the colposcopy quality indicators as questions to be rated on a seven-point scale (1=disagree and 7=agree) according to the association of the indicator with quality and patient outcomes. Participants are given the opportunity to provide written comments and suggest additional indicators that warrant consideration by the panel which may not have been included in the original questionnaire. Following completion of the first questionnaire with identification of candidate indicators, a consensus conference is useful to allow for group discussion to further revise selected indicators. The indicators requiring further evaluation would then be included in the second questionnaire. Once the results of the second questionnaire are reviewed, the expert panel prioritizes the selected indicators. A feasibility assessment follows, where indicators are further defined and the data sources from which these indicators can be collected are identified. Should the data collection for a particular indicator be too costly or cumbersome, exclusion of a certain indicator may take place at this stage. The indicators are then tested in the field, with the opportunity for colposcopy practices to review the preliminary results of the analysis. If the results are found to be valid, the chosen indicators can then be applied more broadly, and begin to be implemented to monitor the performance of colposcopy programs regionally and possibly nationally.

Conclusion

In this chapter, we have systematically reviewed the published literature for all available quality indicators for the performance of colposcopy. The establishment of quality indicators for colposcopy is an essential step to allow for performance evaluation and quality improvement in the diagnostic and treatment phases of the management of cervical neoplasia. We have identified several quality indicators which fit into the established quality framework described by Donabedian: structure, process and outcomes [6].

Possible quallty indicators related to structure include: the presence of a formal colposcopy program, the presence of a registry or database to capture and track patient results, formal training and (re)certification for colposcopists along with continuing medical education, regular audits of practice, minimum numbers of new cases per year, and programs for upgrading skills when remediation is required.

Quality indicators related to process include: the appropriateness of colposcopy referrals, time from cytology to colposcopy, the presence of a satisfactory practice setting, a standardized reporting form, comprehensive reports sent to the family physician, follow-up of referrals to oncology services to ensure compliance, performance of the majority of procedures under local anaesthetic, participation in multi-disciplinary colposcopy team meetings with clinico-pathologic correlation of colposcopic findings, regular assessment of patient perspectives and satisfaction, routine counselling and education of patients, reminder letters for patients who do not attend, and case-analysis for all patients with a diagnosis of invasive cervical cancer.

Finally, quality indicators related to outcomes include: correlation between colposcopy, cytology and histology, biopsy rate, colposcopic detection rate of CIN2+, sensitivity of colposcopy, specificity of colposcopy, positive and negative predictive values of colposcopy, incidence of cervical cancer in women enrolled in the colposcopy program, proportion of cancers diagnosed in stage I, proportion of women with CIN2+ who receive treatment, proportion of women with less than CIN 2 who receive treatment, compliance with follow-up guidelines, and adequacy of treatment.

It is clear that there are many possible quality indicators in use in the published literature. However, quality indicators, especially when used for quality improvement as performance measures, require collaboration and consensus in order to become accepted by key stakeholders. The Delphi method is useful to achieve these goals in an evidence-based, stakeholder-led fashion. The Delphi method should be considered for the future development of colposcopy quality indicators for widespread use in policy and practice.

References

[1]   International Agency for Research on Cancer [homepage on Internet]. Globocan 2008 [updated 2010, cited 2013 May]. Available from: *http://globocan.iarc.fr*

[2]   Zeferino LC, Derchain SF. Cervical cancer in the developing world. *Best Pract Res Clin Obstet Gynaecol.* 2006;20(3):339-54.

[3]   Benedet JL. Progress in gynecologic cancer detection and treatment. *Int J Gynaecol Obstet.* 2000;70(1):135-47.

[4]   Lohr KN, Schoreder SA. A strategy for quality assurance in Medicare. *N Engl J Med.* 1990;322(10):707-12.

[5]   Gagliardi, A. *Hospital Report Research Collaborative Procedure Manual. The development of indicators using a modified Delphi process.* University of Toronto. Revised 29 July, 2005.

[6]   Donabedian A. The quality of care. How can it be assessed? *JAMA.* 1988;260 (12):1743-8.

[7]   Seow H, Snyder CF, Mularski RA et al. A framework for assessing quality indicators for cancer care at the end of life. *J Pain Symptom Manage.* 2009;38(6):903-12.

[8]   Jones J, Hunter D. Consensus methods for medical and health services research. *BMJ.* 1995;311:376–80.

[9]   NHS Cancer Screening Programmes [homepage on the Internet]. Colposcopy and Programme Management: Guidelines for the NHS Cervical Screening Programme, Second edition [updated 2010 May; cited 2013 May]. Available at: *http://www. cancerscreening.nhs.uk/cervical/publications/nhscsp20.html*

[10]   Canadian Partnership Against Cancer [homepage on the Internet]. Guidelines on Performance Measurement for Organized Cancer Screening Programs [updated 2008 April, cited 2013 May]. Available from:*http://www.partnershipagainstcancer.ca/wp-content/uploads/Guidelines_on_Performance_Measurement_for_Organized_Cancer_S creening_Programs_2008-04-10_Final_20_3__0.pdf*

[11]   Canadian Partnership Against Cancer [homepage on the Internet]. Cervical Cancer Screening in Canada: Monitoring Program Performance (2006 – 2008) [updated 2011

December; cited 2013 May]. Available from: *http://www.partnershipagainstcancer. ca/resources-publications/screening/cervical-cancer-control/*

[12] Cancer Care Ontario [homepage on the Internet]. Ontario Cervical Screening Program 2003 – 2008 Evaluation Report [cited 2013 May]. Available from: *https://www.cancercare.on.ca/common/pages/UserFile.aspx?fileId=117127*

[13] Cancer Care Ontario [homepage on Internet]. The Optimum Organization for the Delivery of Colposcopy Services in Ontario 2008 [updated 2008 Feb, cited 2013 May]. Available from: *https://www.cancercare.on.ca/common/pages/UserFile.aspx?fileId= 32292*

[14] Ghazal-Aswad S, Badrinath P, Sidky I, Gargash H. Colposcopy services in the United Arab Emirates. *J Low Genit Tract Dis*. 2006;10(3):151-5.

[15] Jolley S. *Quality in colposcopy. Nurs Stand*. 2004;18(23):39-44.

[16] Lukman H, Bevan JR, Greenwood E. Direct booking colposcopy clinic – the Portsmouth experience. *Cytopathology*. 2004;15(4):217-20.

[17] Arbyn M, Anttila A, Jordan J, Ronco G, Schenck U, Segnan N, et al. European Guidelines for Quality Assurance in Cervical Cancer Screening. Second edition-- summary document. *Ann Oncol*. 2010;21(3):448-58.

[18] Jordan J, Martin-Hirsch P, Arbyn M, Schenck U, Baldauf JJ, Da Silva D, et al. European guidelines for clinical management of abnormal cervical cytology, part 2. *Cytopathology*. 2009;20(1):5-16.

[19] Benedet JL, Matisic JP, Bertrand MA. The quality of community colposcopic practice. *Obstet Gynecol*. 2004;103(1):92-100.

[20] Brenner BN, Donoghue AM. Quality assurance in colposcopy using video capture and the internet for individual audit. *N Z Med J*. 2000;113(1103):41-2.

[21] Bulten J, Horvat R, Jordan J, Herbert A, Wiener H, Arbyn M. European guidelines for quality assurance in cervical histopathology. *Acta Oncol*. 2011;50(5):611-20.

[22] Dexeus S. Colposcopy carried out by experts in multidisciplinary teams provides the best results. *Cytopathology*. 2008;19(6):337-8.

[23] Ferris DG, Spitzer M, Werner C, Dickman ED, Shiver RL. Colposcopy quality control for clinical trials: the positive effects from brief, intensive educational intervention. J Low Genit Tract Dis. 2002;6(1):11-6.

[24] Jeronimo J, Massad LS, Castle PE, Wacholder S, Schiffman M; National Institutes of Health (NIH)-American Society for Colposcopy and Cervical Pathology (ASCCP) Research Group. Interobserver agreement in the evaluation of digitized cervical images. *Obstet Gynecol*. 2007;110(4):833-40.

[25] Nazeer S, Shafi MI. Objective perspective in colposcopy. *Best Pract Res Clin Obstet Gynaecol*. 2011;25(5):631-40.

[26] Shehmar M, Cruikshank M, Finn C, Redman C, Fraser I, Peile E. A validity study of the national UK colposcopy objective structured clinical examination--is it a test fit for purpose? *BJOG*. 2009;116(13):1796-9.

[27] Thangaratinam S, Walker P, Freeman-Wang T, Luesley D, Cruickshank M, Redman CW. Identifying the performance criteria for appraisal of colposcopists: benchmarking Delphi. *BJOG*. 2007;114(10):1288-91.

[28] Redburn J, Sundar S, Usherwood M, Roche M; Four Counties Colposcopy Group. Trends in compliance with the national colposcopy guidelines. *J Obstet Gynaecol*. 2004;24(5):552-6.

[29] Ferris DG, Litaker MS; ASCUS/LSIL Triage Study (ALTS) Group. Colposcopy quality control by remote review of digitized colposcopic images. *Am J Obstet Gynecol.* 2004;191(6):1934-41.

[30] Ferris DG, Litaker M; ALTS Group. Interobserver agreement for colposcopy quality control using digitized colposcopic images during the ALTS trial. *J Low Genit Tract Dis.* 2005;9(1):29-35.

[31] Manopunya M, Suprasert P, Srisomboon J, Kietpeerakool C. Colposcopy audit for improving quality of service in areas with a high incidence of cervical cancer. *Int J Gynaecol Obstet.* 2010;108(1):4-6.

[32] Muwonge R, Mbalawa CG, Keita N, Dolo A, Nouhou H, Nacoulma M, et al. Performance of colposcopy in five sub-Saharan African countries. *BJOG.* 2009;116(6):829-37.

[33] Nooh A, Babburi P, Howell R. Achieving quality assurance standards in colposcopy practice: a teaching hospital experience. *Aust N Z J Obstet Gynaecol.* 2007;47(1):61-4.

[34] Sanghvi H, Limpaphayom KK, Plotkin M, Charurat E, Kleine A, Lu E, et al. Cervical cancer screening using visual inspection with acetic acid: operational experiences from Ghana and Thailand. *Reprod Health Matters.* 2008;16(32):67-77.

[35] Jordan J, Arbyn M, Martin-Hirsch P, Schenck U, Baldauf JJ, Da Silva D, et al. European guidelines for quality assurance in cervical cancer screening: recommendations for clinical management of abnormal cervical cytology, part 1. *Cytopathology.* 2008;19(6):342-54.

[36] Ronco G, van Ballegooijen M, Becker N, Chil A, Fender M, Giubilato P, et al. Process performance of cervical screening programmes in Europe. *Eur J Cancer.* 2009;45(15):2659-70.

[37] Dina R. Recommendations that could improve performance of colposcopy and cytology. *Cytopathology.* 2008;19(6):338-40.

[38] Kietpeerakool C, Manopunya M, Phuprasertsak P, Jaijit T, Srisomboon J. An audit of colposcopy appointment processes in women with abnormal cervical cytology. *Cytopathology.* 2011;22(3):184-8.

[39] Wisniewski M, Wisniewski H. Measuring service quality in a hospital colposcopy clinic. Int J Health Care Qual Assur Inc Leadersh Health Serv. 2005;18(2-3):217-28.

[40] Massad LS. Communicating colposcopy results: opportunities for improvement. *J Low Genit Tract Dis.* 2008;12(2):69-70.

[41] Wensveen C, Kagie M, Nagelkerke N, Trimbos B. Interobserver agreement on interpreting hand drawings of colposcopy in women with borderline cytology to predict high-grade lesions. *Eur J Obstet Gynecol Reprod Biol.* 2007;135(1):123-6.

[42] Moss EL, Byrom J, Owen G, Pearmain P, Douce G, Todd R, et al. Multidisciplinary colposcopy clinicopathology correlation meetings: an activity review. *J Low Genit Tract Dis.* 2009;13(3):169-73.

[43] Benedet JL, Anderson GH, Matisic JP, Miller DM. A quality-control program for colposcopic practice. *Obstet Gynecol.* 1991;78(5 Pt 1):872-5.

[44] Bucchi L, Falcini F, Schincaglia P, Desiderio F, Bondi A, Farneti M, et al. Performance indicators of organized cervical screening in Romagna (Italy). *Eur J Cancer Prev.* 2003;12(3):223-8.

[45] Bowring J, Strander B, Young M, Evans H, Walker P. The Swede score: evaluation of a scoring system designed to improve the predictive value of colposcopy. *J Low Genit Tract Dis.* 2010;14(4):301-5.

[46] Cagle AJ, Hu SY, Sellors JW, Bao YP, Lim JM, Li SM, et al. Use of an expanded gold standard to estimate the accuracy of colposcopy and visual inspection with acetic acid. *Int J Cancer.* 2010;126(1):156-61.

[47] Raab SS, Grzybicki DM, Zarbo RJ, Jensen C, Geyer SJ, Janosky JE, et al. Frequency and outcome of cervical cancer prevention failures in the United States. *Am J Clin Pathol.* 2007;128(5):817-24.

[48] Volante R, Giubilato P, Ronco G. Quality of colposcopy and treatment: data from the national survey of Italian organised cervical screening programmes. *Epidemiol Prev.* 2007 Mar-Jun;31(2-3 Suppl 2):61-8.

[49] Volante R, Giubilato P, Ronco G. Quality of colposcopy and treatment: data from the national survey of Italian organised cervical screening programmes. *Epidemiol Prev.* 2008 Mar-Apr;32(2 Suppl 1):69-76.

[50] Gage JC, Hanson VW, Abbey K, Dippery S, Gardner S, Kubota J, et al. ASCUS LSIL triage Study (ALTS) Group. Number of cervical biopsies and sensitivity of colposcopy. *Obstet Gynecol.* 2006;108:264–72.

[51] Pretorius RG, Zhang WH, Belinson JL, Huang MN, Wu LY, Zhang X, et al. Colposcopically directed biopsy, random cervical biopsy, and endocervical curettage in the diagnosis of cervical intraepithelial neoplasia II or worse. *Am J Obstet Gynecol* 2004;191(2):430–4.

[52] Pretorius RG, Bao YP, Belinson JL, Burchette RJ, Smith JS, Qiao YL. Inappropriate gold standard bias in cervical cancer screening studies. *Int J Cancer.* 2007;121(10):2218-24.

[53] Cox JT. More questions about the accuracy of colposcopy: what does this mean for cervical cancer prevention? *Obstet Gynecol.* 2008;111(6):1266-7.

[54] Nocon M, Mittendorf T, Roll S, Greiner W, Willich SN, von der Schulenburg JM. Review on the medical and health economic evidence for an inclusion of colposcopy in primary screening programs for cervical cancer. *GMS Health Technol Assess.* 2007;3:Doc07.

[55] Wulan N, Rasool N, Belinson SE, Wang C, Rong X, Zhang W, et al. Study of the diagnostic efficacy of real-time optical coherence tomography as an adjunct to unaided visual inspection with acetic acid for the diagnosis of preinvasive and invasive neoplasia of the uterine cervix. *Int J Gynecol Cancer.* 2010;20(3):422-7.

[56] Sjøborg KD, Vistad I, Myhr SS, Svenningsen R, Herzog C, Kloster-Jensen A, et al. Pregnancy outcome after cervical cone excision: a case-control study. *Acta Obstet Gynecol Scand* 2007;86(4):423-8.

[57] Albrechtsen S, Rasmussen S, Thoresen S, Irgens LM, Iversen OE. Pregnancy outcome in women before and after cervical conisation: population based cohort study. *BMJ.* 2008;337:a1343.

[58] Castanon A, Brocklehurst P, Evans H, Peebles D, Singh N, Walker P, et al. Risk of preterm birth after treatment for cervical intraepithelial neoplasia among women attending colposcopy in England: retrospective-prospective cohort study. *BMJ* 2012;345:e5174.

[59] Arbyn M, Kyrgiou M, Simoens C, Raifu AO, Koliopoulos G, Martin-Hirsch P, et al. Perinatal mortality and other severe adverse pregnancy outcomes associated with treatment of cervical intraepithelial neoplasia: meta-analysis. *BMJ.* 2008;337:a1284.

[60] Noehr B, Jensen A, Frederiksen K, Tabor A, Kjaer SK. Loop electrosurgical excision of the cervix and subsequent risk for spontaneous preterm delivery: a population-based study of singleton deliveries during a 9-year period. *Am J Obstet Gynecol* 2009; 201(1):33.e1-6.

[61] Werner CL, Lo JY, Heffernan T, Griffith WF, McIntire DD, Leveno KJ. Loop electrosurgical excision procedure and risk of preterm birth. *Obstet Gynecol* 2010; 115:605.

[62] Jakobsson M, Gissler M, Paavonen J, Tapper AM. Loop electrosurgical excision procedure and the risk for preterm birth. *Obstet Gynecol.* 2009;114(3):504-10.

[63] Bruinsma F, Lumley J, Tan J, Quinn M. Precancerous changes in the cervix and risk of subsequent preterm birth. *BJOG* 2007;114(1):70-80.

[64] Kyrgiou M, Koliopoulos G, Martin-Hirsch P, Arbyn M, Prendiville W, Paraskevaidis E. Obstetric outcomes after conservative treatment for intraepithelial or early invasive cervical lesions: systematic review and meta-analysis. *Lancet* 2006;367(9509):489-98.

[65] Smith MC, Broadhead TJ, Hammond RH. 'See and treat' at colposcopy--achieving the standard. *J Obstet Gynaecol.* 2001 Jan;21(1):62-3.

In: Cervical Cancer   ISBN: 978-1-62948-062-6
Editor: Laurie Elit   © 2014 Nova Science Publishers, Inc.

Chapter VII

Treatment of Cervical Disease: Review of the Current Data

A. C. Freitas, A. L. S. Jesus and F. C. Mariz

Department of Genetics, Federal University of Pernambuco, Brazil

Abstract

Persistent infection involving oncogenic Human Papillomavirus (HPV) types, is the most common sexually transmissible disease and is associated with 5% of all cancers in people of both sexes. Although efficient, the currently licensed anti-HPV vaccines do not have therapeutic potential to treat established lesions. Other immunizing approaches directed to the E6 and E7 viral oncoproteins, have been tested with varying degrees of success to stimulate immune responses to the regression of pre-malignant and malignant lesions. On the other hand, the current therapeutic treatment is not virus-specific and consists of the physical removal of the lesions or the induction of inflammatory responses to cause the regression of established lesions. Hence, recently attempts have been made to identify and characterize the potential molecular antagonists against the viral proteins and their respective cellular targets. The use of lead compounds, which can disturb the viral replication, as well as the inhibitors of the viral carcinogenesis, have proved to be an attractive approach due to their high affinity and specificity. However, these studies are still in their early stages and it is unlikely that new anti-HPV chemotherapeutic agents can be developed for clinics in the next 10-20 years.

Keywords: Cervical cancer, HPV, therapies

Introduction

It is estimated that 5% of all human cancers are caused by HPV infection [1]. Together with cervical intraepithelial lesions of all grades and warts, this scenario represents a huge burden to the health services [2].

Since 2008, two prophylactic vaccines have been licensed to provide protection against HPV. Both have high efficacy against HPV-16 and -18 [3, 4], which are the most common viral types linked to cervical cancer [5], and have the potential to prevent 70% of carcinomas and 90% of genital warts in the next 10-20 years [6].

However, the estimated impact of these vaccines may be compromised due their high costs which prevent them from being available in developing countries, where more than 80% of deaths result from HPV infection [5]. In other words, a large section of the unvaccinated public will still be affected by HPV-related diseases and, thus high priority must be given to producing virus-specific therapies.

The objective of the treatment against HPV clinical infection is the removal of the clinically-visible disease through the destruction of condyloma by physical removal or by the induction of inflammatory responses [2]. Since these alternatives are not virus-specific, these therapeutic approaches have had varying degrees of success [7]. Hence, a great effort has been made to identify and characterize molecules that might be antagonistic to HPV proteins and their cellular targets so that anti-HPV drugs can be produced. However, these studies are still at an early stage and it is unlikely that a chemotherapeutic agent against cervical cancer be developed for clinical use in the next 10-20 years [2].

The Treatment of HPV-Related Lesions: What Makes it Difficult?

The Infectious Cycle X the Host Immunity against HPV

Although the suggestion that HPV plays a role in cervical carcinogenesis was first proposed three decades ago [8], there has been slow progress in the development of effective anti-HPV therapies, largely due to the difficulty of conducting studies into the biology and pathogenesis of HPV, which possess a unique and complex replication cycle [2].

HPV has access to the basal keratinocytes of the stratified squamous epithelium through micro-lesions and/or micro-abrasions. The small viral genome - 8 kb double-stranded DNA - has 8 ORFs (open-reading frames), six of which encode non-structural and early proteins (E1, E2, E4, E5, E6 and E7), while the other two remaining ORFs encode structural or late proteins (L1 and L2) [9]. The gene expression pattern of the virus depends on epithelial differentiation and occurs through a complex network of events involving splicing sites within the virus genome [10].

There are no easily handled animal models for HPV infection and the experimental reproduction of the viral life-cycle can only be achieved by *in vivo* culture systems, which are technically demanding, extremely complex and only capable of producing small amounts of infectious viral particles [11].

As a result of a number of sequential stages, the first sign of cervical carcinogenesis is the HPV infection, but its progress mainly depends on the persistence of this infection [12]. In this context, despite the immunity of the female genital tract, HPV is highly adapted to its host, which allows the persistence of infection. Although they are entirely intraepithelial, HPV infections occur in "privileged" sites in which the number of antigen-presenting cells (APCs), which are basically Langerhans cells (LC), is significantly reduced [13, 14]. In addition, the intraepithelial non-lytic cycle is able to prevent the stimulation of molecular signals which are essential for the immune response, such as those that lead to the production of pro-inflammatory cytokines that result in the migration of APCs [15, 16].

Apart from causing the transformation of infected cells, viral oncoproteins also assist viral evasion of the immune system. The combined action of E5 and E6 proteins has a significant effect on the recognition of infected cells by the immune cells, either by inhibiting contact between infected and immune cells [17], down-regulating MHC/HLA-I [18-23], or preventing an appropriate molecular signaling being employed for the immune system, such as the inhibition of cytokine expression [24, 16, 21].

Another complication of HPV infection is viral latency. This phenomenon is characterized by an infection that is restricted to the basal keratinocytes because the viral genome is maintained in episomal form which significantly lowers the expression of the viral proteins [25]. Latent infection is kept under control by a responsive immunological memory [26], but does not necessarily result in viral clearance [27]. These lesions are unlikely to recur in immunocompetent individuals, but possible factors suppressing the immune system can allow viral reactivation and lesion formation [25, 28].

A correct understanding of this scenario is of great importance for the development of therapeutic strategies against HPV-induced lesions. As a means of bypassing the viral evasion mechanisms and activating effective responses, the most promising approaches to immunization have explored different ways of effectively introducing viral oncoprotein-based antigens to the immune system. However, as these strategies are still in the early stages of being tested, the current therapeutic options consist of ablative therapies or are based on cytotoxic agents, as will be shown in the following sections.

Current Therapeutic Alternatives

Why to Treat, When to Treat and How to Treat?

The vast majority of individuals are able to react against HPV and eliminate viral infection. However, there are a few infected individuals that cannot combat the virus; some of them develop clinical lesions and will be further submitted to the treatment that is currently available; others will remain infected although without HPV-related diseases [29, 30]. Since there is no virus-specific therapy for HPV, the treatment against human papillomatosis is based on an attempt to eliminate lesions which might lead to cancer in association with the stimulus of the immune response in order to resolve the viral infection. Furthermore, as they represent a sexually transmissible disease, the elimination of HPV-related lesions is a means of preventing viral dissemination. It is up to the doctor to assess the need for treatment and which therapeutic option is most suitable, in the light of the following factors: confirmation of virus presence, the type of infecting virus (whether low or high risk), characteristics of the lesions (whether localized or disseminated), the type of infection (clinical, subclinical or latent) [31].

When deciding on the most appropriate treatment the following factors should be taken into account [31]:

1. A molecular biology diagnosis carried out through a genital swab. This kind of diagnosis can reveal the presence of viral DNA although it does not specify the existence and/or location of the lesions, or their characteristics (size, extent etc). It is thus necessary to submit the patient to genitoscopy to carry out a proper mapping of the lesions. In cases where the findings of the research are HPV-positive through the use of a swab without any association with clinically lesions, the patient may be latently infected. As a result, there is no confirmation regarding either whether it might lead to transmission of the disease or if there are any therapeutic indications.

2. The examination by genital swab is HPV-negative. In this case, there is no certainty that the patient is not infected with HPV due to the possible presence of keratinized or old genital lesions, which have a small amount of viral DNA but might permit viral transmission. It is necessary to establish the presence of these lesions to avoid an erroneous diagnosis which might suggest that there is no need for treatment.

3. Treatment of clinical lesions. It is not uncommon to observe warty lesions, called satellite lesions, which are only detectable by genitoscopy. Likewise, there are significant papular lesions which are only visible upon application of acetic acid and further examination with magnification (usually resulting from infection involving high-risk types). These situations may explain, for example, why cases are sometimes wrongly assessed as recurrence, when in fact they represent intraepithelial lesions that have been incorrectly located and treated in an inappropriate way.

4. Diagnosis by genitoscopy (colposcopy). This is the most suitable approach for allowing the correct mapping of lesions and evaluating their characteristics, such as size, location and extent.

For this reason, common sense should prevail when planning the treatment schedule. Radical decisions – which are only favorable for the treatment of clinical lesions or, alternatively, which proposes the treatment of all clinical and subclinical cases, as well as the need to take preventive treatment based on topical preparations – should not be recommended. The effectiveness of current available therapies depends on this analysis, since the alternative forms of treatment can lead to excellent results or be contraindicated, depending on the nature of the HPV infection.

Table 1. The alternative forms of treatment for intra-epithelial lesions caused by HPV are categorized by levels of clinical recommendation. Adapted from American Society for Colposcopy and Cervical Pathology [94]

Category	Method	Mechanism of action	Efficacy rate	Recurrence rate
First line	Imiquimod 5%	Immunomodulatory	72-84%	5-19%
	Podophyllotoxin	Cytotoxic agent	45-88%	31-60%
	Cryoteraphy	Ablative/excisional	68-90%	38%
Second line	Laser therapy	Ablative/excisional	27-82%	7-72%
	Electrosurgery	Ablative/excisional	70-80% *	25-39% *
Other therapies	TCA	Cytotoxic agent	70-81%	30-60% **
	Interferon	Immunomodulatory	32-60% (intralesional)	65-67%
			17-21% (systemic)	Non reported
	Polyphenon E	Immunomodulatory	53.6%	6.8%

* Maw, 2004 [38].

** de Carvalho, 2005 [31]

Another important factor is the progress of the treatment, with regard to the frequency with which recurrence occurs associated with exuberant lesions. This means that, treatment should be more intensive and bring together the different therapeutic options at an early stage.

Table 1 categorizes the alternative forms of treatment for the intraepithelial lesions in accordance with clinical recommendations. In the following section, these therapies will be discussed in the light of the methods employed: non-surgical treatment, ablative/excisional treatment, immunomodulators and combination therapy.

Non-Surgical Treatment

Topical preparations based on cytotoxic agents result in cell death through contact, either by antiproliferative or chemidestructive action, regardless of viral status [2]. The use of podophyllotoxin as a solution or cream is the first line of treatment for genital warts and promotes the destruction of verrucous lesions without major alterations to the normal skin [31, 32]. The resulting necrotic action is thought to be based on its ability to bind to the microtubule proteins with subsequent cell cycle arrest in metaphase [2]. The disadvantages of using podophyllotoxin in therapy include systemic absorption, potential mutagenic action in the epithelium and the recurrence of the condition in 65% of cases. Furthermore, bone marrow suppression, liver disorders and neurological impairment have been reported [33-35]. An alternative treatment is the topical use of trichloroacetic acid (TCA) which involves a local caustic and keratolytic activity that causes corrosion of warts without serious systemic effects [32]. TCA is as effective as podophyllotoxin, although it has drawbacks such as the ulceration of adjacent normal areas, dermal abrasions and secondary infections [31, 32]. As in the case of podophyllotoxin, the rate of recurrences may reach 60% [31].

Ablative/Excisional Therapies

Currently ablative or excisional therapies represent the vast majority of anti-HPV therapeutics for genital lesions [36], which include cryotherapy, excision by scalpel or scissors (also called cold surgery), laser therapy and electro-surgery [31, 37]. These methods are suitable for treating lesions at any site. In the presence of intraepithelial neoplasia, the procedure that is most widely recommended is conization (designation resulting from the conical shape of the removed tissue) or loop electrosurgery (LOOP). The latter, together with cryotherapy and laser therapy, employ physical ablative methods – i.e. the application of extreme heat or freezing for epidermal, dermal and vascular damage, leading to the induction of an effective inflammatory response [31, 32] – which generally offer a highly effective form of protection in the short term, with the disappearance of 70-80% of the lesions [38]. In general, cryotherapy assists the treatment of large or grouped lesions, while laser therapy has beneficial cosmetic results by allowing rapid healing without forming scars [32].

The main drawback is the recurrence rate which can reach almost 40% of cases [38], although the procedures entail the removal of a safety margin of 3-5 mm of healthy tissue beyond the injured area [31]. Alternative treatment in cases of exuberant lesions include the excision of lesions with cold surgery followed by the application of laser therapy in the wound bed, a method which results in a lower recurrence rate [31]. In addition, intraepithelial lesions are often multifocal, which makes the ablation procedure impractical or ineffective [39].

Immunomodulators

The treatment of genital warts based on immunomodulatory agents is able to assist in stimulating an innate immune response. The polyphenon E, or sinecatechins, is an extract obtained from the tea leaves of *Camellia sinensis* administered as a topic ointment. It has an effect on the regression of warty lesions because of the epigallocatechin gallate molecule, which operates under different signaling pathways, and induces apoptosis via caspase activation and inhibition of telomerase [40, 41].

Imiquimod is a topical drug that is capable of inducing the secretion of pro-inflammatory cytokines, interleukins and type I interferons (IFN-I), through its agonist action on the toll-like receptor 7 in macrophages, dendritic cells and keratinocytes [42, 32]. Immunomodulation which is based on the secretion of IFN has integral action on the resolution of warty lesions and also indirectly carries out an antiviral activity [43, 44]. Thus, in addition to its proven efficacy and safety, the use of imiquimod leads to reduced recurrence rates (12%) [45].

However, special attention should be paid to imiquimod and other agents that induce immune responses based on IFN-I. It has been reported that treatment of intraepithelial lesions infected with high risk HPV through the use of IFN-α and IFN-β is highly effective in cells containing the viral DNA in episomal form, by arresting growth and inducing the loss of episomes, but no effect has been reported on cells that are carriers of integrated viral DNA [24, 46]. As a result, repeated use of preparations that can produce high local concentrations of IFN-I may result in the selection of cells containing integrated HPV DNA that allow the disease to become malignant [2].

Combination Therapy

It should be stressed that none of the available therapies is superior to the others and there is no ideal treatment for all cases. Other factors apart from those already discussed with regard to the treatment schedule, should also be taken into account: the cost of treatment and its practicality, side effects and the professional experience of the medical staff. Some patients require a series of treatment sessions rather than just one and, in this respect, the therapeutic modality should be changed if the patient has not made substantial improvement after a complete course of treatment (most genital warts respond within 3 months of therapy) or if side effects are severe [47].

Although relatively recent, the studies which have assessed the effectiveness of combined therapy for the treatment of genital warts have shown promising results. Combination therapy, which generally establishes the association between cytotoxic and immunomodulator modalities, represents an interesting alternative for the treatment of patients with both recurrent and new warty lesions. The recurrence rates observed from a comparison of 5% imiquimod monotherapy, surgical excision of residual warts after partial response to treatment with imiquimod and surgical treatment alone, were respectively: 15% (after 17 months), 20% (after 19 months) and 65% (after 5 months) [48]. Similarly, the use of imiquimod after laser therapy for treatment of genital condylomas has shown recurrence of lesions in only 7.3% of patients (138) [49].

Finally, better therapeutic results can be achieved even in cases where distinct therapies are combined, but with the same purpose (for example, by combining two cytotoxic methods). The remission rates of genital warts (new or recurrent) that were observed from a comparison between the employment of 25% podophyllin, TCA, cryoteraphy, TCA/podophyllin or cryotherapy/podophyllin were, respectively, 82.1%, 84.5%, 92.4%, 94% and 100% [50]. In addition, fewer sessions were needed for the complete remission of warts among patients undergoing the combination therapy in comparison with those submitted to monotherapy [50].

Special attention should be paid to the fact that the concomitant use of imiquimod and cytotoxic agents is not recommended because of the risk that it might exacerbate the inflammatory processes [51].

Special Situations

A rapid growth of friable genital warts has been observed in pregnant women, probably as a result of the higher serum levels of steroid hormones – which act as cofactors in the epithelial proliferation of HPV [52-55] – and the relative state of maternal immune-suppression which is peculiar to this physiological condition [31]. Large or extensive lesions can cause obstruction of the birth canal, laceration of tissue and/or profuse bleeding during vaginal delivery. Thus, treatment of genital warts should be performed during pregnancy to reduce the risk of obstetric and/or neonatal complications, as well as some unforeseen discomfort caused to the mother [31]. The third trimester is considered to be the ideal period for the treatment of infection since at this time there is a lower risk of recurrence [56].

Table 2. Therapies currently available for the treatment of genital warts and their recommended application during pregnancy and puerperal period. Adapted from Maluf & Perin, 2005 [7]

Method	Mechanism of action	Safety during pregnancy	Safety during breastfeeding
Podophylotoxin	Cytotoxic agent	Unknown	Contra-indicated
TCA	Cytotoxic agent	Yes	Indicated
Imiquimod 5%	Immunomodulatory	Unknown	Contra-indicated
Cryotherapy	Ablative/excisional	Yes	Indicated
Electrosurgery	Ablative/excisional	Yes	Indicated
Laser therapy	Ablative/excisional	Yes	Indicated
Interferon	Immunomodulatory	No	Contra-indicated

The use of podophyllotoxin and imiquimod is contra-indicated during pregnancy (Table 2). Although the teratogenic potential of podophyllotoxin has not been confirmed for humans, this cytotoxic agent has been classified as category C by the FDA (Food and Drug Administration). The reason for this is its potential absorption and toxicity to the fetus, since it has neuro and myelotoxicity, as already reported [32, 57]. The administration of imiquimod during pregnancy is also classified as category C by the FDA because there have been no clinical trials conducted with pregnant women with this drug. Even though the teratogenic effects of imiquimod are unknown, it should only be prescribed during pregnancy in cases where its benefits outweigh the possible risk to the fetus [31].

The treatment of genital warts in HIV-infected patients should follow the same line of reasoning. Attention must be paid, however, to immunocompromised patients since their warty lesions have more serious features (they are larger and more numerous), they are not responsive to therapy and there are more frequent recurrences [58, 59]. The use of imiquimod in immunosuppressed patients is safe, although in some circumstances the use of combined therapy is needed to achieve better results and a longer disease-free period [60-63].

Perspectives on New Forms of Treatment

Specific therapies against HPV infection are able to treat both non-apparent infections and visible clinical diseases. These antiviral drugs are the only alternative, for a significant section of the population who are already infected with HPV, and comprise immunosuppressed individuals, who cannot be treated by immunotherapy. In addition, multifocal genital lesions are not sensitive to ablative therapy and do not respond to immunotherapy [2].

The challenges for the development of anti-HPV drugs are proportional to their degree of effectiveness. Papillomaviruses only encode one enzyme, E1 helicase, which considerably constrains the adoption of traditional approaches. The other early genes E2, E4, E5, E6 and E7 act through molecular interactions with DNA and proteins of the host cell, but these interactions have not been suitably characterized for drug design or the identification of candidate molecules [2].

Targeting the Replication of HPV

The replication of the HPV genome is dependent upon E1 and E2 protein interaction [64, 65] in the viral origin of replication (*ori*) [66]. Once the E1-E2 complex is assembled, these proteins recruit the DNA polimerase α to the *ori* for the initiation of viral DNA replication [67]. However, the assembly of this complex is sequential and depends on the binding of ATP to E1 [68], which is a helicase with ATPase activity.

Small inhibitory molecules of the ATPase activity of HPV-6 E1 were identified by high-throughput screening [69]. These lead molecules probably inhibit ATP binding by allosteric mechanisms [70] but, unfortunately, they were not active in cell culture assays [71]. At the same time, two series of inhibitory molecules of the cooperative interaction between E1-E2 and *ori* were identified for genotypes -6 and -11 [69]. These compounds are able to bind to the overlapping sites on the interface between E1-E2 [72]. The mechanism of interaction is illustrated in the figure 1. Unfortunately, the studies involving this class of inhibitors were discontinued after the efficacy of the prophylactic vaccines had been demonstrated in the control tests [2].

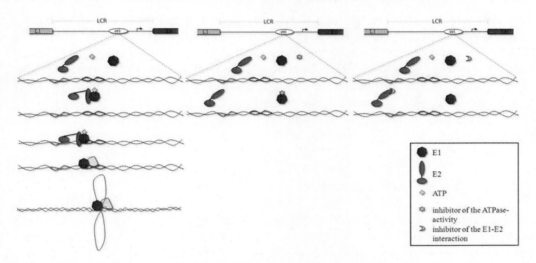

Figure 1. HPV E1 and E2 proteins as antiviral targets. (A) HPV genome replication is dependent upon the interaction of the E1 and E2 proteins in the ori, which is located on the viral LCR (Long Control Region). In turn, the formation of E1-E2 complex depends of ATP binding. Once formed, the E1-E2 complex recruits the DNA pol α to the ori. (B) Molecule inhibitors compete allosterically for the ATP-binding site and prevent the formation of the E1-E2 complex in the HPV-6 ori. (C) Other molecules are also capable of interfering with the formation of E1-E2 complex of HPV-6 and -11 targeting sites which are located in the interaction interfaces of these viral proteins.

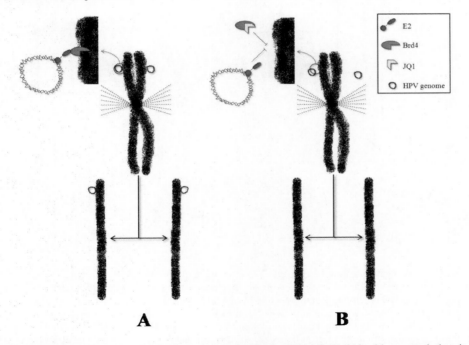

A   **B**

Figure 2. HPV E2 protein as an antiviral target. (A) By interacting with E2, Brd4 is able to attach the viral episome to the host chromosome since it is bound to the acetylated histones of the chromatin. The cooperation between E2-Brd4 allows the viral genomes to be equally partitioned at the mitoses. (B) JQ1 is a small molecule capable of inhibiting the binding of Brd4 to the chromatin and thus represents a potential target for the development of anti-HPV drugs.

Finally, recent evidence has shown the interaction between Brd4 – a bromodomain protein that binds to acetylated histones – and E2 protein of both high and low risk HPV types [73]. Given the role of E2 in the maintenance of the viral episome [74], the E2-Brd4 interaction is likely to be responsible for attaching the viral episome to the mitotic spindle, and thus allow an equal partition of the viral genome during mitosis [75, 76]. The discovery of a molecule capable of inhibiting the binding of Brd4 to chromatin, called JQ1 [77], provides a prospect for producing drugs that can inhibit the interaction between E2 and Brd4. Figure 2 illustrates the role of HPV E2 protein.

Targeting the HPV Carcinogenesis

The combined action of E6 and E7 oncoproteins of high-risk genotypes is essential for the maintenance of the neoplastic phenotype and uncontrolled cell cycle [78]. As a result, different strategies have been employed to investigate the interruption of the activity of these oncoproteins: siRNA, antisenseRNA, ribozymes and peptide aptamers [79]. However, the major progress has been made in the case of E6.

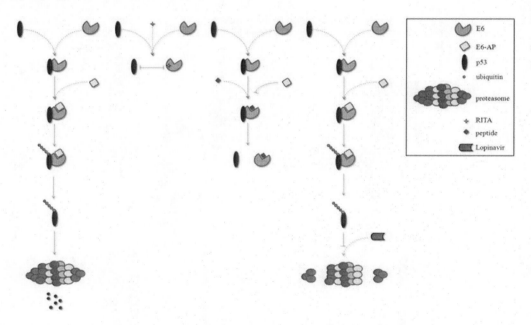

Figura 3. HPV E6 protein as antiviral target. (A) The interaction of p53 with E6 forms a stable complex that recruits the E6/AP ubiquitin ligase. The p53 protein is then ubiquitinated and signaled for degradation via proteasome. (B) The p53 reactivation and induction of apoptosis (RITA) can be achieve in cervical cancer cells through the use of small molecule inibitors capable of interact directly with E6 and prevents its binding to p53. (C) The inhibition of p53-mediated degradation by E6 has also been achieved through the use of small peptides capable of binding to E6 and prevents its interaction with E6-AP, which results in p53 reactivation and subsequently promotion of apoptosis. (D) The degradation of p53 in cervical carcinoma cells can be achieved through the use of Lopinavir, which is a protease inhibitor molecule used in anti-HIV therapy due to its ability to block the viral proteasome activation.

The deregulation of the cell cycle caused by HPV is due, in part, to the E6-mediated degradation of p53. After interacting with p53, the E6 oncoprotein recruits ubiquitin ligase E6/AP, which ubiquitinates the complex and signals to proteolytic degradation [80]. Three different molecular strategies have been employed to prevent E6-mediated degradation: (i) interference with the direct p53-E6 interaction; (ii) interference with the binding of E6/AP to E6; (iii) selective inhibition of proteasome. These molecular strategies are illustrated in the figure 3. With regard to the first alternative, cervical cancer cells can be suppressed *in vitro* by small molecules that cause the reactivation of p53 and induction of apoptosis (RITA) [81]. RITA interacts with p53, by blocking the binding of this molecule to E6 and its subsequent ubiquitination [2]. In the second strategy, small peptides that are capable of inhibiting the formation of E6/AP-E6 complex, were developed in parallel and have been shown to promote cell cycle arrest and/or apoptosis by p53 reactivation [82, 83], but these studies are still in an early stage of evaluation [2].

The third strategy probably represents the most practical alternative from the standpoint of clinical viability. The use of Lopinavir, an antiretroviral protease used in anti-HIV therapy, is able to block the activation of proteasome caused by HIV, stabilize p53 and induce apoptosis of HPV-infected cells *in vitro* [84-86]. The effectiveness of Lopinavir in the clearance of lesions caused by HPV was evaluated without success [87], but it is worth noting that the concentration of the drug used in *in vitro* assays is greater than that achieved by oral administration [84]. The cervico-vaginal concentration of the drug was probably suboptimal. Lopinavir is a licensed drug and thus the formulation of topical preparations for anti-HPV therapeutics may be used in clinical trials within a few years [2], since their efficacy and safety have already been proven.

Immunotherapy

Both the HPV vaccines that are currently available have proved to be effective against the HPV types that were targeted by each vaccine in clinical trials. The vaccines are targeted at adolescent girls but their precise ages vary from country to country. In spite of these differences, vaccination should ideally be performed before the onset of sexual activity, since neither vaccine has demonstrated therapeutic activity for preexisting infections [88].

However, vaccination with these prophylactic vaccines could support the treatment of HPV-related diseases. The use of quadrivalent HPV vaccine has been linked to a reduced incidence of subsequent cervical, vulvar and vaginal intraepithelial neoplasia and genital warts in women who had been diagnosed and treated for cervical and vulvar or vaginal disease [89]. Those women who had been given prior vaccination, had a significantly reduced risk (64.9%) of subsequent high-grade cervical lesions, as well as a reduced risk (35.2%) of developing any subsequent disease related to the HPV vaccine types (-6, -11, -16 and -18), in comparison with the placebo recipients. Although the exact underlying mechanism is not fully known, these observed reduction rates are clinically significant [89].

Despite the effectiveness of prophylactic vaccines, anti-HPV therapeutic interventions based on immunotherapy could make it possible to treat unapparent infections and/or diseases. As the regression of HPV-caused diseases is the result of a Th1 cellular response [16], the more attractive immunotherapeutic approaches have explored the immunization with

E6 and E7 antigens, which are essential for the progression and maintenance of the malignant phenotype and are constitutively expressed in all the cervical intraepithelial lesions [2, 12].

Although studies of immunization with HPV-16 and -18 E6 and E7 have shown they are successful against HPV-expressing cancers in mice, the same results have not been observed in humans [90]. All the vaccines tested in human clinical trials have proved to be safe and capable of inducing antigen-specific cellular immune response, but cancers and high-grade lesions induced by HPV have been highly refractory to the same immunotherapies explored in the mouse model [91]. The attempts that are currently being employed to circumvent these problems have investigated immunomodulators and/or adjuvants that are capable of enhancing the immunogenicity of therapeutic vaccines and/or manipulating the local immunity [2]. Some discrete, but significant, advances have been made in this direction [91-93].

Conclusion

Despite the advances in prevention strategies against cervical cancer, the 'unknowns' regarding the mechanisms for the viral evasion of the host immunity, impose significant challenges for the development of antiviral therapeutic approaches. For this reason, even though several alternatives are available for the treatment of cervical lesions, they are all limited in regard to the clearance of the diseases caused by HPV.

Great progress has been made in carrying out various programs to identify and characterize both molecular targets and antagonist molecules for HPV proteins. However, marketing considerations have prevented the pharmaceutical companies from making progress in producing antiviral drugs and improving chemotherapy for the treatment of cervical cancer. These companies have been afraid that these drugs would have reduced market face to the prophylactic vaccines that have recently been licensed. Despite their proven effectiveness, the optimistic forecasts and the amount of lobbying for the currently available HPV vaccines, the success of immunization is below expectations. The reality is that over the next two or three decades a large section of the public will remain unvaccinated, and it is necessary to develop appropriate treatment for these people, either by antiviral drugs and/or immunotherapy.

References

[1]   De Martel C, Ferlay J, Franceschi S, Vignat J, Bray F, Forman D, et al. The global burden of cancers attributable to infections in the year 2008: a review and synthetic analysis. *Lancet Oncol* 2012;13:607-15.

[2]   Stanley MA. Genital human papillomavirus infections: current and prospective therapies. *J Gen Virol* 2012;93:681–691.

[3]   Paavonen J, Naud P, Salmeron J, Wheeler CM, Chow SN, Apter D, et al. Efficacy of human papillomavirus (HPV)-16/18 AS04-adjuvanted vaccine against cervical infection and precancer caused by oncogenic HPV types (PATRICIA): final analysis of a double-blind, randomised study in young women. *Lancet* 2009;374:301–314.

[4]   Kjaer SK, Sigurdsson K, Iversen OE, Hernandez-Avila M, Wheeler CM, Perez G, et al. A pooled analysis of continued prophylactic efficacy of quadrivalent human papillomavirus (types 6/11/16/18) vaccine against high-grade cervical and external genital lesions. *Cancer Prev Res* 2009;2:868–878.

[5]   WHO/ICO. Information Centre on HPV and Cervical Cancer (HPV Information Centre). Human papillomavirus and related cancers in world. Summary Report. [09/26/2011]. Available in: <*www.who.int/hpvcentre*>, 2010.

[6]   Kaufmann AM, Scheneider A. New paradigm for prevention of cervical cancer. *Eur J Obstet Gynecol Reprod Biol* 2007;130:25-29.

[7]   Maluf M, Perin PM. HPV e gestação. In: Rosenblatt C, editor. *HPV na pratica clinica. Atheneu: Brazil Press*; 2005. p. 193–225.

[8]   zur Hausen H, de Villiers EM, Gissmann L. Papillomavirus infections and human genital cancer. *Gynecol Oncol* 1981;12:S124–S128.

[9]   Doorbar J. Molecular biology of human papillomavirus infection and cervical cancer *Clin Sci* 2006;110:525–541.

[10]   Schwartz S. HPV-16 RNA processing. *Front Biosci* 2008;13:5880–5891.

[11]   Meyers C, Mayer TJ, Ozbun MA. Synthesis of infectious human papillomavirus type 18 in differentiating epithelium transfected with viral DNA. *J Virol* 1997;71:7381–7386.

[12]   Venuti A, Paolini F, Nasir L, Corteggio A, Roperto S, Campo MS, et al. Papillomavirus E5: the smallest oncoprotein with many functions. *Mol Cancer* 2011;10:140.

[13]   Lehtinen M, Rantala I, Toivonen A, Luoto H, Aine R, Lauslahti K, et al. Depletion of Langerhans cells in cervical HPV infection is associated with replication of the virus. *APMIS* 1993;101:833–837.

[14]   Connor JP, Ferrer K, Kane JP, Goldberg JM. Evaluation of Langerhans' cells in the cervical epithelium of women with cervical intraepithelial neoplasia. *Gynecol Oncol* 1999;75:130-135.

[15]   Kupper TS, Fuhlbrigge RC. Immune surveillance in the skin: mechanisms and clinical consequences. *Nat Rev Immunol* 2004;4:211–222.

[16]   Stanley M. Immune responses to human papillomavirus. *Vaccine* 2006;24:S16–22.

[17]   Matthews K, Leong CM, Baxter L, Inglis E, Yun K, Bäckström BT, et al. Depletion of Langerhans cells in human papillomavirus type 16-infected skin is associated with E6-mediated down regulation of E-cadherin. *J Virol* 2003;15:8378–85.

[18]   Schapiro F, Sparkowski J, Adduci A, Schlegel R, Grinstein S. Golgi alkalinization by the papillomavirus E5 oncoprotein. *J Cell Biol* 2000;148:305–315.

[19]   Ashrafi GH, Haghshenas MR, Marchetti B, O'Brien PM, Campo MS. The E5 protein of human papillomavirus type 16 selectively down-regulates surface HLA class. *Int J Cancer* 2005;113:276–283.

[20]   Ashrafi GH, Haghshenas M, Marchetti B, Campo MS. E5 protein of human papillomavirus 16 downregulates HLA class I and interacts with the heavy chain via its first hydrophobic domain. *Int J Cancer* 2006;119:2105–2112

[21]   Stanley MA, Pett MR, Coleman N. HPV: from infection to cancer. *Biochem Soc Trans* 2007;35:1456–1460.

[22]   Bottley G, Watherston OG, Hiew YL, Norrild B, Cook GP, Blair GE. High-risk human PV E7 expression reduces cell-surface MHC class I molecules and increases susceptibility to natural killer cells. *Oncogene* 2008;27:1794–1799.

[23] Kim SH, Oh JM, No JH, Bang YJ, Juhnn YS, Song YS. Involvement of NF-kappaB and AP-1 in COX-2 upregulation by human papillomavirus 16 E5 oncoprotein. *Carcinogenesis* 2009;30:753–757.

[24] Herdman MT, Pett MR., Roberts I, Alazawi WO, Teschendorff AE, Zhang XY, et al. Interferon-beta treatment of cervical keratinocytes naturally infectedwith human PV 16 episomes promotes rapid reduction in episome numbers and emergence of latent integrants. *Carcinogenesis* 2006;27:2341–2353.

[25] Maglennon GA, McIntosh P, Doobar J. Persistence of viral DNA in the epithelial basal layer suggests a model for papillomavirus latency following immune regression. *Virology* 2011;414:153–163.

[26] Schmook T, Nindl I, Ulrich C, Meyer T, Sterry W, Stockfleth E. Viral warts in organ transplant recipients: new aspects in therapy. *Brit J Dermatol* 2003;149:20–24.

[27] Abramson AL, Nouri M, Mullooly V, Fisch G, Steinberg BM. Latent human papillomavirus infection is comparable in the larynx and trachea. *J Med Virol* 2004;72:473–477.

[28] Gravitt PE. The known unknowns of HPV natural history. *J Clin Invest* 2011;121:4593–4599.

[29] Syrjänen KJ. Natural history of genital HPV infections. *Papillomavirus Rep* 1990;1:1-5.

[30] Syrjänen KJ, Syrjänen S. *Papillomavirus infections in human pathology*. Winchester: John Wiley & Sons; 2000.

[31] de Carvalho JJM. Tratamento. In: Rosenblatt C, editor. *HPV na pratica clinica. Atheneu: Brazil Press;* 2005. p. 105-115.

[32] Viera MH, Amini S, Huo R, Konda S, Block S, Berman B. Herpes simplex virus and human papillomavirus genital infections: new and investigational therapeutic options. *Int J Dermatol* 2010;49:733–749.

[33] Moher LM, Maurer SA. Podophyllum toxicity: case report and literature review. *J Fam Pract* 1979;9:237–240.

[34] Leslie KO, Shitamoto B. The bone marrow in systemic podophyllin toxicity. *Am J Clin Pathol* 1982;77:478–480.

[35] Petersen CS, Weismann K. Quercetin and kaempherol: an argument against the use of podophyllin? *Genitourin Med* 1995;71:92–93.

[36] von Krogh G, Lacey CJ, Gross G, Barrasso R, Schneider A. European course on HPV associated pathology: guidelines for primary care physicians for the diagnosis and management of anogenital warts. *Sex Transm Infect* 2000;76:162–168.

[37] Sonnex C, Lacey CJ. The treatment of human papillomavirus lesions of the lower genital tract. *Best Pract Res Clin Obstet Gynaecol* 2001;15:801–816.

[38] Maw R. Critical appraisal of commonly used treatment for genital warts. *Int J STD AIDS* 2004;15:357–364.

[39] Jones RW. Vulval intraepithelial neoplasia: current perspectives. *Eur J Gynaecol Oncol* 2001;22:393–402.

[40] Yang GY, Liao J, Kim K, Yurkow EJ, Yang C S. Inhibition of growth and induction of apoptosis in human cancer cell lines by tea polyphenols. *Carcinogenesis* 1998;19:611–616.

[41] Beltz LA, Bayer DK, Moss AL, Simet IM. Mechanisms of cancer prevention by green and black tea polyphenols. *Anticancer Agents Med Chem* 2006;6:389–406.

[42] Stanley MA. Imiquimod and the imidazoquinolones: mechanism of action and therapeutic potential. *Clin Exp Dermatol* 2002;27:571–577.

[43] Arany I, Tyring SK, Brysk MM, Stanley MA, Tomai MA, Miller RL, et al. Correlation between pretreatment levels of interferon response genes and clinical responses to an immune response modifier (Imiquimod) in genital warts. *Antimicrob Agents Chemother* 2000;44:1869–1873.

[44] Wagstaff AJ, Perry CM. Topical imiquimod: a review of its use in the management of anogenital warts, actinic keratoses, basal cell carcinoma and other skin lesions. *Drugs* 2007;67:2187–2210.

[45] Beutner KR, Tyring SK, Trofatter KF Jr, Douglas JM Jr, Spruance S, Owens ML, et al. Imiquimod, a patient-applied immune response modifier for treatment of external genital warts. *Antimicrob Agents Chemother* 1998;42:789–794.

[46] Pett MR, Herdman MT, Palmer RD, Yeo GS, Shivji MK, Stanley MA, et al. Selection of cervical keratinocytes containing integrated HPV16 associates with episome loss and an endogenous antiviral response. *Proc Natl Acad Sci USA* 2006;103:3822–3827.

[47] Centers for Disease Control and Prevention. Sexually transmitted diseases treatment guidelines . *MMWR* 2010;59(RR12):69–78.

[48] Carrasco D, Straten M, Tyring SK. Treatment of anogenital warts with imiquimod 5% cream followed by surgical excision of residual lesios. *J Am Acad Dermatol* 2002;4:S212–6.

[49] Hoyme UB, Hagedorn M, Schindler AE, Schneede P, Hopfenmüller W, Schorn K, et al. Effect of adjuvant imiquimod 5% cream on sustained clearance of anogenital warts following laser treatment. *Infect Dis Obstet Gynecol* 2002;2:79–88.

[50] Sherrard J, Riddell L. Comparison of the effectiveness of commonly used clinic-based treatments for external genital warts. *Int J STD AIDS* 2007;18:365–368.

[51] Parellada CI, Pereyra EAG. Novas terapêuticas. In: Rosenblatt C, editor. *HPV na pratica clinica. Atheneu: Brazil Press*; 2005. p. 117-130.

[52] Chen YH, Huang LH, Chen TM. Differential effects of progestins and estrogens on long control regions of human papillomavirus types 16 and 18. *Biochem Biophys Res Commun* 1996; 224:651-9.

[53] Gloss B, Bernard HU, Seedorf K, Klock G. The upstream regulatory region of the human papilloma virus-16 contains an E2 protein-independent enhancer which is specific for cervical cervical carcinoma cells and regulated by glucocorticoid hormones. *EMBO J* 1987; 6:3735-43.

[54] Michelin D, Gissmann L, Street D, Potkul RK, Fisher S, Kaufmann AM, et al. Regulation of human papillomavirus type 18 in vivo: effects of estrogen and progesterone in transgenic mice. *Gynecol Oncol* 1997; 66:202-8.

[55] Mittal R, Tsutsumi K, Pater A, Pater MM. Human papillomavirus type 16 expression in cervical keratinocytes: role of progesterone and glucocorticoid hormones. *Obstet Gynecol* 1993; 81:5-12.

[56] Ferenczy A. Treating genital condyloma during pregnancy with the carbon dioxide laser. *Am J Obstet Gynecol* 1984;148:9–12.

[57] Chamberlain MJ, Reynolds AL, Yeoman WB. Toxic effect of podophyllum application in pregnancy. *Br Med J* 1972;3:391–392.

[58] Silverberg MJ, Ahdieh L, Munoz A, Anastos K, Burk RD, Cu-Uvin S, et al. The impact of HIV infection and immunodeficiency on human papillomavirus type 6 or 11 infection and on genital warts. *Sex Transmit Dis* 2002;29:427–435

[59] De Panfilis G, Melzani G, Mori G, Ghidini A, Graifemberghi S. Relapses after treatment of external genital warts are more frequent in HIV-positive patients than in HIV-negative controls. *Sex Transmit Dis* 2002; 29: 121–125.

[60] Conant MA. Immunomodulatory therapy in the management of viral infections in patients with HIV infection. *J Am Acad Dermatol* 2000;43:S27–30.

[61] Gayed SL. Topical imiquimod cream 5% for resistant perianal warts in a renal transplant patient. *Int J STD AIDS* 2002;13:501–503.

[62] Gilson RJ, Shupack JL, Friedman-Kien AE, Conant MA, Weber JN, Nayagam AT, et al. A randomized, controlled, safety study using imiquimod for the topical treatment of anogenital warts in HIV-infected patients. Imiquimod Study Group. *Int J STD AIDS* 1999;13:2397–2404.

[63] Hagman JH, Bianchi L, Marulli GC, Soda R, Chimenti S. Successful treatment of multiple filiform facial warts with imiquimod 5% cream in a patient infected by human immunofeficiency virus. *Clin Exp Dermatol* 2003;28:260–261.

[64] Yang L, Li R, Mohr IJ, Clark R, Botchan MR. Activation of BPV-1 replication in vitro by the transcription factor E2. *Nature* 1991;353:628–632.

[65] Chiang CM, Ustav M, Stenlund A, Ho TF, Broker TR, Chow LT. Viral E1 and E2 proteins support replication of homologous and heterologous papillomaviral origins. *Proc Natl Acad Sci USA* 1992;89:5799–5803.

[66] Sanders CM, Stenlund A. Recruitment and loading of the E1 initiator protein: an ATP-dependent process catalysed by a transcription factor. *EMBO J* 1998;17:7044–7055.

[67] Masterson PJ, Stanley M A, Lewis AP, Romanos MA. A C-terminal helicase domain of the human papillomavirus E1 protein binds E2 and the DNA polymerase alpha-primase p68 subunit. *J Virol* 1998;72:7407–7419.

[68] Titolo S, Pelletier A, Sauvé F, Brault K, Wardrop E, White PW, et al. Role of the ATP-binding domain of the human papillomavirus type 11 E1 helicase in E2-dependent binding to the origin. *J Virol* 1999;73:5282–5293.

[69] White PW, Faucher AM, Goudreau N. Small molecule inhibitors of the human papillomavirus E1-E2 interaction. *Curr Top Microbiol Immunol* 2011;348:61–88.

[70] White PW, Faucher AM, Massariol MJ, Welchner E, Rancourt J, Cartier M, et al. Biphenylsulfonacetic acid inhibitors of the human papillomavirus type 6 E1 helicase inhibit ATP hydrolysis by an allosteric mechanism involving tyrosine 486. *Antimicrob Agents Chemother* 2005;49:4834–4842.

[71] Faucher AM, White PW, Brochu C, et al. Discovery of small molecule inhibitors of the ATPase activity of human papillomavirus E1 helicase. *J Med Chem* 2004; 47: 18-21.

[72] Yoakim C, Ogilvie WW, Goudreau N, Naud J, Haché B, O'Meara JA, et al. Discovery of the first series of inhibitors of human papillomavirus type 11: inhibition of the assembly of the E1-E2-origin DNA complex. *Bioorg Med Chem Lett* 2003;13:2539–2541.

[73] Gagnon D, Joubert S, Senechal H, Fradet-Turcotte A, Torre S, Archambault J. Proteasomal degradation of the papillomavirus E2 protein is inhibited by overexpression of bromodomain containing protein 4. *J Virol* 2009;83:4127–4139.

[74] Smith JA, White EA, Sowa ME, Powell ML, Ottinger M, Harper JW et al. Genome-wide siRNA screen identifies SMCX, EP400, and Brd4 as E2-dependent regulators of human papillomavirus oncogene expression. *Proc Natl Acad Sci USA* 2010;107:3752–3757.

[75] McBride AA, McPhillips MG, Oliveira JG. Brd4: tethering, segregation and beyond. *Trends Microbiol* 2004;12:527–529.

[76] Abbate EA, Voitenleitner C, Botchan MR. Structure of the papillomavirus DNA-tethering complex E2:Brd4 and a peptide that ablates HPV chromosomal association. *Mol Cell* 2006;24:877–889.

[77] Filippakopoulos P, Qi J, Picaud S, Shen Y, Smith WB, Fedorov O, et al. Selective inhibition of BET bromodomains. *Nature* 2010;468:1067–1073.

[78] Moody CA, Laimins LA. Human papillomavirus oncoproteins: pathways to transformation. *Nat Rev Cancer* 2010;10:550–560.

[79] Govan VA. Strategies for human papillomavirus therapeutic vaccines and other therapies based on the E6 and E7 oncogenes. *Ann N Y Acad Sci* 2005;1056:328–343.

[80] Talis AL, Huibregtse JM, Howley PM. The role of E6AP in the regulation of p53 protein levels in human papillomavirus (HPV)-positive and HPV-negative cells. *J Biol Chem* 1998;273:6439–6445.

[81] Zhao CY, Szekely L, Bao W, Selivanova G. Rescue of p53 function by small-molecule RITA in cervical carcinoma by blocking E6-mediated degradation. *Cancer Res* 2010;70:3372–3381.

[82] Be X, Hong Y, Wei J, Androphy EJ, Chen JJ, Baleja JD. Solution structure determination and mutational analysis of the papillomavirus E6 interacting peptide of E6AP. *Biochemistry* 2001;40:1293–1299.

[83] Liu Y, Liu Z, Androphy E, Chen J, Baleja JD. Design and characterization of helical peptides that inhibit the E6 protein of papillomavirus. *Biochemistry* 2004;43:7421–7431.

[84] Hampson L, Kitchener HC, Hampson IN. Specific HIV protease inhibitors inhibit the ability of HPV16 E6 to degrade p53 and selectively kill E6-dependent cervical carcinoma cells in vitro. *Antivir Ther* 2006;11:813–825.

[85] Kim DH, Jarvis RM, Xu Y, Oliver AW, Allwood JW ,Hampson L, et al. Combining metabolic fingerprinting and footprinting to understand the phenotypic response of HPV16 E6 expressing cervical carcinoma cells exposed to the HIV anti-viral drug lopinavir. *Analyst* (Lond) 2010;135:1235–1244.

[86] Batman G, Oliver AW, Zehbe I, Richard C, Hampson L, Hampson IN. Lopinavir up-regulates expression of the antiviral protein ribonuclease L in human papillomavirus-positive cervical carcinoma cells. *Antivir Ther* 2011;16:515–525.

[87] De Vuyst H, Lillo F, Broutet N, Smith JS. HIV, human papillomavirus, and cervical neoplasia and cancer in the era of highly active antiretroviral therapy. *Eur J Cancer Prev* 2008;17:545–554.

[88] Campo MS, Roden RBS. Papillomavirus Prophylactic Vaccines: Established Successes, New Approaches. *J Virol* 2010;84:1214.

[89] Joura EA, Garland SM, Paavonen J, Ferris DG, Perez G, Ault KA, et al. Effect of the human papillomavirus (HPV) quadrivalent vaccine in a subgroup of women with cervical and vulvar disease: retrospective pooled analysis of trial data. *BMJ* 2012;344:1401.

[90] Su JH, Wu A, Scotney E, Ma B, Monie A, Hung CF, et al. Immunotherapy for cervical cancer: research status and clinical potential. *BioDrugs* 2010;24:109–129.

[91] Trimble CL, Frazer IH. Development of therapeutic HPV vaccines. *Lancet Oncol* 2009;10:975–980.

[92] Kenter GG, Welters MJ, Valentijn AR, Lowik MJ, Berends-van der Meer DM, Vloon AP, et al. Vaccination against HPV-16 oncoproteins for vulvar intraepithelial neoplasia. *N Engl J Med* 2009;361:1838–1847.

[93] Daayana S, Elkord E, Winters U, Pawlita M, Roden R, Stern PL, et al. Phase II trial of imiquimod and HPV therapeutic vaccination in patients with vulval intraepithelial neoplasia. *Br J Cancer* 2010;102:1129–1136.

[94] American Society for Colposcopy and Cervical Pathology. Web site available at: *http://www.asccp.org/PracticeManagement/Vulva/HPVInfectionsandVIN/HPVTreatme nts/tabid/7457/Default.aspx*. Accessed April 29, 2013.

In: Cervical Cancer
Editor: Laurie Elit

ISBN: 978-1-62948-062-6
© 2014 Nova Science Publishers, Inc.

Chapter VIII

Vaginal Treatment of Early-Stage Cervical Cancer

Erasmo Bravo[*,1,2,3], *Catalina Alonso*[1,3], *Jaime Cartagena*[1,3],
Sergio Rojas[1,3] *and Carolina Opazo*[1]

[1]Gynecologic Oncology Unit, Gustavo Fricke Hospital, Viña del Mar, Chile
[2]Gynecologic Oncology Unit, Carlos van Buren Hospital, Valparaíso, Chile
[3]Department of Obstetrics and Gynecology, Universidad de Valparaíso, Chile

Abstract

The treatment of early-stage cervical cancer (IA2-IIA1) consists of surgery or radiochemotherapy, with similar oncological outcomes for either option. However, for young patients who want to preserve their sexual and ovarian functioning, and avoid the complications of radiation therapy, surgery is the preferred option. Surgery for early-stage cervical cancer consists of a radical hysterectomy in which, in addition to the removal of the uterus, parametrial or paracervical tissue is removed along with the vaginal cuff. This procedure may be performed by the abdominal route (Wertheim-Meigs operation) or by the vaginal route (Schauta's operation), and may be a laparoscopy-assisted or it maybe completed totally by the laparoscopic route with vaginal or abdominal extraction of the specimen. In young patients who want to preserve their fertility, it is possible to perform a radical vaginal trachelectomy (Dargent's operation). This consists of the removal of the uterine cervix along with the parametria and the vaginal cuff, preserving the corpus uteri, which maintains the patient's potential fertility. This may be performed either by the abdominal or vaginal route, depending on the experience of the surgical team. In exceptional situations in which cervical cancer coincides with the initial stages of pregnancy, it is possible to perform this techinique while preserving the pregnancy and maintaining fetal viability. The vaginal route for completing the hysterectomy has been proven to be safer, with faster recovery time, less postoperational pain, lower cost, fewer complications, and better cosmetic outcomes.

---

[*] Correspondence concerning this article should be addressed to Dr Erasmo Bravo. Email: erasmobravo@gmail.com.

Hence, our units opt for the vaginal approach in the treatment of early-stage cervical cancer, performing Schauta's operation combined with laparoscopic pelvic lymphadenectomy. Using this as the starting point, and based on our unit's extensive experience in vaginal surgery, we then perform a radical vaginal trachelectomy. We believe that with adequate training and experience in vaginal surgery, it is feasible to treat early-stage cervical cancer this way, thereby providing patients the advantages that this technique offers.

Keywords: Vaginal, radical, hysterectomy, trachelectomy

Introduction

The treatment of early-stage cervical cancer is a challenge for modern oncologic gynecology. It is well known that the oncologic outcomes for stages IA2 to IIA1 are similar for surgery or radiochemotherapy. Thus, the choice of treatment depends on factors related to the patient and with their wish to preserve their fertility.

Over the past few decades, new concepts for the management of cervical cancer have forced the teams charged with the treatment and care of these patients to acquire surgical skills and abilities (e.g., vaginal laparoscopic surgery) that require a long learning curve. This has deterred many specialists from acquiring these skills. Hence, progress in this area has remained in the hands of a few gynecologic oncology centers that have decided to offer such alternatives to cervical cancer patients who fit the profile.

In this chapter, we will analyze, address, and describe the surgical treatment of early-stage cervical cancer from the vaginal perspective, beginning with simple vaginal hysterectomy for benign uterine pathology, radical vaginal hysterectomy, radical vaginal trachelectomy, and radical vaginal trachelectomy in pregnant patients, accompanied by laparoscopic lymphadenectomy, a requirement for adequate management of this oncologic pathology.

Simple Vaginal Hysterectomy

A simple vaginal hysterectomy for benign uterine pathology constitutes the most basic competence for the vaginal approach of early-stage cervical cancer. This technique, which consists of the removal of the uterus, can be performed either by the abdominal route, laparoscopically, with laparoscopic assistance, or by the vaginal route. The abdominal route has been the classic technique to treat benign uterine pathology and has yielded good outcomes. The predominance of the abdominal route over the vaginal route is due to preference of the surgical teams, who have been trained in and have extensive experience with this technique, and the progressive loss of the teaching and learning of vaginal surgery. The introduction of the laparoscopic approach has shown limitations with regard to operating time, a higher incidence of complications, a longer and more complex learning curve, and higher cost. The vaginal route has, according to several European studies, shown advantages with regard to such factors as a lower index of complications, lower cost, faster recovery, early return to work, enhanced cosmetics, and the possibility of being incorporated into outpatient surgery programs.

The history of vaginal hysterectomy dates back to the 2nd century BCE, when Soranus of Ephesus removed a prolapsed, gangrened uterus by the vaginal route. Giaccome Berengario DaCapi (1480-1550) was the first to make reference to sexual activity after vaginal hysterectomy.

The indications for vaginal hysterectomy do not differ markedly from the abdominal approach. Uterine myomatosis and adenomyosis are the most frequent, followed by preneoplastic pathology of the cervix and endometrial hyperplasia. Severe endometriosis and vaginal narrowness are considered as formal contraindications. The size of the uterus, or a history of scarring from cesarean or pelvic surgery, do not necessarily constitute a contraindication for using that approach. The fundamental conditions to perform the vaginal hysterectomy are the following: uterine decent, sufficient vaginal width, and an experienced surgical team. Assessments of both the vaginal width and uterine descent must be carried out in the operating room under the effect of anesthesia. The third condition, an experienced team, requires learning the technique in training centers with expertise and extensive case-based practice, combined with a progressive and ongoing training.

The surgical technique requires two assistants who are familiar with the vaginal approach. Regional anesthesia is preferred over general anesthesia due to the faster recovery and lithotomy positioning. As a first step, a vaginal retractor is placed into the vagina and the cervix is pulled down with Pozzi forceps to to check the uterine mobility and the width of the vagina.

A circular incision is made in the vagina with a scalpel or scissors, opening both the anterior and posterior fornices, if possible. The uterosacral and cardinal ligaments, along with the uterine vessels and utero-ovarian pedicles, are divided and ligated. If necessary, one or both of the pedicles are removed, dividing and ligating the infundibulopelvic ligaments. The closing of the vaginal vault is performed through the apposition of the uterosacral and cardinal ligaments, without requiring peritoneal closing.

In order to facilitate the removal of the uterus by the vaginal route the following techniques of uterine reduction have been described:

Trachelectomy: this involves the removal of the cervix after uterine artery ligation, which allows the corpus uteri to approach the operating field, facilitating its extraction.

Bisection: this is the division of the corpus uteri in half in order to create easier access to the utero-ovarian pedicles. Special care must be taken not to damage the urinary bladder when performing this procedure.

Myomectomy: this involves the enucleation of the myomas that appear as the surgery progresses. This is reserved for myomas of a small or moderate size.

Morcellation: this is carried out by cutting the myomas that were too large to enucleate into smaller pieces and removing them.

Coring: This is the removal of the central portion of the uterus, in concentric block form while the trachelectomy is being performed. Care must be taken not to inadvertently transfix the uterine walls.

The role of videolaparoscopy in vaginal hysterectomy is limited but must be considered in some cases for the diagnostic confirmation of adnexal tumors, as well as to ensure access to the respective infundibulopelvic ligament. It should also be considered for use in some cases of severe pelvic endometriosis and inflammatory processes of the pelvis where there is the suspicion of the existence of adhesions that would make access by the vaginal route difficult.

Both of the major regional hospitals (Gustavo Fricke Hospital of Viña del Mar and Carlos van Buren Hospital of Valparaiso) simultaneously began using vaginal hysterectomy in benign uterine pathology (except for prolapse) starting in 1997. Having performed approximately 9,000 hysterectomies, the percentage of vaginal hysterectomies is 81% for these two hospitals.

Once adequate skill and experience in this technique has been acquired, the oncologic surgeon is able to perform a radical vaginal hysterectomy, in which most of the surgical steps are similar to a simple vaginal hysterectomy, previous to performing a laparoscopic pelvic and lumbo-aortic lymphadenectomy.

Laparoscopic Lymphadenectomy

Since the introduction of laparoscopy in gynecology in the 1970s and videolaparoscopy in the 1990s, this technique has gradually replaced laparotomy, owing to the obvious benefits for the patient and the expanded training of gynecological surgeons in this technique. In the mid-1990s, the first publications dealing with laparoscopic surgery in oncologic gynecology appeared, especially with respect to the use of this technique to perform pelvic and lumbo-aortic lymphadenectomy. Dargent and Querleu in France, and Childers in the United States are considered the precursors of laparoscopy in oncology. These techniques gained rapid acceptance and advanced quickly, such that Sert et al. published the first case of radical hysterectomy by robot-assisted surgery in 2006.

Laparoscopic surgery has various roles in oncology. The main ones are to identify whether nearby organs have been compromised, to evaluate lymph nodes and identify the presence of intra-abdominal disease. Systematic lymphadenectomy in cervical cancer is a fundamental part of the surgery, since pelvic lymph node status is one of the most important prognostic factors for disease recurrence. It also determines the need for adjuvant treatments or changes in the treatment that was initially planned for the patient. Since the introduction of pelvic lymphadenectomy in the surgical treatment of cervical cancer by Meigs in 1944, this procedure has changed with regard to surgical technique and the route of the approach, principally due to the need to perform more conservative surgeries with reduced morbidity.

Depending on the profile of the patient and their wish to retain fertility, laparoscopic lymphadenectomy may be used in conjunction with several techniques, such as: laparoscopic radical hysterectomy, laparoscopic assisted radical hysterectomy, radical vaginal hysterectomy (Schauta's operation), radical trachelectomy (vaginal or laparoscopic), cone biopsy, and even robot-assisted radical hysterectomy.

The transperitoneal and the retroperitoneal laparoscopic approach have been described in the literature. The latter has the advantage of decreasing bowel morbidity and adhesions, but does not permit a complete evaluation of the pelvis or permit a laparoscopic hysterectomy. Studies that have compared the abdominal route with laparoscopy have not shown differences in the overall rates of survival, but they have reported reduced morbidity associated with radical techniques performed by laparoscopy.

The most frequently described complications of laparoscopic lymphadenectomy are ureteral, vascular, and neural lesions (due to the radicality of the technique). These occur with less frequency that in the laparotomic approach.

The sentinel lymph node biopsy technique has been used to identify lymph nodes that are the first barrier facing the tumoral tissue. Its use in radical cervical surgery has increased in recent years without being standardized. Lymphatic dissemination in cervical cancer follows a sequential order, so the injection of patent blue v and/or Technetium-99m peritumoral can be used to identify the compromised lymph nodes and to decide whether to continue or to stop the radical surgery. Given the risk of lymph node metastasis in the early stages, which vary from 0% to 16%, the identification of the compromised sentinel lymph nodes avoids the complications of performing a systematic lymphadenectomy and reduces the complications associated with double therapy (ie., when postoperative adjuvant radiotherapy is required). Current evidence shows no difference in outcomes between laparoscopy or laparotomy. Therefore, the use of laparoscopy to identify sentinel lymph nodes is the preferred technique, owing to the advantage of being less invasive.

The indications of laparoscopic lymphadenectomy are:

- Early stages of cervical cancer: IA2, IB1, and IIA1.
- Together with surgery to preserve fertility (cone, trachelectomy)
- As a complement to radical vaginal techniques (radical vaginal hysterectomy)
- Reduction of lymph node tumors
- Study of lumbo-aortic lymph node to determine the extension of the field of the radiotherapy (with the presence of positive pelvic lymph nodes)

Radical Vaginal Hysterectomy

The first description of a radical vaginal hysterectomy (RVH) was carried out by Anton Pawlik and was popularized by Frederik Schauta in the treatment of cervical cancer at the beginning of the twentieth century. It resulted in a decline in postsurgical mortality in comparison with the abdominal technique of Wertheim. Subsequently, Schauta's operation was modified by Amreich and Stockel. When Meigs demonstrated an increase in the survival by performing a pelvic lymphadenectomy together with a radical abdominal hysterectomy (RAH), Schauts's operation was practically forgotten, given the impossibility of removing lymph nodes by the vaginal route. But when laparoscopic lymphadenectomy appeared in the 1980s, there was a revival of the RVH technique, which has been increasing accepted in medical centers throughout the world.

RAH is a surgery that involves slow recovery and significant morbidity with respect to vesical and bowel dysfunction. The advantages of laparoscopic surgery are widely recognized: fast recovery, less postoperative pain, the absence of laparotomy and its complications, and enhanced vision of the anatomical structures. Using the vaginal route instead of the abdominal route demonstrates similar advantages: faster and enhanced recovery, fewer complications, lower cost, a shorter postoperative hospital stay, and better cosmetic outcome, leaving no visible scar. Videolaparoscopy-assisted RVH brings both techniques together, in addition to the advantage of entailing only a single surgery. Over the past decade, it has been shown that, compared with RAH, RVH offers advantages with regard to the loss of blood, the rates of blood transfusions, the length of stay, and recovery time for spontaneous vesical functioning. The only advantage of RAH is the shorter time required for the operation. The overall survival rate and the postoperative complications are similar for both techniques. It is important to bear in mind that, due to the learning curve, it will take some time before these benefits are fully realized, but this is inherent in the implementation of any new surgical technique. The technique employed in our centers, as well as those described in the recent literature, entails, firstly, a laparoscopic inspection to identify sentinel lymphs nodes and other suspicious lymph nodes, which are removed for histopathological study. If the biopsies are negative with regard to metastasis, we proceed with the pelvic lymphadenectomy and the hysterectomy. Otherwise, the planned surgery is suspended and a lumbo-aortic lymphadenectomy is performed to evaluate la extension of the treatment field of radiotherapy.

Once metastastic compromise of the lymph nodes has been discarded and the systematic laparoscopic pelvic lymphadenectomy has been completed, the pararectal and paravesical spaces are opened, the proximal and distal parts of the parametrium are dissected, and the uterine arteries are divided from their origin in the hypogastric arteries. In these cases the ovaries are preserved or they are ligated to the infundibulopelvic ligaments.

The second step proceeds initially by delineating the extension of the vaginal cuff. Then a circular incision is made, dissecting the vagina up to the cervix, and holding it in place with Chroback clamps. The bladder is separated by introducing a vaginal retractor (Diver) in the vesico-uterine space without opening the peritoneum. The paravesical space is opened, exposing the vesical pillar and enabling the identification and dissection of the ureters. Next, the base of the posterior fornix is opened and the pararectal space is identified, exposing it to the uterosacro ligament, which is divided near the rectum. In this way the uterus remains connected to the pelvic wall by the para-cervix, which is cut and ligated as near as possible to the pelvic wall.

Finally, the uterus and the parametrial tissue are pulled down and extracted from the vagina. The hemostasis is completed and the vaginal vault is closed with a polyglycolic acid suture. The third step entails the laparoscopic inspection of the hemostasis and allowing for drainage at the base of the fornix. The indications of RVH are the same as those for the abdominal route: patients with cervical cancer in FIGO stages IA2, IB1, IIA1, and endometrial cancer with cervical compromise.

On the other hand, there are situations that absolutely or relatively contraindicate the vaginal route or laparoscopy, such as: the presence of a significant abdominal adhesions secondary to an inflammatory pelvic process, endometriosis, and other causes, previous reconstructive pelvic surgery, cervical effacement without the possibility of dissection by the vaginal route, significant vaginal atrophy, or genital prolapse (which can significantly alter the anatomy).

Conceptually we can say that for a medical center where RVH is the standard technique, it is unusual to encounter patients who have indication of radical surgery and cannot be treated by the vaginal route. Starting in 2005, we introduced radical vaginal hysterectomy with systematic pelvic laparoscopic lymphadenectomy for the surgical treatment of early-stage cervical cancer, with 108 cases having been performed to date. The index of complications, which stands at 18.5%, is less than that for the Wertheim Meigs operation and the recurrence-free and overall survival rates are similar to those reported in the literature. The average length of stay in hospital is 2.9 days, recovery is rapid, and there is a high degree of user satisfaction.

Radical Vaginal Trachelectomy

Carcinoma of the cervix continues to be the leading cause of gynecologic cancer death in the world. In developed countries, however, the strategy of screening has dramatically reduced the incidence of this disease and, in turn, the mortality associated with it. Of the cancers that are diagnosed, an increasing percentage of them occur among young women, with a growing number occurring before 40 years of age. In addition and related to the social profile and the growing role of women in the professional fields, and with the significant delay in maternity, there has been a rise in the frequency of cervical cancer among nulliparous women and women who have given birth to a single child. Another important aspect is that the majority of women with cancer in this age range are diagnosed in the early stages of the disease. And when detected in the early stages, there is a high probability of cure, with an overall five-year survival rate of around 95%.

In light of this, in 1994 Dr. Daniel Dargent described the technique of radical vaginal trachelectomy, which removes the cervix, the parametria, and the vaginal cuff, in conjunction with a systematic laparoscopic pelvic lymphadenectomy, preserving the corpus uteri and its pedicles. This technique is currently widely accepted as being oncologically safe, without affecting the recurrence-free and overall survival rates, with more than 700 cases described in the literature, including 250 pregnancies and 100 births. Other options currently described include radical abdominal trachelectomy and robot-assisted laparoscopy.

The selection of patients is critical for the success of this intervention. Patients who express a desire to preserve their fertility and exhibit a real medical possibility of becoming pregnant will all qualify if they have early-stage cervical (squamous), adenocarcinoma and adenosquamous carcinoma histological types, as well as those with FIGO stage IA1 with lymphovascular invasion, FIGO stage IA2, and FIGO stage IB1. With respect to the macroscopic stage, efforts should be made to eliminate those patients with a high risk of failure, principally obese patients with a higher probability of compromise of the lymph nodes. That is why the assessment of sentinel lymph nodes and the determination of the area of the surgery is important. Magnetic Resonance at the time of pre-surgical planning is mandatory in some centers.

First stage laparoscopy: classical systematic pelvic lymphadenectomy preceded by the detection of bilateral sentinel lymph nodes, ideally via mixed technique, Technetium-99 y azul patente v in conjunction with biopsy. If this is not available, a rapid biopsy is performed on suspicious lymph nodes. If these are found to be positive, the surgery is cancelled and an evaluation of the lumbo-aortic and common iliac lymph nodes is carried out to determine the field of radiation.

If the laparoscopy is completed and no positive lymph nodes are found, we proceed to the vaginal stage with a circumferential incision of the vagina and the removal of a vaginal cuff of approximately 2 cms. Without opening the peritoneum, the bladder base is mobilized until the anterior bladder pillars are exposed and the base of the posterior vaginal fornix is opened. Then, pararectal spaces are opened and both uterosacral ligaments (posterior parametrium) are divided. Next, the paravesical spaces are formed and the anterior vesical pillar is dissected, with both ureters being moved away from the operative field toward the head or anterior section, which allows the anterior and lateral parametrium to be grasped. Next comes the ligation of the cervical branch of the uterine artery, followed by the division of the cervix at the level of its attachment with the uterine isthmus. A rapid biopsy of the edge of the upper section is performed to ensure a free margin of at least 5 mm and a Shirodkar cerclage is set in place. Finally, vaginal closure is carried out around the isthmus with laparoscopic confirmation of hemostasis.

This technique requires a long learning curve and demands refined techniques in vaginal surgery. It is preferably practiced in medical centers where complex vaginal surgery is performed. From the point of view of perioperative outcomes, this technique is quite similar to the conventional radical techniques. Its oncologic outcomes are are also similar to the radical techniques, with an average 5-year recurrence rate of between 5 and 10%, without affecting overall survival with respect to historical controls. Recurrences are concentrated in cases with tumors of more than 2 cms, lymphovascular invasion, and deep stromal invasion of the cervix, as well as cases of positive lymph nodes, and adenocarcinoma histological type, the same manner as in conventional techniques. With respect to the last point, there is a controversy regarding whether the histological type is a dependent variable of the other risk factors mentioned above.

Another complex topic is the indication of adjuvant treatment, since many patients reject such treatment in order to improve the probability of pregnancy, hence increasing the risk of local recurrence.

With respect to post-trachelectomy follow-up, a majority of the recurrences of early-stage cervical cancer occur within the first 2 years. Thus, our center applies the clinical practice guidelines for radical hysterectomy, which includes Pap smears and colposcopy every 3 months for the first 2 years, every 6 months up to the 5th year, and on an annual basis after that.

Between 45 and 70% of the patients who attempt to become pregnant are able to do so. This group has a percentage of first trimester loss similar to that in the general population, a second trimester loss probability double that of the general population (8 to 10%), and a considerably increased risk of premature birth (20 to 30%). In sum, the probability that a patient subjected to a radical vaginal trachelectomy will conceive and carry the pregnancy to term is approximately 40%.

Radical Vaginal Trachelectomy during Pregnancy

Cervical cancer is one of the most frequent neoplasia diagnoses during pregnancy. It is diagnosed in 0.5 to 1.5% of pregnant patients and increases the rates of maternal morbidity and neonatal morbimortality. The estimated rate of incidence runs from 0.8 to 1.5 per 1000 to 10,000 live births. The diagnosis is significantly higher in stage I due to the greater obstetric control at that stage.

The survival of patients does not seem to be affected by pregnancy. However, the scarcity of cases and the poor methodological quality of the studies do not permit a categoric judgment at this time. The form of treatment to be administered must consider the desire of the patient to be pregnant, the status of the cancer, and the stage of the pregnancy. Therefore, we believe that the treatment to be chosen must be individualized for each patient. In general the guidelines for treatment of pregnant women with cervical cancer are similar to those for non-pregnant women. The treatment of choice for patients with IA1 cervical cancer without lymphovascular invasion is cervical conization, which has demonstrated excellent maternal and perinatal outcomes.

Indicating the most suitable treatments for stages IA1 with lymphovascular invasion, IA2, IB1, and IIA1 is more difficult and should be carried out by a multidisciplinary team. When the diagnosis involves a pregnancy with fetal lung maturity, the indication is for labor to be induced and the respective postpartum oncologic care administerred. If the pregnancy is approaching fetal lung maturity, it is recommended that corticoids be administered and a short waiting period be observed before inducing labor.

The most common problem occurs in patients with previable pregnancies (less than 22-24 weeks) in which the wait for fetal maturity will take a longer time and will theoretically become risky. In these cases various treatment alternatives are offered depending on the status of the individual, including the interruption of the pregnancy, neoadjuvant chemotherapy, and radical trachelectomy. In Chile the former is automatically excluded, as the law prohibits and penalizes the interruption of a pregnancy. Platinum-based neoadjuvant chemotherapy is indicated in patients over 20 weeks pregnant for whom a period of from 6 to 10 weeks will provide the time needed to acquire fetal lung maturity. In pregnancies of less than 20 weeks, chemotherapy treatment becomes quite risky given the amount of time it will have to be administered, without clear benefit and with higher maternal and fetal risks.

Immediate and definitive treatment is recommended independent of the length of the pregnancy for patients with locally advanced disease, lymphatic metastasis, the insistence of the patient, and disease progression during the pregnancy.

Radical vaginal trachelectomy is a surgical technique that allows early-stage cervical cancer to be treated while preserving the fertility of the patient. Introduced by Daniel Dargent in 1994, it was subsequently used as a timely treatment that allowed pregnant patients to preserve the pregnancy. The evaluation of the status of the lymph nodes was performed with a bilaterial pelvic lymphadenectomy, which from our perspective is the best route of approach for videolaparoscopy, given the minimal uterine manipulation, which theoretically results in less uterine irritation and less possibility of miscarriage. Several cases have been published regarding these techniques but the results have been inconclusive. The first case reporting successful outcomes with radical trachelectomy and abdominal lymphadenectomy was published by Ungar in 2006. The first case reporting a successful outcome with radical vaginal trachelectomy with abdominal lymphadenectomy in a patient with 16 weeks of pregnancy was published by Van de Nieuwenhoe in 2008. Subsequently several authors have published their outcomes: one case by Mandic in 2009, one case by Abu-Rustum in 2010, three cases by Sioutas in 2011, and one case by Iwami in 2011. All of them reported good maternal-perinatal outcomes, except for three of Ungar's patients, who presented postoperative fetal loss. The abdominal route lymphadenectomy approach was used in these three patients. In 2012 our team published, as in two cases of Sioutas, a case of radical vaginal trachelectomy with pelvic laparoscopic lymphadenectomy with a successful outcome.

It involved a patient who was operated on in 2008 with stage IB1 cervical cancer and whose pregnancy was in its 11th week. In total thirteen cases have been reported in the literature, ten with successful maternal and perinatal outcomes. All of these operations were performed on patients with less than 20 weeks of pregnancy.

Complications may arise in the surgical technique described above when the size of the uterus is large and when there is increased bleeding due to the staus of the pregnancy. Once the cervix has been removed, along with the parametrial tissue and the vaginal cuff, treatment calls for a cerclage made of nonabsorbable material to be placed around the uterine isthmus. When the surgery has finished, fetal vitality is tested via obstetric echography and close monitoring by the perinatology team.

The indications that we consider sufficient to carry out this treatment in these patients are the following: the desire of the patient to continue their pregnancy, a nuclear magnetic resonance evaluation to eliminate parametrial and lymphatic compromise, cervical tumors less than or equal to 30 mm. in stage I or IIA1, and with fewer than 20 weeks of pregnancy.

Conclusion

Treating early-stage cervical cancer with the vaginal approach provides advantages for patients. However, this requires that the surgical team have adequate training and experience in vaginal surgery. This training should be acquired progressively, starting with simple vaginal hysterectomy, accompanied by laparoscopic surgery, and advancing to the point where systematic pelvic and lumbo-aortic lymphadenectomy can be performed.

References

Abu-Rustum NR, Tal MN, DeLair D et al. 2010. Radical abdominal trachelectomy for stage IB1 cervical cancer at 15-week gestation. *Gynecol. Oncol.* 116:151–152.

Alouini S, Rida K, Mathevet P. 2008. Cervical cáncer complicating pregnancy: Implications of laparoscopic lymphadenectomy. *Gynecologic Oncology*: 108: 472-477.

Angioli R, Martin J, Heffernan T, Massi G. Radical vaginal hysterectomy: classic and modified. *Surg Clin. North Am.* 2001;81:829-40.

Beiner ME, Hauspy J, Rosen B, Murphy J, Laframboise S, Nofech-Mozes S, et al.2008. Radical vaginal trachelectomy vs. radical hysterectomy for small early stage cervical cancer: a matched case-control study. *Gynecol. Oncol.*;110:168–71.

Bennett C,. Bravo E. y cols. Histerectomía vaginal en útero de gran tamaño y en ausencia de prolapso. *Rev. Chil. Obstet. Ginecol.* 1998;43(4):263-267.

Bravo E, Parry S, Alonso C, Rojas S. 2011. Histerectomía Radical Vaginal En Cáncer Cérvicouterino De Estadio Precoz. *Rev. Chil. Obstet. Ginecol.*; 76(5): 334 – 337.

Bravo E., Bennett C. y cols. Histerectomía vaginal en ausencia de prolapso. *Rev. Chil. Obstet. Ginecol.* 1998;43(4):257-261.

Bravo E., Parry S., Alonso C., Rojas S. 2012. Radical vaginal trachelectomy and laparoscopic pelvic lymphadenectomy in IB1 cervical cancer during pregnancy *Gynecologic Oncology Reports* 2 : 78–79.

Childers J, Hatch K, Tran A, Surwit E. 1993. Laparoscopic para-aortic lymphadenectomy in gynecologic malignancies. *Obstet. Gynecol.*; 82:741-7.

Childers JM, Brzechffa PR. Laparoscopically assisted surgical staging (LASS) of endometrial cancer., *Gynecol. Oncol.* 1993;51(1):33-8.

Cosson M., Querleu D., Subtil D. y cols. The feasibility of vaginal hysterectomy . *Eu. J. Obstet. Gynaecol. Reprod. Biol.* 1996;62(1):95-99.

Coulam C., Prott J. Vaginal hysterectomy: Is previous pelvic operation a contraindication? *Am. J. Obstet. Gynaecol.* 1973;116(2):252-260.

Covens A, Rosen B, Murphy J, Laframboise S, Depetrillo A, Lickrish G, et al. 2001. Changes in the demographics and perioperative care of stage Ia(2)/Ib(1) cervical cancer over the past 16 years. *Gynecol. Oncol.*;81:133–7.

Dargent D, Brun J, Roy M, Mathevet P, Remy I. 1994. La trachelectomie elargie (te), une alternative a l'hysterectomie radicale dans le traitement des cancers in!ltrants developpes sur la face externe du col uterin. *J. Obstet. Gynecol.*;2:285–92.

Dargent D, Martin X, Sacchetoni A, Mathevet P. 2000. Laparoscopic vaginal radical trachelectomy: a treatment to preserve the fertility of cervical carcinoma patients. *Cancer*;88:1877–82.

Dargent D, Mathevet P. Schauta's vaginal hysterectomy combined with laparoscopic lymphadenectomy. *Baillieres Clin. Obstet. Gynaecol.* 1995;9(4):691-705.

Dargent D. A new future for Schauta`s operation through pre-surgical retroperitoneal pelviscopy. *Eur. J. Gynecol. Oncol.* 1987;8:292-6.

Davies A., O,Connor H., Magos A. A prospective study to evaluate oophorectomy at the time of vaginal hysterectomy. *Br. J. Obstet. Gynaecol.* 1996;103(9):915-920.

Dicker R., Greenspan J., Strauss L. y cols. Complications of abdominal and vaginal hysterectomy among women of reproducive age in the United States. *Am. J. Obstet. Gynecol.* 1982;114(7):841-848.

Dorsey J., Holtz P., Griffiths R. et al. Costs and charges associated with three alternative techniques of hysterectomy. *N. Engl. J. Med.* 1996;335:477-482.

Doucette R., Scott J. Comparison of laparoscopically assisted vaginal hysterectomy with abominal and vaginal hysterectomy. *J Reprod. Med.* 1996;41(1):1-6.

Dursun P, LeBlanc E, Nogueira MC. Radical vaginal trachelectomy (Dargent's operation): a critical review of the literature. *Eur. J. Surg. Oncol.* 2007;33(8):933-41.

Fernandez C., Duque G., Fernandez E. Cirugía endoscópica en ginecología. Nuestra experiencia en histerectomía total. *Rev. Chil. Obstet. Ginecol.* 1994;59(4):261-267.

Gien L, Covens A. 2010. Fertility-sparing options for early stage cervical cancer. *Gynecol. Oncol.;* 117: 350 – 357.

Gien L., Covens A. 2009. Lymph node assessment in cervical cancer: Prognostic and therapeutic implications. *Journal of Surgical Oncology,* 2009; 99(4):242–247.

Hopkins MP, Morley GW. 1992. The prognosis and management of cervical cancer associated with pregnancy. *Obstet. Gynecol.*;80(1):9.

Ingram J., Withers R., Wright H. .Vaginal hysterectomy after previous pelvic surgery. *Am. J. Obstet. Gynaecol.* 1957;74(6):1181-1186.

Jones R. Complications of laparoscopic hysterectomy: 250 cases. *Gynaecological endoscopy* 1995;4:95-99.

Kalogirou D., Antoniou G., Karalitsos P. y cols. Comparison of abdominal and vaginal hysterectomy. Study of complications. *Clin. Exp. Obstet. Gynaecol.* 1996;23(3):161-167.

Lopez J., Briones H. Estado actual de la histerectomía vaginal. *Rev. Chil. Obstet. Ginecol.* 1982;47(6):393-404.

Mandic A., Novakovic P., Nincic D., Zivaljevic M, Rajovic J. 2009. Radical abdominal trachelectomy in the 19th gestationweek in patients with early invasive cervical carcinoma: case study and overview of literatura. *American Journal of Obstetrics & Gynecology*

Marchiole P, Benchaib M, Buenerd A, Lazlo E, Dargent D, Mathevet P.2007. Oncological safety of laparoscopic-assisted vaginal radical trachelectomy (LARVT or Dargent's operation): a comparative study with laparoscopic-assisted vaginal radical hysterectomy (LARVH). *Gynecol. Oncol.*;106:132–41.

Marchiole P, Benchaib M. Oncological safety of laparoscopic-assisted vaginal radical trachelectomy (LARVT or Dargent's operation): a comparative study with laparoscopic-assisted vaginal radical hysterectomy (LARVH). *Gynecol. Oncol.* 2007;106(1):132-41.

Michels W., Possover M, Tozzi R, Schneider A. 2003. Laparoscopic-assisted radical vaginal hysterectomy (LARVH): prospective evaluation of 200 patients with cervical cancer. *Gynecologic Oncology*; 90:505-11.

Milliken DA, Shepherd JH. 2008. Fertility preserving surgery for carcinoma of the cervix. *Curr. Opin. Oncol.*;20:575–80.

MINSAL Chile. Guían clínica GES Cáncer cervicouterino. 2010.

Moen M. Using morcellation for vaginal hysterectomy. *Contemporary Obs Gyn.* 1996;41(10):33-45.

Morgan D, Hunter D, McCracken G, McClelland HR, Price JH, Dobbs SP. 2007. Is laparoscopically assisted radical vaginal hysterectomy for cervical carcinoma safe? A case control study with follow up. *BJOG;* 114:537-42.

Munro M., Deprest J. Laparoscopic hysterectomy. Does it work?. A bicontinental review of the literature and clinical commentary. *Clinical Obstetrics and Gynaecology* 1995;38(2):401-425.

Nanako Iwami, Shinichi Ishioka , Toshiaki Endo, Tsuyoshi Baba, Kunihiko Nagasawa ,Madoka Takahashi, Asuka Sugio, Sakura Takada, Tasuku Mariya, Masahiro Mizunuma, Tsuyoshi Saito. First case of vaginal radical trachelectomy in a pregnant Japanese woman. *International Journal of Clinical Oncology* © *Japan Society of Clinical Oncology 201110.1007/s10147-011-0209-3.*

Newman T., Lopez J., Miranda C. y cols. Experiencia en histerectomía total laparoscópica. *Rev. Chil. Obstet. Ginecol.* 1997;62(1):3-8.

Pahisa J, Martinez-Román S, Torné A, Fusté P, Alonso I, Lejárcegui JA, Balasch J. 2010. Comparative study of laparoscopically assisted radical vaginal hysterectomy and open Wertheim-Meigs in patients with early stage cervical cancer. *Int. J. Gynecol. Cancer*;20:173-7.

Pellegrino A, Vizza E. Total laparoscopic radical hysterectomy and pelvic lymphadenectomy in patients with Ib1 stage cervical cancer: analysis of surgical and oncological outcome. *Eur. J. Surg. Oncol.* Jan 2009;35(1):98-103.

Pelosi M., Pelosi M III. A comprehensive approach to morcellation of the large uterus. *Contemporary Ob. Gyn.* 1997:106-125.

Peppercorn PD, Jeyarajah AR, Woolas R, Shepherd JH, Oram DH, Jacobs IJ, et al. 1999. Role of MR imaging in the selection of patients with early cervical carcinoma for fertility-sparing surgery: initial experience. *Radiology*; 212:395–9.

Querleu D, LeBlanc E, Castellain B. Laparoscopic pelvic lymphadenectomy in the staging of early cervical carcinoma of the cervix. *Am. J. Obstet. Gynecol.* 1991;164:579-81.

Richardson R., Bournos N., Magos A. Is laparoscopic hysterectomy a waste of time? *The Lancet* 1995;345:36-41.

Roy M, Plante M. 2011. Place of Schautas radical vaginal hysterctomy. *Best Practice and Research Clinical Obstetrics and Gynaecology.* 25; 227-237.

Sarrouf J. , Sarrouf M. C. Laparoscopía en cáncer de cuello uterino. *Rev. Per. Ginecol. Obstet.* 2009;55:105-112.

Sert BM, Abeler VM. Robotic assisted laparoscopic radical hysterectomy (Piver type III) with pelvic node dissection- case report. *Eur. J. Gynecol. Oncol.* 2006; 27 (5):531-533.

Sheth SS. The place of opherectomy at vaginal hysterectomy. *Br. J. Obstet. Gynecol.* 1991;98:662-67.

Sioutas A, Schedvins K, Larson B, Gemzell-Danielsson K. 2011. Three cases of vaginal radical trachelectomy during pregnancy. *Gynecol Oncol*; 121(2):420.

Smith L, Dalrymple J, Leiserowitz G, Danielsen B, Gilbert W. 2001. Obstetrical deliveries associated with maternal malignancy in California, 1992 through 1997. *Am. J. Obstet. Gynecol.*;184(7):1504.

Sonoda Y, Abu-Rustum N. Schauta radical vaginal hysterectomy. *Gynecologic Oncologic.* 2007;104:20-4.

Takushi M, Moromizato H, Sakumoto K, Kanazawa K. 2002. Management of invasive carcinoma of the uterine cervix associated with pregnancy: outcome of intentional delay in treatment.. *Gynecol. Oncol.*; 87(2):185.

Ungar, L., Smith, J., Pálfalfi, I., Del Priore, G. 2006. Abdominal radical trachelectomy during pregnancy to preserve pregnancy and fertility. *Obstet. Gynecol.* 108, 811–814.

Valdivia H., Álvarez M. La cirugía laparoscópica en ginecología oncológica y experiencia en el Instituto Nacional de Enfermedades Neoplásicas de Lima, Perú, *Rev. Per. Ginecol. Obstet.* 2009;55:58-64.

Van de Nieuwenhof, H., Van Ham, M., Lotgering, F., Massuger, L. 2008. First case of vaginal radical trachelectomy in a pregnant patient. *Int. J. Gynecol. Cancer.* 18 (6), 1381–1385.

Yahata T, Numata M, Kashima K, Sekine M, Fujita K, Yamamoto T, Tanaka K. 2008. Conservative treatment of stage IA1 adenocarcinoma of the cervix during pregnancy. *Gynecol. Oncol.*; 109(1):49.

Zemlickis D, Lishner M, Degendorfer P, Panzarella T, Sutcliffe SB, Koren G. 1991. Maternal and fetal outcome after invasive cervical cancer in pregnancy. *J. Clin. Oncol.*; 9(11):1956.

In: Cervical Cancer
Editor: Laurie Elit

ISBN: 978-1-62948-062-6
© 2014 Nova Science Publishers, Inc.

Chapter IX

Neoadjuvant Chemotherapy in Locally Advanced Cervical Cancer: Current Concepts and Future Challenges

P. Estevez-Garcia[1,2], E. Calvo[1], I. Duran[1,2] and I. Diaz-Padilla[3]*

[1]Gynecologic Cancer Program. Medical Oncology Department. University Hospital
Virgen del Rocio. Seville, Spain
[2]Instituto de Biomedicina de Sevilla, Universidad de Sevilla. Seville, Spain
[3]Gynecologic Cancer Program. Division of Medical Oncology, Centro Integral
Oncologico Clara Campal. University Hospital HM Sanchinarro. Madrid, Spain

Abstract

Cervical cancer is the third most common cancer in females worldwide. In developing countries, cervical cancer represents a major health problem, where it is responsible for more than 10% of cancer-related deaths and is associated with significant morbidity. Around 30% of newly diagnosed cases encompass the category of locally advanced cervical cancer (LACC), a broad group comprising early-stage bulky disease and tumor spreading outside the uterus. Treatment with concurrent chemo-radiotherapy is the standard of care in these patients. Limited access to high-quality radiation therapy in developing countries, long-term comorbidity associated with radiotherapy and a modest control of distant recurrences may challenge this therapeutic approach. These concerns have led to the investigation of new treatment strategies, such as the incorporation of neoadjuvant chemotherapy (NACT). In this chapter, we will summarize the results of the main clinical studies of NACT in locally advanced disease and discuss the potential clinical role of NACT in the current management of cervical cancer.

* Corresponding author: Ivan Diaz-Padilla, M.D., Gynecologic Cancer Program, Division of Medical Oncology, Centro Integral Oncologico Clara Campal, University Hospital HM Sanchinarro, 10 Ona, 28050 Madrid, Spain, Tel: +34 91 756 78 00, Fax: +34 91 750 02 02, E-mail: drdiazpadilla@me.com.

1. Introduction

Cervical cancer (CC) is the third most common cancer in women, with over 530,000 new cases diagnosed every year worldwide, accounting for approximately 8% of the total cancer deaths among females (Ferlay et al., 2010). There are marked differences in incidence and mortality between developed countries, where CC is a rare malignancy, and developing countries, where it represents a major health problem. Africa, South-Central Asia and South America account for more than 85% of the CC cases and related deaths (Jemal et al., 2011).

CC develops from non-invasive premalignant lesions to infiltrative tumors in a well-known natural history. Persistent infection by oncogenic types of human papilloma virus (HPV) is the most important causative factor in the development of CC (Kjaer et al., 2010; Rodriguez et al., 2010). Other risk factors involved in CC pathogenesis are the same as those for sexually transmitted diseases, including having sexual intercourse at an early age, several sexual partners, other sexually transmitted diseases such as chlamydia or herpes simplex virus, and immunosuppressed states underlining HIV infection (Randall et al., 2009). Screening programs using cervical cytology have been established in western countries over the last decades, leading to a significant decrease both in incidence and mortality due to a high diagnostic rate of premalignant lesions and early-stage disease, where treatment is curative. In contrast, many low-resource countries with high prevalence of HPV infection unfortunately lack well-established screening programs and modern treatment modalities (e.g. laparoscopic surgery, radiation therapy) are not accessible to a majority of women suffering CC.

Treatment recommendations for CC are based on the Federation Internationale de Gynecologie et d'Obstetrique (FIGO) stage of the disease (Figure 1). Taking into consideration the limited access to imaging and surgical staging in low-resource countries, the latest update in FIGO classification is still based in clinical staging, limiting radiographic imaging to chest radiography, intravenous pyelography and barium enema and not incorporating surgical findings in staging (Pecorelli et al., 2009).

Therapeutic management of CC is complex. It generally involves surgery, chemotherapy and/or radiotherapy, depending on the stage of the disease at diagnosis and patient characteristics. For early-stage non-bulky (< 4 cm) disease surgery and/or radiotherapy are the preferred options. New conservative approaches (e.g. trachelectomy) are currently advocated for fertility preservation or in tumors diagnosed during pregnancy (Gien & Covens, 2010; Shepherd, 2012). For metastatic and/or recurrent disease, palliative platinum-based chemotherapy represents the standard of care (Eifel et al., 2008).

Locally advanced cervical cancer (LACC) is a broad disease category, compromising early-stage bulky (> 4cm) disease and tumors extending beyond the uterus that involve adjacent organs and/or pelvic wall (stages IB2-IVA). Locally advanced tumors are clinically heterogeneous, have higher local failure rates and worse survival compared to early-stage non-bulky tumors (Al-Mansour and Verschraegen, 2010). Treatment recommendations for management of LACC can also vary depending on the stage and patient's clinical characteristics. Generally, a multidisciplinary approached is needed, involving either primary chemo-radiation or primary surgery followed by adjuvant chemoradiotherapy. The role of neoadjuvant chemotherapy (NACT) for the treatment of LACC is a common practice in certain clinical settings although its role is still under debate.

In this chapter we will review the current evidence supporting NACT for the management of LACC, including published and ongoing clinical trials. We will also discuss the most appropriate clinical indications where NACT could be effectively integrated with the current therapeutic strategies for CC.

2. Concurrent Chemo-Radiation in LACC

The use of radiotherapy (RT) as a single treatment modality has been the most common recommended treatment for LACC in the past. With this approach, local control and survival were both directly related to the size of the primary tumor (Eifel et al., 1994). Five-year survival rates of RT for the treatment of LACC were over 60%, with local failure rates of 18-39% (Randall et al., 2009). During the late 1990s, several studies evaluated if the addition of chemotherapy (CT) to RT (concurrent chemo-radiation, CRT) would be of benefit. Several cytotoxic drugs have been tested as radiosensitizers for the treatment of LACC (i.e. 5-fluoruracil, mitomycin, carboplatin, cisplatin, paclitaxel, epirubicin) (Eifel, 2006), being cisplatin the most effective drug across all published randomized trials (Whitney et al., 1999; Morris et al., 1999; Rose et al., 1999; Keys et al., 1999; Peters et al., 2000; Thomas et al., 1999) (Table 2).

Table 1. FIGO staging of cervical cancer

FIGO	Description
0	Carcinoma *in situ*
I	Cervical carcinoma limited to the uterus (Extension to the corpus should be disregarded)
IA	Invasive carcinoma only diagnosed by microscope.
IA1	Stromal invasion 3.0 mm or less in depth and 7.0 mm or less in horizontal spread
IA2	Stromal invasion more than 3.0 mm in depth and not more than 5.0 mm and horizontal spread of 7.0 mm or less
IB	Clinically visible lesion limited to the cervix or microscopic lesion larger than IA2.
IB1	Clinically visible lesion 4.0 cm or less in greatest dimension.
IB2	Clinically visible lesion larger than 4.0 cm in greatest dimension.
II	Cervical carcinoma extended beyond uterus but not pelvic wall or lower third of vagina.
IIA	Cervical carcinoma without parametrial extension.
IIA1	Tumor 4.0 cm or less in greatest dimension.
IIA2	Tumor larger than 4.0 cm in greatest dimension
IIB	Cervical carcinoma with parametrial extension.
III	Tumor extended to the pelvic wall and/or involves lower third of vagina and/or presenting hydronephrosis or non-functioning kidney.
IIIA	Tumor involvement of the lower third of vagina without extension to the pelvic wall.
IIIB	Tumor extended to the pelvic wall and/or causes hydronephrosis or non-functioning kidney.
IVA	Tumor involvement of rectal and/or bladder mucosa and/or with extension beyond true pelvis.
IVB	Distant metastases.

Table 2. Prospective randomized trials of concurrent radiotherapy and chemotherapy for patients with locally advanced cervical cancer

Reference	Eligible FIGO stages	Number of patients	Treatment	Relative risk of recurrence (90% CI)	p value
Rose (1999)	IIB-IVA	526	CDDP 40 mg/m2/wk vs HU 3 g/m2 (22 x wk) or	0.57 (0.42-0.78)	<0.001
			CDDP 50 mg/m2, 5FU 4 g/m2/ 96h, HU 2 g/m2 (2 x wk) vs HU 3 g/m2 (22 x wk)	0.55 (0.40-0.75)	<0.001
Morris (1999)	IB-IIA (≥5cm), IIB-IVA	403	CDDP 75 mg/m2 + 5FU 4 g/m2/96h (3 cycles) vs None	0.48 (0.35-0.66)	<0.001
Keys (1999)	IB (≥4cm)	369	CDDP 40 mg/m2/wk (up to 6 cycles) vs None	0.51 (0.34-0.75)	0.001
Whitney (1999)	IIB-IVA	368	CDDP 50 mg/m2 + 5FU 4g/m2/96h (2 cycles) vs HU 3g/m2 (22 x week)	0.79 (0.62-0.99)	0.03
Peters (2000)	I-IIA after RHT with nodes, margins or parametrium positives	268	CDDP 70 mg/m2 + 5FU 4g/m2/96h (2 concurrent + 2 adjuvant cycles) vs None	0.50 (0.29-0.84)	0.01
Thomas (1999)	IB-IIA (≥5cm), IIB-IVA	234	5FU 4g/m2/96h x 2 cycles vs None	-	Not stated

CDDP: cisplatin; 5FU: 5-fluoruracil; HU: hydroxyurea; wk: week; RHT: radical hysterectomy.

A meta-analysis of 18 randomized trials of CRT in LACC has recently been published (Chemoradiotherapy for Cervical Cancer Meta-Analysis Collaboration [CCMAC], 2008). Cisplatin-based CRT was used in 85% of the patients, either as a single agent (eight trials) or in combination regimens (three trials). An absolute benefit of 8% in disease-free survival (HR of 0.78 [95% CI 0.70-0.87]; p<0.000005) and 6% in 5-year overall survival (HR=0.81 [95% CI 0.71-0.91] p<0.0006) was demonstrated for cisplatin-based regimens. Consistent with previous studies of RT alone, the higher benefit with CRT was mostly achieved in early-stage patients (I-II), with an estimated survival benefit at 5 years of 10% (stage IA-IIA), 7% (IIB) and 3% (III-IVA) (CCMAC, 2008). The results of this meta-analysis further confirm that the addition of CT to RT significantly improves survival in LACC.

However, treatment with CRT is associated with substantial toxicity and distant relapses still occur. Common complications of CRT mainly involve the gastrointestinal and urologic tracts. Acute toxicity typically includes diarrhea and bladder irritation, and usually can be managed effectively with conservative treatment. Rates of major late sequelae range from 5% to 10% in stage I and II-IVA respectively, and the majority of late toxicities appear within the first 3 years after CRT. Risk increases with several factors, essentially volume treated and radiation dose, with a higher incidence of pelvic complications found in patients who receive above 40 to 50 Gy to the whole pelvis. (Randall et al., 2009).

Chronic genitourinary complications are the most frequent late toxicities, with a reported incidence of 26% in patients treated with RT alone for CC (Parkin et al., 1988). The latency period between RT administration and sequelae manifestations is considerably long, with a 0.3% risk of appearance per year beyond 20 years, and a reported actuarial risk of 14% of major complications at 20 years (Eifel et al., 1995). Severe toxicities include hemorrhagic cystitis and fistula in 2-3% of cases (Perez et al., 1996; Perez et al., 1999).

Bowel injury is the most frequent gastrointestinal late toxicity of RT for CC, ranging from 5% to 15%, with a reported median latency period of 10 months (Iraha et al., 2007). Intestinal major complications include stenosis/fibrosis causing obstruction, severe bleeding, fistula or radiation proctitis/enteritis with treatment refractory diarrhea. However, these events are fortunately infrequent, and the risk of appearance decreases over time. The risk of rectal complications after the first two years of follow-up declines to 0.06% per year. (Randall et al., 2009).

RT can alter also vaginal function by reducing length, caliber and lubrication, but symptoms can usually be managed with hormonal replacement and vaginal dilatation. A recent study reported a 20.2% of severe vaginal late toxicity at 3 years in patients treated with RT alone and 35.1% for CRT (p=0.026). Moderate (HR 3.6, 95% CI 2.0-6.5, p<0.001) or poor dilator compliance (HR 8.5, 95% CI 4.3-16.9, p<0.001) compared to high compliance, and age older than 50 years (HR 1.8, 95% CI 1.1-3.0, p=0.013) were significantly related to higher severe vaginal late toxicity. (Gondi et al., 2012)

Lumbosacral plexopathy, lymphedema or pelvic insufficiency fractures are less frequent but quite debilitating side effects.

3. Neoadjuvant Chemotherapy in LACC

The toxicities associated with CRT and the limited access to modern radiation techniques in countries with low economic resources has led to consider alternative therapeutic approaches that can be implemented globally. Neoadjuvant chemotherapy (NACT) has been evaluated as a potential treatment option for women with LACC over the last two decades.

The use of pre-operative chemotherapy in locally advanced disease has demonstrated to be an effective therapeutic approach in other solid tumors (e.g. breast cancer, head and neck cancer, non-small cell lung cancer, osteogenic sarcoma) where NACT followed by local treatment with RT or surgery have improved loco-regional control rates (DeVita and Chu, 2008).

The potential advantages of NACT may include the down-staging of the tumor and reduction of lymph node positivity making radical surgery feasible in cases judged unresectable due to either adverse tumor or patient characteristics. Advocates of NACT argue for its role in helping eradicate occult micrometastasis, thus preventing a significant proportion of distant relapses (Tierney et al., 2008). Tumor size reduction and node negativity would result in less aggressive surgery procedures and decreased use postoperative RT or CRT, which would consequently ameliorate the rate of treatment-related toxicities, especially in young and sexually-active women.

Neoadjuvant Chemotherapy Followed by Surgery

Response to NACT has been identified as an important prognostic factor in several solid tumors becoming a well-accepted surrogate endpoint for survival (Kong et al., 2011). In CC, response rates over 75% to NACT have been reported in retrospective studies. Furthermore, those women who achieved a complete pathologic response to NACT had better outcomes (Benedetti et al., 1998; Buda et al., 2005, Fossati et al., 2005).

A systematic review and meta-analysis of the role of NACT followed by surgery compared with radiotherapy alone in LACC was published in 2003 (Chemoradiotherapy for Cervical Cancer Meta-analysis Collaboration [CCCMAC], 2003) based on data from five trials including 872 patients. Three of the five trials (Sardi et al., 1996; Sardi et al. 1998; Kigawa et al., 1996) only included FIGO stages IIB-III, one trial only included early-stage IB2-IIA patients (Chang et al., 2000) and the other study included a wider range of patients from stage IB2 to stage III (Benedetti-Panici et al., 2002). Overall, the majority of the patients analyzed had FIGO stages IIB-III (64.5%; 563 patients), and 35.5% (309 patients) had stages IB2-IIA. Cisplatin-based regimens were used for 2 to 7 cycles before radical surgery. Radiotherapy schemes in control arms were similar across studies. A highly significant 35% reduction in the risk of death (HR 0.65; CI 95% 0.53-0.80; p=0.0004) and an absolute improvement of 14% in 5-year survival favoring NACT was demonstrated in the combined analysis of all trials. This effect was independent of age, stage, histology, grade or performance status. (CCCMAC, 2003).

More recently, The Cochrane Collaboration reviewed the evidence supporting the use of NACT followed by surgery compared to surgery alone in LACC (Rydzewska et al., 2010). Pooled analysis of six trials including 1072 individual patient data was undertaken (Table 3). Progression-free survival (PFS) data were available in all trials for the great majority of the patients (1036 women), although data on overall survival (OS) were only available for five of the six trials (909 to 938 women). NACT significantly improved PFS (HR 0.76, CI 95% 0.62-0.94, p=0.01), without benefit observed in OS (HR 0.85, CI 95% 0.67-1.07, p=0.17).. Estimates for local and distant recurrence showed a non-significant trend towards better outcome for trials incorporating NACT (OR 0.76, CI 95% 0.49-1.17, p = 0.21; and OR = 0.68, CI 95% 0.41-1.13, p = 0.13, respectively). An interesting subgroup exploratory analysis was performed evaluating the impact of pathological response after NACT in poor prognosis patients presenting with positive lymph node and parametrial infiltration at diagnosis. The use of NACT in such subgroups revealed a positive effect with a significant decrease in both (OR 0.54, CI 95% 0.39-0.73, p=0.0001 for lymph node status; OR 0.58, CI 95% 0.41-0.82, p=0.002 for parametrial infiltration). No differences according to total cisplatin dose, NACT cycle length or FIGO stage were observed.

An update of this meta-analysis has been recently published, reporting mature data from 1078 patients (Rydzewska et al., 2012). The authors described greater consistency between outcomes of OS and PFS in the trials after adding supplementary data, with significant improvements in outcomes supporting the use of NACT. Cisplatin-based chemotherapy was administered in all the trials, but total doses ranged from 140 mg/m^2 to 300 mg/m^2 given in 2 to 4 cycles at 10 to 21 days intervals. Radical hysterectomy was also comparable across the six trials but lymphadenectomy was variable, with three studies performing pelvic dissection, while another two added para-aortic lymph node dissection and one did not provide such information. Some of the patients also underwent post-operative RT depending on the risk factors of recurrence considered in each study. Some heterogeneity was observed regarding the distribution of FIGO stage (the evaluated studies randomized 107 to 291 women presenting FIGO stages IB to IIIB). However, three trials only recruited patients with stage IB disease and, in the remaining three, most patients early-stage disease (IB-II).

In summary, NACT followed by surgery significantly decreased both the risk of death compared to surgery alone (HR 0.77, CI 95% 0.62-0.96, p=0.02) and the risk of disease progression (HR 0.75, CI 95% 0.45-0.99, p=0.04). The risk of distant recurrence (OR 0.72, CI 95% 0.45-1.14, p=0.16) and the likelihood of achieving a complete resection (OR 1.55, CI 95% 0.96-2.50, p=0.07) showed a trend favoring the use of NACT, although heterogeneity also limited this analysis. Interestingly, despite underscored differences in the studies, patients who received NACT prior to surgery showed a significant decrease in adverse pathological findings including lymph node involvement and parametrial infiltration (OR 0.54, CI 95% 0.40-0.73, p=0.0001; and OR 0.58, CI 95% 0.41-0.82, p=0.002, respectively) compared to those who underwent surgery alone.

Table 3. Characteristics of selected randomized trials of neoadjuvant chemotherapy plus surgery compared to surgery

Reference	Eligible FIGO stages	Number of patients	Comparison	Treatment
Sardi (1997)	IB	210	NACT+RS or RT vs RS or RT	CDDP+VCR+BLM
Napolitano (2003)	IB-III	156	NACT+RS or RT vs RS or RT	CDDP+VCR+BLM
Cai (2006)	IB	106	NACT+RS vs RS	CDDP+5FU
Katsumana (2006)	Bulky I-II	134	NACT+RS vs RS	CDDP+VCR+BLM
Eddy (2007)	Bulky IB	291	NACT+RS vs RS	CDDP+VCR
Chen (2008)	IB2-IIB	133	NACT+RS (+/-RT) vs RS (+/-RT)	CDDP+Mito+5FU
Zanaboni (2013)	IB2-IIB	92	NACT+RS	CDDP+Topo

CDDP: cisplatin; VCR: vincristine; BLM: bleomycin; Mito: mitomycin-C; 5FU: 5-fluoruracil; Topo: topotecan; NACT: neoadjuvant chemotherapy; RS: radical surgery; RT: radiotherapy.

Taken together, available data would suggest that either NACT followed by surgery or CRT are better treatment options for LACC than radiotherapy alone. However, these two treatment options have not been compared prospectively yet. A large-scale retrospective study has been recently published by Yin et al. to compare the long-term survival of 426 stage IB2-IIB LACC patients treated with NACT followed by radical surgery (hysterectomy plus pelvic lymph node dissection) with those treated with radical surgery alone or CRT. This study is the current reference for NACT followed by surgery in LACC. However, as a retrospective study, it shows some limitations that cannot be eliminated such as selection bias. Statistically significant differences were found between the three treatments groups NACT plus surgery, surgery alone and CRT in some features that may affect the survival evaluation such as age, tumor size, FIGO stage, and differentiation degree. To minimize this effect, a multivariate Cox regression analysis adjusting these variables was performed. NACT followed by radical surgery had improved survival than radical surgery alone or CRT. Five-year DFS rates for NACT and surgery, surgery alone, and CRT were 85%, 77.4% and 52.9% respectively. Five-year OS was also favorable for NACT and surgery (88.6%) compared to surgery alone (80.2%) and CRT (64.7%) (Yin et al., 2011).

To further confirm the long-term efficacy of NACT followed by surgery, a randomized phase III study comparing NACT followed by surgery versus primary CRT was initiated in 2002 by the European Organization for Research and Treatment of Cancer (EORTC) and it is currently underway (NCT00039338). Results are eagerly awaited. Two other trials in Asia are currently comparing standard cisplatin CRT with NACT followed by surgery. Chemotherapy regimens include carboplatin plus paclitaxel (NCT00193739) and cisplatin plus gemcitabine (NCT01000415).

Neoadjuvant Chemotherapy Followed by RT

Based on the positive results of NACT followed by surgery over RT alone, the role of NACT followed by radical RT was subsequently evaluated. Seven randomized trials using a variety of cisplatin-based regimens as NACT have been published. Five of these studies could not demonstrate benefit from NACT (Chauvergne et al., 1990; Kumar et al., 1994; Leborgne et al. 1997; Sundfør et al. 1996; Tattersall, 1995), and the other two confirmed a statistically significant improvement in survival in the radiotherapy alone arm (Souhami et al., 1991; Tattersall et al. 1992). A potential explanation for these results in NACT is based on the rapid proliferation rate of CC cells, with a median doubling time of 4-4.5 days and high growth fraction. Tumor shrinkage would be accomplished by the use of NACT, but if the drug and/or timing are not optimal tumors could regrowth quickly between cycles (Al-Mansour and Verschraegen, 2010). Moreover, development of cross-resistance between platinum compounds and radiotherapy could facilitate the progressive development of radio-resistant cellular clones (Ozols et al., 1988; Gonzalez-Martin et al., 2008).

In 2003 the Neoadjuvant Chemotherapy for Locally Advanced Cervical Cancer Meta-Analysis Collaboration (CCCMAC) published a systematic review and meta-analysis in an attempt to clarify the role of NACT followed by radical RT versus RT alone in LACC. Individual data from 2074 patients IB-IVA FIGO stage were obtained from 18 randomized trials. The majority of the patients (69%) had advanced-stage II-III FIGO stage tumors, but some IB stage women were also included (12%). A small number of patients underwent surgery as an alternative treatment to radical RT, and most of the women in another trial experienced RS followed by radical RT (Leborgne et al., 1997; MRCCeCa unpublished). Cisplatin was the most frequently used drug in NACT regimens. However, there were variations in the treatment schemes administered across the studies, with doses of cisplatin ranging from 100 to 320 mg/m^2 in cycles from 10 to 28 days. External beam and intracavitary RT received by the patients varied substantially, with total doses ranging from 55 to 80 Gy. Such differences in design and the heterogeneous results observed in individual studies made difficult to reach a definitive conclusion as to whether the addition of NACT followed by RT adds value to RT alone or not. A highly significant level of statistical heterogeneity was evident (p<0.001) across the included studies. Thus, a pooled analysis combining all trials showed no evidence of an effect of NACT on survival. A pre-specified analysis separated included studies in two groups, based on the CT schedule and the dose intensity. The administration of cycles of 14 days or shorter in duration (HR=0.83, 95% CI 0.69-1.00, p=0.046) and doses of cisplatin $\geq$ 25 mg/m^2/week (HR 0.91, 95% CI 0.78-1.05, p=0.20) suggested a benefit of NACT in survival, as opposed to CT cycles lasting more than 14 days (HR 1.25, 95% CI 1.07-1.46, p=0.005) or cisplatin doses below 25 mg/m^2/week (HR 1.35, 95% CI 1.11-1.14, p=0.002). Authors concluded that overall results did not support cisplatin-based NACT followed by radical RT in LACC. (CCCMAC, 2003).

Adjuvant Chemotherapy after NACT Followed by Surgery

The potential benefit of adding adjuvant chemotherapy after NACT and surgery has also been investigated. To date, there is scant evidence to recommend this therapeutic option. On the one hand, the addition of a *consolidation* scheme could help in reducing relapse rates after primary treatment in high-risk patients; on the other hand, extending chemotherapy duration can undoubtedly cause significant morbidity and lower patient's adherence to the treatment. Therefore, an accurate identification of patients who would benefit most from adjuvant chemotherapy needs to be established.

Parametrial infiltration, positive surgical margins and lymph node metastases are the most important adverse prognostic factors in CC (Sedlis et al., 1999; Mohar and Frias-Mendivil, 2000; Angioli et al., 2012). Thus, adjuvant chemotherapy has been traditionally considered in this high-risk patient population, and it was administered to the 9-21% of these patients in some reported series including FIGO stages IB bulky and II (Chen et al., 2008; Eddy et al., 2007; Cai et al., 2006, Gong et al., 2012).

Only two trials have been reported evaluating the efficacy of adjuvant chemotherapy after prior NACT and surgery. In 1998, a pilot phase II trial compared three treatment groups in 56 LACC patients with IB-IIIB FIGO stage: i) NACT followed by surgery and RT; ii) NACT followed by surgery and adjuvant chemotherapy; and iii) a control arm with RT alone. NACT included cisplatin 50 mg/m^2 on day 1, vincristine 1 mg/m^2 on day 1, and bleomycin 25 mg/m^2 on days 1-3. Treatment was administered was given every 10 days for 3 cycles. Adjuvant chemotherapy consisted of cisplatin 50 mg/m^2, methotrexate 30 mg/m^2 and cyclophosphamide 500 mg/m^2 for 3 cycles every 21 days. Overall survival for stage IB patients was 88% after a median follow-up of 75 months, 78% for stage IIB and 50% for IIIB. When residual tumor volume was less than 2 cm in the surgical specimen, pelvic recurrences significantly decrease compared to residual tumor larger than 2 cm (3 versus 6, respectively; p<0.001) (Sananes et al., 1998). More recently, Angioli and colleagues evaluated the feasibility of administering adjuvant cisplatin 100 mg/m^2 plus paclitaxel 175 mg/m^2 every 3 weeks for 4 cycles after NACT (with the same regimen for 3 cycles) and surgery in 115 LACC patients (Angioli et al., 2012). Stable or progressive disease patients after NACT were excluded of the protocol (13%; 15 patients), as well as patients with positive aortic nodes found during surgery and those with resection margins close to vagina (2 and 3 patients, respectively). Adjuvant chemotherapy was generally well tolerated. The most frequent toxicities were G1-2 nausea and vomiting (39%) and myelosuppression (41%). There were no treatment-related deaths, but G3-4 reported toxicity included hematologic (15%), nausea and vomiting (11%), neuropathy (2%), hepatic (3%) and 1 patient developed stroke and cerebral hemorrhage. Of note, consistent data corroborating the relevance of nodal status in prognosis were obtained. Patients with pelvic node metastasis presented 60% 5-year OS compared to

87% in negative pelvic nodes. Global five-year OS and disease-free survival (DFS) were 77% and 61% respectively in the intention-to-treat analysis. These data seem to be comparable to that reported in the CRT in LACC meta-analysis (CCMAC, 2008), suggesting that the addition of adjuvant CT to the approach of NACT followed by surgery is worth investigating further in LACC.

Conclusion

The standard treatment of LACC was established more than a decade ago and consists of concurrent CRT. This approach has consistently demonstrated improved clinical outcomes across many randomized trials compared with radiation as a single-modality treatment. Despite its improved efficacy, CRT does have short and long-term toxicities.

The use of NACT has proven beneficial in other solid tumors, which prompted its evaluation as an alternative treatment in LACC. The main advantages of NACT would be represented by its potential in decreasing tumor volume and extension, thus making surgery and/or radiotherapy more feasible. The rationale of administering NACT relies on its ability to eliminate micrometastatic disease. Therefore, the incorporation of NACT has been evaluated in different clinical scenarios for the management of LACC. Based on encouraging phase II data, the use NACT prior to surgery holds promise as an alternative therapeutic strategy in LACC, with results comparable to CRT. A currently active phase III randomized study is comparing NACT followed by surgery with the standard CRT in LACC. The results of such a trial will definitively clarify the role of NACT in the management of locally-advanced diseases. In the meantime, the use of NACT remains investigational.

Moving forward, the best chemotherapeutic regimen to use in NACT needs to be elucidated, as well as the role of NACT in special situations, such as pregnancy and fertility-sparing treatments.

References

Al-Mansour, Z; Verschraegen, C. Locally advanced cervical cancer: what is the standard of care? *Curr Op Oncol*, 2010, 22, 503-512.

Angioli, R; Plotti, F; Montera, R; et al. Neoadjuvant chemotherapy plus radical surgery followed by chemotherapy in locally advanced cervical cancer. *Gynecol Oncol*, 2012, 127, 290-296.

Basile, S; Angioli, R; Manci, N; Palaia, I; Plotti, F; Benedetti-Panici, P. Gynecological cancers in developing countries: the challenge of chemotherapy in low-resources setting. *Int J Gynecol Cancer*, 2006, 16, 1491–7.

Benedetti-Panici, P; Greggi, S; et al. Long-term survival following neoadjuvant chemotherapy and radical surgery in locally advanced cervical cancer. *Eur J Cancer*, 1998, 34, 341–6.

Benedetti-Panici, P; Greggi, S; Colombo, A; et al. Neoadjuvant chemotherapy and radical surgery versus exclusive radiotherapy in locally advanced squamous cell cervical cancer: results from the Italian multicenter randomized study. *J Clin Oncol*, 2002, 20, 179-188.

Buda, A; Fossati, R; Colombo, N; et al. Randomized trial of neoadjuvant chemotherapy comparing paclitaxel, ifosfamide, and cisplatin with ifosfamide and cisplatin followed by radical surgery in patients with locally advanced squamous cell cervical carcinoma: the SNAP01 (Studio Neo-Adiuvante Portio) Italian Collaborative Study. *J Clin Oncol*, 2005, 23, 4137–45.

Cai, HB; Chen, HZ; Yin, HH. Randomized study of preoperative chemotherapy versus primary surgery for stage IB cervical cancer. *J Obstet Gynaecol Res*, August 2006, 32, 315-323.

Chang-Ting, C; Lai, CH; Hong, JH; et al. Randomized trial of neoadjuvant cisplatin, vincristine, bleomycin, and radical hysterectomy versus radiation therapy for bulky stage Ib and IIA cervical cancer. *J Clin Oncol*, 2002, 20, 179-188.

Chauvergne, J; Rohart, J; Héron, JF; et al. Essai randomisé de chimiothérapie initiale dans 151 carcinomes de col utérin localement étendus (T2b-N1, T3b, MO). *Bull cancer*, 1990, 77, 1007.

Chemoradiotherapy for Cervical Cancer Meta-analysis Collaboration. Neoadjuvant chemotherapy for locally advanced cervical cancer: a systematic review and meta-analysis of individual patient data from 21 randomized trials. *Eur J Cancer*, 2003, 39, 2470-86.

Chemoradiotherapy for Cervical Cancer Meta-analysis Collaboration. Reducing uncertainties about the effects of chemoradiotherapy for cervical cancer: a systematic review and meta-analysis of individual patient data from 18 randomized trials. *J Clin Oncol*, 2008, 26, 5802-5812.

Chen, H; Liang, C; Zhang, L; et al. Clinical efficacy of modified preoperative neoadjuvant chemotherapy in the treatment of locally advanced (stage IB2 to IIB) cervical cancer: a randomized study. *Gynecol Oncol*, 2008, 110, 308-315.

Choi, CH; Kim, TJ; Lee, LW; et al. Phase II study of neoadjuvant chemotherapy with mitomycin-C, vincristine and cisplatin (MVC) in patients with stages IB2-IIB cervical carcinoma. *Gynecol Oncol*, 2007, 104, 64-69.

DeVita, VT; Jr. Chu, E. Principles of Medical Oncology. In: DeVita VT, Lawrence TS, Rosenberg SA (Editors). Cancer principles and practice of oncology. 8th ed., 2008 Philadelphia, Pennsylvania: Lippincott Williams & Wilkins: 337-350.

Duenas-Gonzalez, A; Lopez-Graniel, C; Gonzalez, A; et al. A phase II study of gemcitabine and cisplatin combination as induction chemotherapy for untreated locally advanced cervical carcinoma. *Ann Oncol*, 2001, 12, 541-547.

Eddy, GL; Bundy, BN; Creasman, WT; et al. Treatment of ("bulky") stage IB cervical cancer with or without neoadjuvant vincristine and cisplatin prior to radical hysterectomy and pelvic/para-aortic lymphadenectomy: a phase III trial of the gynecologic oncology group. *Gynecol Oncol*, 2007, 106, 362-369.

Eifel, PJ. Chemoradiotherapy in the treatment of cervical cancer. *Semin Radiat Oncol*, 2006, 16, 177-185.

Eifel, PJ; Berek, JS; Markman, MA. Cancer of the cervix, vagina, and vulva. In: DeVita VT, Lawrence TS, Rosenberg SA (Editors). Cancer principles and practice of oncology. 8th ed., 2008 Philadelphia, Pennsylvania: Lippincott Williams & Wilkins: 1496-1543.

Eifel, PJ; Morris, M; Wharton, JT; et al. The influence of tumor size and morphology on the outcome of patients with FIGO stage IB squamous cell carcinoma of the uterine cervix. *Int J Radiat Oncol Biol Phys*, 1994, 29, 9-16.

Ferlay, J; Shin, HR; Bray, F; Forman, D; Mathers, C; Parkin, DM. GLOBOCAN, 2008 v1.2, Cancer Incidence and Mortality Worldwide: IARC CancerBase No. 10 [Internet]. Lyon, France: International Agency for Research on Cancer: 2010. http://globocan.iarc.fr, accessed on 30/04/2013.

Fossati, R; Buda, A; Rulli, E; et al. Randomized trial of neoadjuvant chemotherapy followed by radical surgery in locally advanced squamous cell cervical carcinoma (LASCCC). Comparison of paclitaxel, cisplatin (TP), versus paclitaxel, ifosfamide, cisplatin (TIP): the SNAP-02 Italian Collaborative study., 2005 ASCO annual meeting proceedings. *J Clin Oncol*, 2005, 23(16S, Part I), 5026.

Gien, LT; Covens, A. Fertility-sparing options for early stage cervical cancer. *Gynecol Oncol*, 2010, 117(2), 350-7.

Gondi, V; Bentzen, SM; Sklenar, KL; Dunn, EF; Petereit, DG; Tannehill, SP; et al. Severe late toxicities following concomitant chemoradiotherapy compared to radiotherapy alone in cervical cancer: an inter-era analysis. *Int J Radiat Oncol Biol Phys*, 2012, 84(4), 973-82.

Gong, L; Lou, JY; Wang, P; et al. Clinical evaluation of neoadjuvant chemotherapy followed by radical surgery in the management of stage IB2-IIB cervical cancer. *Int J Gynaecol Obstet*, 2012, 117, 23-26.

Gonzalez-Martin, A; González-Cortijo, L; Carballo, N; et al. The current role of neoadjuvant chemotherapy in the management of cervical carcinoma. *Gynecol Oncol*, 2008, 110, S36-S40.

Jemal, A; Bray, F; Center, M; et al. Global Cancer Statistics. *CA Cancer J Clin*, 2011, 61, 69-90.

Katsumata, N; Yoshikawa, H; Hirakawa T; et al. Phase III randomized trial of neoadjuvant chemotherapy (NAC) followed by radical hysterectomy (RH) versus RH for bulky stage I/II cervical cancer (JCOG 0102). *J Clin Oncol*, 2006 ASCO Annual Meeting proceedings (Post-Meeting edition), 2006, 24(18S), 5013.

Keys, HM; Bundy, BN; Stehman, FB; et al. Cisplatin, radiation, and adjuvant hysterectomy compared with radiation and adjuvant hysterectomy for bulky stage IB cervical carcinoma. *N Engl J Med*, 1999, 340, 1154-1161.

Kigawa, J; Minagawa, Y; Ishihara, H; Itamochi, H; Kanamori, Y; Terawaka, N. The role of neoadjuvant intra-arterial infusion chemotherapy with cisplatin and bleomycin for locally advanced cervical cancer. *Am J Clin Oncol*, 1996, 19, 255-259.

Kjaer, SK; Frederiksen, K; Munk, C; et al. Long-term absolute risk of cervical intraepithelial neoplasia grade 3 or worse following human papillomavirus infection: role of persistence. *J Natl Inst*, 2010, 102, 1478-1488.

Kong, X; Moran, MS; Zhang, N; Haffty, B; Yang, Q. Meta-analysis confirms achieving pathological complete response after neoadjuvant chemotherapy predicts favourable prognosis for breast cancer patients. *Eur J Cancer*, 2011, 47(14), 2084-90

Kumar, L; Kaushal, R; Nandy, M; et al. chemotherapy followed by radiotherapy versus radiotherapy alone in locally advanced cervical cancer: a randomized study. *Gynecol Oncol*, 1994, 54, 307.

Leborgne, F; Leborgne, JH; Doldán, R; et al. Induction chemotherapy and radiotherapy of advanced cancer of the cervix: a pilot study and phase III randomized trial. *Int J Radiat Oncol Biol Phys*, 1997, 37, 343.

Lissoni, AA; Colombo, N; Pellegrino, A; et al. A phase II, randomized trial of neo-adjuvant chemotherapy comparing a three-drug combination of paclitaxel, ifosfamide, and cisplatin (TIP) versus paclitaxel and cisplatin (TP) followed by radical surgery in patients with locally advanced squamous cell cervical carcinoma: the Snap-02 Italian Collaborative Study. *Ann Oncol*, 2009, 20, 660-665.

Mohar, A; Frias-Mendivil, M. Epidemiology of cervical cancer. *Cancer Invest*, 2000, 18, 540-590.

Morris, M; Eifel, PJ; Lu, J; et al. Pelvic radiation with concurrent chemotherapy compared with pelvic and para-aortic radiation for high-risk cervical cancer. *N Engl J Med*, 1999, 340, 1137-1143.

Napolitano, U; Imperato, F; Mossa, B; et al. The role of neoadjuvant chemotherapy for squamous cell cervical cancer (Ib-IIIb): a long-term randomized trial. *Eur J Gynecol Oncol*, 2003, 24, 51-59.

Ozols, RF; Masuda, H; Hamilton, TC. Mechanisms of cross-resistance between radiation and antineoplastic drugs. *NCI Monogr*, 1988, 6, 159-165.

Pecorelli, S; Zigliani, L; Odicino, F. Revised FIGO staging for carcinoma of the cervix. *Int J Gynaecol Obstet*, 2009, 105, 107-108.

Peters, WA ; 3rd. Lui, PY; Barrett, RJ ; 2nd. et al. Concurrent chemotherapy and pelvic radiation therapy compared with pelvic radiation therapy alone as adjuvant therapy after radical surgery in high-risk early-stage cancer of the cervix. *J Clin Oncol*, 2000, 18, 1606-1613.

Randall, ME; Michael, H; Long, III, H; et al. Uterine cervix. In: Barakat RR, Markman M, Randall ME (editors). Principles and practice of gynecologic oncology 5th edition, 2009. Lippincott-Williams and Wilkins: 622-681.

Rodriguez, AC; Schiffman, M; Herrero, R; et al. Longitudinal study of human papillomavirus persistence and cervical intraepithelial neoplasia grade 2/3: critical role of duration of infection. *J Natl Cancer Inst*, 2010, 102, 315-324.

Rydzewska, L; Tierney, J; Vale, CL; et al. *Neoadjuvant chemotherapy plus surgery for cervical cancer (Review) Cochrane Database Sys Rev*, 2010, 1. CD 007406.

Rydzewska, L; Tierney, J; Vale, CL; et al. Neoadjuvant chemotherapy plus surgery versus surgery for cervical cancer (Review). *Cochrane Database Sys Rev*, 2012, 12. CD007406.

Rose, PG; Bundy, BN; Watkins, EB; et al. Concurrent cisplatin-based radiotherapy and chemotherapy for locally advanced cervical cancer. *N Engl J Med*, 1999, 340, 1144-1153.

Sananes, C; Giaroli, A; Soderini, A; et al. Neoadjuvant chemotherapy followed by radical hysterectomy and postoperative adjuvant chemotherapy in the treatment of carcinoma of the cervix uteri, long-term follow-up of a pilot study. *Eur J Gynaecol Oncol*, 1998, 19, 368-73.

Sardi, J; Giaroli, A; Sananes, C; et al. Randomized trial with neoadjuvant chemotherapy in stage IIIB squamous carcinoma cervix uteri: an unexpected therapeutic management. *Int J Gynecol Cancer*, 1996, 6, 85-93.

Sardi, J; Sananes, CE; Giaroli, AA; et al. Neoadjuvant chemotherapy in cervical carcinoma stage IIB: a randomized controlled trial. *Int J Gynecol Cancer*, 1998, 8, 441-450.

Sedlis, A; Bundy, BN; Rotman, MZ; et al. A randomized trial of pelvic radiation therapy versus no further therapy in selected patients with stage IB carcinoma of the cervix after radical hysterectomy and pelvic lymphadenectomy: a gynecologic oncology group study. *Gynecol Oncol*, 1999, 73, 177-183.

Shepherd, JH. Cervical cancer. *Best Pract Res Clin Obstet Gynaecol.*, 2012, 26(3), 293-309.

Souhami, L; Gil, R; Allan, S; et al. A randomized trial of chemotherapy followed by pelvic radiation therapy in stage IIIB carcinoma of the cervix. *Int J Radiat Oncol Biol Phys*, 1991, 9, 970.

Sundfør, K; Trope, CG; Hogberg, T; et al. Radiotherapy and neoadjuvant chemotherapy for cervical carcinoma: A randomized multicenter study for sequential cisplatin and 5-fluorouracil and radiotherapy in advanced cervical carcinoma stage 3B and 4A. *Cancer*, 1996, 77, 2371.

Sugiyama, T; Nishida, T; Kumagai, S; et al. Combination therapy with irinotecan and cisplatin as neoadjuvant chemotherapy in locally advanced cervical cancer. *Br J Cancer*, 1999, 81, 95-98.

Tattersall, MHN; Larvidhaya, V; Vootiprux, V; et al. Randomized trial of epirubicin and cisplatin chemotherapy followed by pelvic radiation in locally advanced cervical cancer. *Am J Clin Oncol*, 1995, 13, 444.

Tattersall, MHN; Ramirez, C; Coppleson, M. A randomized trial comparing platinum-based chemotherapy followed by radiotherapy alone in patients with locally advanced cervical cancer. *Int J Gynecol Cancer*, 1992, 2, 244.

Tierney, JF; Vale, C; Symonds, P. Concomitant and neoadjuvant chemotherapy for cervical cancer. *Clin Oncol*, 2008, 20, 401-416.

Thomas, GM. Improved treatment for cervical cancer-concurrent chemotherapy and radiotherapy. *N Engl J Med*, 1999, 340, 1198-1200.

Waggoner, SE. Cervical cancer. *Lancet*, 361, 2217-2225.

Whitney, CW; Sause, W; Bundy, BN; et al. Randomized comparison of fluorouracil plus cisplatin versus hydroxyurea as an adjunct to radiation therapy in stage IIB-IVA carcinoma of the cervix with negative para-aortic lymph nodes: a Gynecologic Oncology Group and Southwest Oncology Group study. *J Clin Oncol*, 1999, 17, 1339-1348.

Yin, M; Zhao, F; Lou, G; et al. The long-term efficacy of neoadjuvant chemotherapy followed by radical hysterectomy compared with radical surgery alone or concurrent chemoradiotherapy on locally advanced-stage cervical cancer. *Int J Gynecol Cancer*, 2011, 21, 92-99.

Zanaboni, F; Grijuela, B; Guidici, S; et al. Weekly topotecan and cisplatin (TOPOCIS) as neo-adjuvant chemotherapy for locally-advanced squamous cervical carcinoma: results of a phase II multicentric study. *Eur J Cancer*, 2013, 49, 1065-1072.

Zanetta, G; Lissoni, A; Pellegrino, A; et al. Neoadjuvant chemotherapy with cisplatin, ifosfamide and paclitaxel for locally advanced squamous-cell cervical cancer. *Ann Oncol*, 1998, 9, 977-980.

In: Cervical Cancer
Editor: Laurie Elit

ISBN: 978-1-62948-062-6
© 2014 Nova Science Publishers, Inc.

Chapter X

Surgical Staging of Advanced Cervical Cancer

Cristina Gonzalez-Benitez[1], Patricia Salas[1], Sara Iacoponi[1],
Javier De Santiago[1] and Ignacio Zapardiel[1]
[1]Gynecologic Oncology Unit, La Paz University Hospital, Madrid, Spain

Abstract

Cervical cancer is the second most frequent malignancy worldwide. Its incidence is even greater in developing countries. Prognosis is directly related to the tumor stage at diagnosis, and despite the efforts to make an early diagnosis, 25% of cases are diagnosed in advanced stages (FIGO stages IIB-IVA). For advanced disease the treatment consist in chemoradiation therapy, with or without radiotherapy at para-aortic region depending on nodal involvement. Cervical cancer staging is currently based on clinical characteristics. Although this strategy is usually valid in the assessment of local spread of the disease, it is not valid for node involvement or distant assessment. Clinical exam and primary tumor assessment is often the decisive factor to decide if a patient will undergo primary surgery or chemoradiation therapy. Scientific evidence suggests that surgical staging improves treatment adjustment in comparison to the underestimation caused by FIGO classification. Up to 26% of women without evidence of disease at the preoperative study show postoperative para-aortic involvement. This underestimation of tumor stage could modify treatment in more than 40% of patients, so a precise assessment of the spread of the disease is essential.

Five-year overall survival is 85-90% when node involvement is negative, dropping to 20-75% when it is positive. That's the reason why the presence of metastasis in lymph nodes is considered the most important prognostic factor for cervical cancer patients. The gold standard for assessment of node involvement is para-aortic lymphadenectomy.

The laparoscopic extraperitoneal para-aortic lymphadenectomy could be the most appropriate and less invasive way to staging advanced cervical cancer.

Keywords: Cervical cancer; para-aortic lymphadenectomy; extraperitoneal technique; advanced disease

Introduction

Cervical cancer is the world's second most frequent form of cancer. The incidence of cervical cancer is even greater in developing countries, where 80% of cases are diagnosed, and it is the primary cause of death due to cancer [1]. Prognosis is directly related to the tumor stage at diagnosis, and despite efforts for early diagnosis, 25% of cases are diagnosed at a late stage. Surgery is not part of the routine staging of advanced cervical cancer; rather, treatment consists of radio-chemotherapy for curative intent. Many studies have shown the need to look for extra-pelvic disease when planning appropriate therapy, with or without extending to the para-aortic region, according to its involvement.

Cervical cancer staging is currently based on clinical characteristics (FIGO). FIGO stages IIB-IVA are considered to be advanced cervical cancer [2]. Although this strategy is usually valid in the assessment of local spread of the disease, it is not valid for node involvement or distant assessment. Clinical examination and primary tumor assessment are often the decisive factors in deciding if a patient will undergo primary surgery or chemotherapy for curative intent. Already available scientific evidence posits that postsurgical staging improves treatment adjustment in comparison with the underestimation due to FIGO classification.

Cervical cancer dissemination is usually sequential, first the disease metastasizes to the pelvic nodes and then to the common iliac nodes and lastly to the para-aortic nodes. Dissemination in para-aortic nodes without pelvic involvement is, possible, but is extremely infrequent [3-5]. The possibility of lymphatic dissemination depends on the stage of the cancer (Table 1). We can see that in advanced stage cervical cancer, the probability of node involvement is high. The node involvement is an important prognosis factor, because the five-year survival depends on this. In patients with negative node involvement, this survival rate is 85-90% while in positive cases the survival rate decreases to 20-75%. Other prognostic factors in node positive cases are the size, number and localization of the nodes. For that reason the presence of metastasis in lymph nodes is considered the most important prognostic factor for cervical cancer patients [2].

Table 1. Nodal involvement according to FIGO stage

FIGO STAGE	Pelvic nodes + (%)	Paraaortic nodes + (%)
IA1	0	0
IA2	4.8	<1.0
IB	16	2
IIA	25	11
III	45	30
IVA	55	40

Table 2. Survival according to staging technique

	SURGICAL STAGING	CLINICAL STAGING
4-years survival	49 %	36 %
GLOBAL survival	54 %	40 %

Due to all these factors it is very important to know of the presence of para-aortic metastasis in advanced cervical cancer, and we can carry out the study of this node through surgery (para-aortic lymphadenectomy) or with an imaging test.

Although the FIGO classification does not include the radiologic or histologic evaluation of nodes, approximately 26% of women without disease evidence in the presurgical assessment show para-aortic involvement if surgically staged. This underestimation of the tumor stage could modify the treatment of up to 40% of patients and this could change the overall and 4-year survival rate [3, 7] (Table 2). Thus, we suggest, an assessment of the spread of the disease, expecially the nodal disease, is essential.

Imaging Tests

MRI, CT and PET scans are the most used tests, each having different advantages and disadvantages. CT and MRI are usually used to evaluate the size of the cervix, the evaluation of the pelvic and para-aortic nodes and distant assessment. Both tests can detect nodes larger than 1cm, and these nodes are considered pathological. However these nodes can simply be hyperplasic and nodes smaller than these could be metastasic [8]. The sensitivity and specificity of CT and MRI for node evaluation are 64.7 vs 70.6% and 96.6 vs 89.9% [9]. However MRI is more accurate than CT for the study of parametrium, tumor size and bladder and rectal disease. In conclusion, both tests are similar for node false positive rates, but MRI is more accurate for distant assessment [10].

Another test we can use is FDG-PET, which has demonstrated a higher detection of retroperitoneal nodes than CT and MRI [8]. Recently, PET has emerged as a technique that allows the assessment of lymph node involvement in patients with uterine cervix carcinoma and does not present the inconvenience of MRI regarding the radiation therapy treatment planning.

Since PET is based on physiological processes of cell metabolic activity, it seems more effective than a CT scan and MRI for the detection of metastasis in the retroperitoneal area, showing a greater sensitivity and specificity than MRI in the detection of adenopathies. There are various studies that have compared PET with CT and MRI. For example Sugawara et al. found sensitivity for pelvic and para-aortic nodes to be 86% with PET, and 57% with CT (11). Choi et al. compared the precision of PET scan with MRI in the detection of node metastasis and PET scan was more precise (72.6% vs 85.1%).

On the other hand, both PET and CT scans allowed the assessment of the response to the treatment, but PET scan also seemed to be correlated to disease-free survival and overall survival. In fact, some authors consider PET scan more useful in prognosis than in the evaluation of lymph node involvement.

In conclusion, the use of PET/CT has been demonstrated to be better than CT and MRI for detecting metastatic lymph nodes in patients with cervical cancer. Nonetheless, given its high cost and low availability only in third-level centres, its use as a routine screen in the study of cervical cancer spread may be questioned.

Para-Aortic Lymphadenectomy

The gold standard for the assessment of node involvement is para-aortic lymphadenectomy. This para-aortic lymphadenectomy can be low or high. The low lymphadenectomy consists of the resection of lymph tissue from the common iliac artery to the inferior mesenteric artery.

It should include the lymph tissue above the inferior cava vein, between the aorta and the cava vein, above the aorta and on the left para-aortic space, until the left ureter. High lymphadenectomy retrieves nodes up to the renal vessels. If there is nodal involvement, subsequent the radiotherapy treatment should include para-aortic field. There is no evidence that recommends this side of radiotherapy as profilactic [12].

Surgical staging is the most accurate technique to determine nodal involvement. It has been demonstrated that results are even better than when assessment is done by diagnostic imaging tests [13]. Approximately 26% of women without distant disease in the presurgical study have para-aortic disease in surgical staging, and in this case para-aortic field radiotherapy will be offered [6].

Lymph node debulking has demonstrated a therapeutic benefit due to the resection of macroscopic nodes, and is associated with a survival rate of 50%. This rate of survival is similar for women with microscopic nodes disease and better than for women with macroscopic affectation who have not had the nodes removed [14]. Another study also suggest that lymph node debulking improves the results of future treatment with chemoradiation therapy [15].

Lymphadenectomy might further present a therapeutic role by the removal of lymph nodes with micrometastases, in around 8.3% of the cases. These metastases are noticeable only with ultra-staging by measuring serial sections and using immunohistochemistry, but its clinical role is uncertain [16].

1. Route of Surgery

Over the past few decades, several surgical approaches have been attempted in order to reduce the morbidity of lymphadenectomy. The para-aortic lymphadenectomy approach can be by laparotomy or laparoscopy and the latter can be transperitoneal or extraperitoneal. The laparoscopic extraperitoneal para-aortic lymphadenectomy is the most appropriate way of staging the advanced cervical cancer.

The laparoscopic extraperitoneal approach is associated with less risk of adherences, and due to this, we will have less radiation enteritis and less visceral and vessel lesions. Furthermore, the access to vessels is faster and is not modified by previous abdominal surgery. Another advantage is the lower incidence of paralytic ileus.

1.1. Laparotomy

Lymphadenectomy is a fundamental step of the surgical treatment for cervical carcinoma. Over the past few years, different surgical approaches have been described to perform lymphadenectomy including transperitoneal or extraperitoneal laparotomy and, more recently, the laparoscopic approach has also been introduced. The use of laparoscopy for gynecologic procedures has expanded rapidly: improvements in instrumentation and video technology have allowed the surgeon to perform more complex and major operations through laparoscopy. Recently, several papers have been published about laparoscopic lymphadenectomy in gynecologic malignancies in an effort to determine whether or not laparoscopic lymphadenectomy is comparable to those performed via laparotomy [17].

The first surgical stagings were performed by transperitoneal laparotomy and despite improvements in the assessment of the extent of disease; they were associated with an increased morbidity. The main complications were associated with the surgical procedure or as a result of adhesions associated with the effects of subsequent radiotherapy [16].

The Pfannenstiel incision allowed for improved exposure to bilateral para-aortic and specifically the pelvic lymph node chain; the ability to resect grossly positive lymph nodes that is equivalent to vertical incisions; potentially less risk of damage to epigastric arteries than with paramedian incision and potentially less risk of rectus muscle paralysis as compared to paramedian incisions. The main disadvantage of the Pfannenstiel incision is that it is in the radiation field (18).

1.2. Laparoscopy

1.2.1. General Surgical Technique

Para-aortic lymph node dissection has traditionally been performed through a laparotomy but actually can also be performed laparoscopically through either a transperitoneal or a retroperitoneal approach.

Transperitoneal approach: The patient is placed in a low lithotomy position with their legs abducted and their arms positioned by their side. The monitor is placed at the head on the patient's right while the operator stands between the patient's legs. Five trocars are placed: a 10mm optical trocar is placed in the umbilical position, two 5mm trocars are placed in the right and left lower quadrants 3cm medial to the anterior iliac crest, and a third in the left flank and a 10mm trocar is placed in the low midline suprapubically.

The initial phase is an exploration of the abdominal cavity. The posterior peritoneum is opened above the point where the right ureter crosses the iliac vessels at the origin of the iliac bifurcation; lymph node dissection is performed along the common iliac vessels up to the anterior surface of the aorta [19].

Retroperitoneal approach: This technique always starts with transperitoneal laparoscopy, placing a 10mm trocar in the umbilicus to inspect the peritoneal cavity. The patient is placed in the dorsal decubitus position, the surgeon to the left of patient and the assistant to the left of the surgeon with the monitor to the right of patient. A 15mm incision is performed at the left MacBurney point, 3cm medial to the left anterior superior iliac spine. Skin, subcutaneous fat, fascia and muscles are opened preserving the peritoneum. The surgeon introduces his right forefinger into the incision to develop the extraperitoneal space under the control of transperitoneal laparoscopy. Digital dissection is performed caudally until identification of the anterior surface of the psoas muscle to the level of the iliac crest. After the preparation of the preperitoneal space, a 10mm trocar (Hasson) is introduced and the preperitoneal space is insufflated with a 12mmHg pressure. Two additional trocars are introduced in the midaxillary line in the preperitoneal space. A 5mm trocar is placed above the iliac crest and a 10 mm trocar just below the ribs. The left ureter is identified on the anterior surface of psoas muscles and is retracted with peritoneum. The dissection continues medially and cranially until the identification of the left common iliac artery, the aorta, the inferior mesenteric artery and the left renal vein [20].

1.2.2. Single-Port Extraperitoneal Technique

Although laparoscopic surgery has reduced the mortality directly related to surgery, there are other risks associated with the surgery (blood loss, infection, iatrogenic damage to the viscera, hernias and cosmetic damage). The latest advances in technical expertise and surgical instruments have allowed previously minimally invasive surgery to become even less invasive. This has led to the development of a number of surgical techniques such as laparoscopic-endoscopic single-site surgery (LESS). The advances in optics, instrumentation, and surgical expertise over the last decade have expanded and confirmed the advantages of minimally invasive surgery in the treatment of many gynecologic malignancies.

1.2.3. Transperitoneal Approach

A single 2-3cm vertical incision is made at the base of the umbilicus via an open Hasson approach. A multichannel single port device is positioned through the incision. The abdomen is insufflated with 15 mmHg of carbon dioxine gas and a 5mm 30-degree laparoscope is inserted through the most cephalad port. The patient is placed in the steep Trendelenburg. The descending colon is either dissected and mobilized medially through the white line of Told or left in situ for a transmesenteric approach to the aorta. Nodal tissue is dissected away from the aorta and vena cava from the aortic bifurcation to the left renal vein.

1.2.4. Extraperitoneal Approach

For the extraperitoneal approach, only one 3-4cm incision is necessary on the patient's left side between the iliac crest and the last rib. The skin, fascia, transverse muscles, and deep fascia are incised, with care taken not to open the peritoneum. The landmarks for finger dissection are well-known and include iliac fossa, the psoas muscle and, more medially, the left common iliac artery. When the dissection is complete, the single port dispositive is introduced into the extraperitoneal space. The peritoneal cavity is deflated, whereas the extraperitoneal space is inflated with carbon dioxide up to a maximum pressure of 10 mmHg. The procedure is conducted using the same landmarks of conventional laparoscopy. At the end of the procedure a marsupialization of the peritoneum is performed to reduce the risk of symptomatic lymphocele [21]. Several studies have demonstrated that laparoscopic approaches to various gynecologic oncology conditions, particularly for cervical cancer are feasible and result in shorter hospital stays, improved quality of life and a surgical and oncologic outcome comparable to abdominal staging [22, 23]. Limited data have been published about the clinical benefits of single porto versus conventional multi-port laparoscopy, including better cosmesis from a relatively hidden umbilical scar and improved postoperative pain management [24]. Curcillo et al. report that after a 297 cases of single-port access cholecystectomy, no umbilical site hernias have been reported [25].

2. Surgery Complications

2.1. Vascular Complications

Vascular complications are the most frequent perioperative complications. They represent 1-10% depending on the series, with an overall average between 0.5 and 5%. They are located preferentially at the external iliac vein, in the junction between the hypogastric artery and external iliac artery and at the umbilical artery. Twenty-five percent of vascular wounds are caused by the introduction of the trocars, especially the umbilical trocar [26]. There is evidence that the open technique protects from vascular lesions when its compared with a Veress needle technique, therefore the question of which technique for initial port placement is safest has not been definitively answered to date.

Vascular complications are higher in paraaortic lymphadenectomy. However, contrary to what was previously described, the extraperitoneal approach is not correlated with a greater conversion rate to laparotomy due to difficult to control bleeding (vena cava inferior mesenteric artery) and does not influence the vascular complications rate [26].

2.2. Urological Complications

The most common urological injuries are bladder perforation, followed by fistula, ligation and section of the ureter and these can be thermal or mechanical. Bladder injuries are two to three times more common than ureteral injuries. Ureteral wounds represent 0.9% to 2.6% of intraoperative complications [22] depending on the series. Most often they are located at the ureter - common iliac artery junction. Their intraoperative diagnosis is indispensable to decrease the morbidity associated with this type of complication, and allows repair by laparoscopy [26].

2.3. Visceral Injuries

Visceral complications represent 0.6% to 1.6% of laparoscopic lymphadenectomy complications. Intraoperative complications occur most often at the beginning of the operative procedure: the introduction of the umbilical trocar needle Veress. They are mostly located in the small intestine, colon and omentum, in order of frequency. The second etiology of visceral wounds is the use of bipolar current and monopolar current. The postoperative course is uneventful. The difficulty of visceral complications intraoperatively is the fact that they go unnoticed in two thirds of cases and intraoperative identification is essential to reduce morbidity [26].

2.4. Nerve Complications

Nerve complications are rare. They are more often associated with bipolar coagulation or monopolar accidents (complete transaction of the nerve or neuralgia) and usually are treat with anti-inflammatory drugs and physiotherapy. The most commonly affected nerve is the obturator nerve [26]. The obturator nerve arises from the anterior division of the second, third, and fourth lumbar nerves; enters the pelvis through the psoas muscle; and runs along the lateral pelvic wall in the obturator fossa to exit the pelvis through the obturator foramen along with the obturator vessels. It is a motor nerve to the adductor muscles of the thigh and is the only motor nerve that arises from the lumbar plexus without innervating any of the pelvic structures. Damage to the obturator nerve produces not only motor impairment to the adductor muscles but also sensory loss along the medial aspect of the thigh.

2.5. Lymphatic Complications

The lymphoceles are the most frequent postoperative complications. Their incidence in pelvic and para-aortic lymphadenectomy range from 0.8% to 58% depending on the series, but they are generally a rare complication (less than 5% of cases): superinfection, obstructive uropathy, venous compression, digestive fistula, lymphedema of the lower limb and external genitalia.

The number of lymph nodes and lymph node invasions are not correlated to the rate of seromas unlike some series which showed that from an average of 12 pelvic lymph nodes the risk of seroma was increased. The extraperitoneal approach is responsible for a higher rate of seroma. This can be explained by the fact that the lymphatic system is the most important, and by the lack of lymph drainage or absorption in the peritoneal cavity. In addition, chylous lymphoceles are mostly found by the extraperitoneal approach. The closure of the peritoneum increases the rate of seroma. Also the association with adjuvant-radiochemotherapy increases the number of seromas. Indeed, radiotherapy removes a number of collateral drainage channels. Even if lymphoceles remains one of the most common complications of lymphadenectomy by laparoscopic, the rate is lower than laparotomy. This can be explained by the fact that there are less postoperative adhesions after laparoscopy [26].

2.6. Gastrointestinal Complications

Aside from common side-effects such as hemorrhage, deep vein thrombosis, embolism, lymphocele and lymphorrea, para-aortic lymphadenectomy is also associated with a high risk of postoperative gastrointestinal (GI) problems, mainly consisting of nausea and vom iting. Although GI side-effects can usually be successfully and conservatively managed, they can cause a significant increase of the median length of hospital stays and a notable readmission rate. In both cases, a significant increase of pathology-related costs and a reduction of the patients' quality of life are probable results. Two main theories have been proposed in order to explain the occurrence of GI symptoms in patients who underwent para-aortic lymphadenectomy: I) the anatomical disruption of the para-aortic autonomic fibers innervating the bowel during the dissection of aortic lymph nodes, and II) the surgical trauma specifically related to extensive intestinal mobilization and/or manipulation, length of the operation, blood loss, and such.

Conclusion

The para-aortic lymph node assessment should be systematic, and, if possible, histologic, with para-aortic lymphadenectomy. If this option is not possible we would have to use imaging testing. MRI, CT and PET are the most used tests, PET/CT has been demonstrated to be better than CT and MRI for detecting metastatic lymph nodes in patients with cervical cancer. Nonetheless, given its high cost and availability only in level three centres, its use as a routine screen in the study of cervical cancer spread may be questioned.

The laparoscopic extraperitoneal para-aortic lymphadenectomy is the most appropriate way of staging the advanced cervical cancer. The laparoscopic extraperitoneal approach is associated with less risk of adherences, and due to this, we will have less radiation enteritis and less visceral and vessel lesions. Furthermore, the access to vessels is faster and is not modified by previous abdominal surgery. Another advantage is the lower incidence of paralytic ileus.

References

[1]   Holschneider C. H. Invasive cervical cancer: Epidemiology, clinical features, and diagnosis. UpToDate, Noviembre 2008.

[2]   FIGO Committee on Gynecologic Oncology. Revised FIGO staging for carcinoma of the vulva, cervix, and endometrium. *International Journal of Gynecology and Obstetrics* 2009; 105:103–104.

[3]   Benedetti-Panici P., Maneschi F., Scambia G., et al.: Lymphatic spread of cervical cáncer: An anatomical and pathological study based on 225 radical hysterectomies with systematic pelvic and aortic lymphadenectomy. *Gynecol. Oncol.* 1996;62:19–24.

[4]   Sakuragi N., Satoh C., Takeda N., et al.: distribution pattern of pelvic and paraaortic lymph node metastasis in patients with stages IB, IIA and IIB cervical carcinoma treated with radical hysterectomy. *Cancer* 1999; 85:1547 – 1554.

[5]   Siu S. S. N., Cheung T. H., Lo K. W. K., et al.: Is common iliac lymph node dissection necessary in early stage cervical carcinoma? *Gynecol. Oncol.* 2006; 103:58 – 61.

[6]   Lai C. H., Huang K. G., Hong J. H., Lee C. L., Chou H. H., Chang T. C., Hsueh S., Huang H. J., Ng K. K., Tsai C. S. Randomized trial of surgical staging (extraperitoneal or laparoscopic) versus clinical staging in locally advanced cervical cancer. *Gynecol. Oncol.* 2003 Apr; 89(1):160-7.

[7]   Gold M. A., Tian C., Whitney C. W., et al. Surgical versus radiographic determination of para-aortic lymph node metastases before chemoradiation for locally advanced cervical carcinoma. *Cancer* 2008May 1;112(9):1954-63.

[8]   Gien L. T., Covens A. Lymph Node Assessment in Cervical Cancer: Prognostic and Therapeutic Implications. *Journal of Surgical Oncology* 2009; 99:242–247.

[9]   Yang W. T., Lam W. W., Yu M. Y., et al.: Comparison of dynamic helical CT and dynamic MR imaging in the evaluation of pelvic lymph nodes in cervical carcinoma. *Am. J. Roentgenol.* 2000;175: 759 – 766.

[10]   Bipat S., Glas A. S., Van Der Velden J., Zwinderman A. H., Bossuyt P. M., Stoker J. Review. Computed tomography and magnetic resonance imaging in staging of uterine cervical carcinoma: a systematic review. *Gynecol. Oncol.* 2003 Oct; 91(1):59-66.

[11]   Sugawara Y., Eisbruch A., Kosud S., et al.: Evaluation of FDG-PET in patients with cervical cancer. *J. Nucl. Med.* 1999; 40:1125 – 1131.

[12]   Rotman M., Pajak T. F., Chol K., Clery M. Et al. Prophylactic extended-field irradiation of para-aortic nodes in stages IIB and Bulky IB-IIA cervical carcinoma. *Ten years treatement results of RTOG 79-20 Jama* 1995; 274:387-393.

[13] Hertel H., Köhler C., Elhawary T., et al. Laparoscopic staging compared with imaging techniques

[14] Cosin J. A., Fowler J. M., Chen M. D., et al. Pretreatment surgical staging of patients with cervical carcinoma

[15] Marnitz S., Köhler C., Roth C., et al. Is there a benefit of pretreatment laparoscopic transperitoneal surgical staging in patients with advanced cervical cancer

[16] Zanvettor P. H., Filho D. F., Neves A. R., Amorim M. J., Medeiros SM, Laranjeiras LC, Morais JA, Araujo IO, Barbosa HS.Laparoscopic surgical staging of locally advanced cervix. *Gynecol. Oncol.* 2011; 120(3):358-361.

[17] Benedetti-Panici P., Plotti F., Zullo M. A., Muzii L., Manci N., Palaia I., Ruggiero A., Angioli R. Pelvic lymphadenectomy for cervical carcinoma *Gynecol. Oncol.* 2006; 103(3):859-864.

[18] Moore K. N., Gold M. A., McMeekin D. S., Walker J. L., Rutledge T., Zorn K. K. Extraperitoneal para-aortic lymph. *Gynecol. Oncol.* 2008; 108(3):466-471.

[19] Ballester M., Chereau E., Werkoff G., Zilberman S., Darai E., Rouzier R. Laparoscopic lumbo-aortic lymph node dissection. *Journal of visceral surgery* 2010; 148:e273-e278.

[20] Dargent D., Ansquer Y., Mathevet P. Technical development and results of left extraperitoneal laparoscopic paraaortic lymphadenectomy for cervical cancer. *Gynecol. Oncol.* 2000; 77:87-92.

[21] Lambaudie E., Cannone F., Bannier M. et al. Laparoscopic extraperitoneal aortic dissection : does single-port surgery offer the same possibilities as conventional laparoscopy' *Surg. Endosc.* 2012; 26: 1920-1923.

[22] Escobar P., fader A., Rasool N. et al.Single-port Laparoscopic pelvic and para-aortic lymph node sampling or lymphadenectomy *Int. J. Gynecological Cancer* 2010; 20 (7):1268-1273.

[23] Childers J., Surwit E., Tran A., et al. Laparoscopic para-aortic lymphadenectomy in gynecologic malignancies. *Obstet. Gynecol.*1993;82:741-747.

[24] Kim T. J., Lee Y. Y., Chan H. H., et al. Single port-access laparoscopic-assisted vaginal hysterectomy: a comparison of perioperative outcomes. *Surg. Endosc.* 2010; 24 (9): 2248-52.

[25] Curcillo P. G. 2nd, Wu A. S., Podolsky E. R., et al. Single-port access cholecystectomy: a multi-institutional report of the first 297 cases. *Surg. Endosc.* 2010 24 (8):1854-60.

[26] G. Cartron. E. Leblanc, G. Ferron, P. Martel, F. Narducci, D. Querleu. Complications of laparoscopic lymphadenectomy in gynaecologic oncology. A series of 1102 procedures in 915 patients. *Gynécologie Obstétrique and Fertilité* 2005; 33:304–314.

In: Cervical Cancer
Editor: Laurie Elit

ISBN: 978-1-62948-062-6
© 2014 Nova Science Publishers, Inc.

Chapter XI

Cervical Carcinoma Metastatic to the Para-Aortic Lymph Node Chain

Mark Ranck, Gene-Fu Liu and Yasmin Hasan*
University of Chicago Department of Radiation and Cellular Oncology,
Chicago, IL, US

Abstract

In 2011, there were 12,000 cases of cervical carcinoma in the US. Despite advances in vaccine prophylaxis and the success of screening programs, cervical cancer will remain a significant cause of morbidity and mortality for many years to come.

Contemporaneously with an understanding of HPV as etiologic, the treatment of cervical cancer has also evolved, most dramatically with the use of concurrent chemoradiation for locally-advanced disease, where a survival benefit has been demonstrated. Additionally, advances in medical imaging have affected cancer management in many disease sites. Currently, positron emission tomography (PET) is recommended as part of the initial workup for cervical cancer of stage IB1 or greater. Consequently, many patients are now found with asymptomatic involvement of the paraaortic lymph node (PA-LN) chain. This is considered metastatic disease based on FIGO staging, but long term survival can be achieved with appropriate therapy. Herein we review the current status of PA-LN positive cervical carcinoma and explore possibilities for future study.

Keywords: Cervical cancer, para-aortic node metastases, PET scan

Introduction

Cervical cancer staging classically relies upon the FIGO system [1], which does not utilize computerized tomography (CT), magnetic resonance imaging (MRI), or positron emission tomography (PET). While these modalities facilitate staging and promote uniformity in reporting outcomes in developing countries where disease prevalence is highest, the FIGO system may suboptimally define disease extent and limit therapeutic options.

Integrating advanced imaging modalities into cervical cancer management may further improve patient outcomes by more accurately defining locoregional and metastatic disease. In particular, detection of para-aortic lymph node (PALN) metastases may identify patients requiring extended field radiotherapy (EFRT). Currently, the National Comprehensive Cancer Network (NCCN) recommends CT or PET-CT as part of the initial evaluation of patients with cervical cancer greater than stage IB1 [2]. With increased adoption of advanced imaging, clinically occult PALN metastases may be more often detected. However, reconciling such data gained from CT or PET-CT with FIGO staging can be problematic. PALN involvement is considered distant disease by FIGO (stage IVB), yet long term survival can be achieved in these patients with appropriate therapy [3, 4]. Herein we review the current management of patients with PALN positive cervical carcinoma and explore possibilities for future study.

Para-Aortic Lymph Node Involvement: Prevalence and Prognosis

Cervical cancer is thought to spread via orderly lymphatic dissemination. Extension can occur laterally along the uterine artery to the external iliac lymph nodes, posterolaterally behind the uterus to the internal iliac lymph nodes or posteriorly to involve the common iliac and presacral lymph nodes. A retrospective surgical series from Austria evaluated 619 patients with Ib1 to IIB cervical carcinoma who underwent hysterectomy and lymph node dissection in an attempt to identify the first site of nodal metastasis [5]. One hundred and twenty patients were found to have at least one involved lymph node with the most common sites being external iliac (43%), obturator (26%), and parametrial (21%). Further dissemination can then involve the PALN chain, though isolated PALN metastases without pelvic involvement is rare (1%).

The likelihood of PALN involvement has been shown to increase with increasing primary tumor stage, and perhaps grade. Much of this data comes from the GOG experience of extended lymph node dissections that often included PALN evaluation as part of initial staging or therapy [6]. This can be considered the gold standard of PALN evaluation as patients underwent surgical exploration through a transabdominal approach prior to definitive therapy and provides us with the most accurate data regarding the risk of PALN involvement as it relates to stage. This data is presented in Table 1. For patients with stage IIA to IIIB disease, this risk is approximately 30% and cannot be considered trivial.

Furthermore, PALN involvement has been shown to be the most significant prognostic factor for disease recurrence [7]. Over 600 patients from 3 GOG trials were compiled in an effort to identify patient and tumor characteristics associated with disease progression. Multi-variable analysis demonstrated that patient age, performance status, tumor size, and lymph node status were significantly associated with progression-free interval (PFI) and survival. Of these variables, lymph node status was found to be most predictive of PFI and there was a stepwise increase in the relative risk (RR) of disease progression with increasing lymph node extension. For pelvic lymph node (PLN) involvement only, the RR was 1.9 as compared to that of node negative patients. For PALN involvement, the RR was 11.0, overwhelming all other variables studied. Furthermore, the patterns of failure differ as patients with PALN involvement are as likely to fail distantly as in the pelvis, and their overall survival is comparatively poor [8].

Table 1. Risk of para-aortic lymph node involvement by stage (GOG 19) [6]

By clinical stage			
Clinical stage	No. of patients with positive para-aortic lymph nodes	No. of patients evaluated	%
IB	8	143	5.6
IIA	4	22	18.2
IIB	19	58	32.8
IIIA	0	2	0
IIIB	19	61	31.1
IVA	1	3	33.3
By histology			
Histologic grade	No. of patients with positive para-aortic lymph nodes	No. of patients evaluated	%
1	6	37	16.2
2	29	172	16.9
3	16	81	19.8

Evaluation of the Para-Aortic Lymph Node Chain

Surgical Staging

As discussed, surgical staging provides the most accurate method of determining lymph node involvement [5, 6]. However, this approach is invasive and can be associated with significant morbidity. Traditionally, a transabdominal approach has been performed and potential morbidities include ureteral injury, bleeding, fistula formation, or intestinal obstruction, though the likelihood of any of these events remains low (<3%). Wound infection or dehiscence are slightly more frequent (8%), while perioperative mortality remains rare [6]. Postoperative adhesions are the most commonly observed complication and have been documented to occur in approximately 60% of patients following laparotomy [9].

A more common and less invasive surgical approach employs the use of laparoscopy to evaluate PALN and PLN. A German series of 84 patients who underwent laparoscopy to identify and localize suspicious lymph nodes confirmed the ability of laparoscopic characteristics to accurately identify abnormal lymph nodes [10]. All patients underwent subsequent transabdominal para-aortic lymphadenectomy, and these results were compared to the earlier laparoscopic assessment. The sensitivity of laparoscopy for identifying PALN and PLN metastases was 92.3%. When combined with frozen section, all patients with involved nodes were correctly identified, and this impacted the patient's primary therapy 15.4% of the time. While considered a significant improvement over transabdominal evaluation, this technique remains invasive and recent efforts have focused on developing non-invasive technologies.

Radiographic and Morphologic Imaging

Imaging may allow accurate PALN evaluation, while avoiding surgical morbidity. Early methods included lymphangiogram (LAG), whereby cannulation of the lymphatic ducts allowed the injection of contrast agents directly into the lymph system. Deviation or obstruction of lymphatic channels and lymph node filling defects are considered positive results. This technique has been compared to cross-sectional radiographic imaging and ultrasonic evaluation in the determination of PALN status [11]. GOG 63 enrolled 323 patients who completed standard FIGO staging and then went on to undergo LAG, CT, and ultrasound of the aortic region (US). All positive findings were confirmed with fine needle aspiration (FNA) or selective para-aortic lymphadenectomy; PALN dissection was mandated for patients with negative LAG, CT, or US. In total, 264 patients were evaluable and most were stage IIB (63%) and III (34%). The overall incidence of PALN involvement was 21% for stage IIB and 31% for stage III. The sensitivities and specificities of these imaging modalities are displayed in Table 2. LAG was found to be the most sensitive technique and had a low false negative rate of 6%; implying that a negative LAG could be considered sufficient to eliminate the need for surgical PALN staging. It is important to realize that the quality of CT scans in this study is inferior to those obtained with modern techniques as they were obtained in 1cm intervals. Modern CT scanners commonly employ 2-5 mm slice thicknesses and may be a more sensitive way to evaluate for lymph node involvement. MRI has also been used to evaluate locoregional nodal involvement but its predominant indication has been in the evaluation of the primary tumor and the extent of local invasion given its superior soft tissue resolution [12]. More recently, a meta-analysis of 17 studies was undertaken to compare the utility of LAG, CT and MRI for evaluation of lymph node involvement in cervical cancer [13]. All three modalities performed similarly in the detection of lymph node metastasis although there was a trend to favor MR imaging. As CT and MRI are less invasive and also allow assessment of the primary tumor, they are felt to be the favored adjunctive modalities to clinical evaluation.

Table 2. Comparison of extended diagnostic modalities of para-aortic lymph nodes (GOG 63) [11]

Technique	Sensitivity	Specificity
Lymphangiogram	79%	73%
Computed tomography	34%	96%
Ultrasound	19%	99%

Metabolic Imaging

The value of PET has been well documented across multiple disease sites [14-16]. Its impact on cervical cancer has been similarly demonstrated for both initial staging and prediction of outcomes after definitive therapy [17, 18]. Initial efforts to evaluate this imaging modality in cervical cancer patients included a surgicopathologic study of 32 patients conducted by the GOG to determine the value of PET in ascertaining PALN status [19]. Patients without evidence of extra-pelvic disease on CT of the abdomen and pelvis underwent

PET followed by lymphadenectomy. Eight patients were found to have PALN involvement on surgical staging, 6 of whom were correctly identified with the use of PET. The sensitivity and specificity of PET was determined to be 75% and 92%, respectively, yielding a positive predictive value of 75% and a negative predictive value of 92%.

Furthermore, PET has been shown to better prognosticate outcomes when compared to CT in patients treated with definitive concurrent chemoradiotherapy [20]. A retrospective series from Washington University evaluated 101 patients with stage Ia-IVb cervical carcinoma. CT was able to identify abnormal PALN in 7%, while PET identified PALN abnormalities in 21%. The 2 year progression free survival (PFS) estimate was 64% if both imaging studies were negative but only 18% if positive on PET only. This poor PFS was likely due to the omission of treatment directed to the para-aortic chain in 10 of 14 patients with PET only PALN involvement.

More recently, metabolic imaging has been combined with cross-sectional imaging to generate PET/CT with improved spatial resolution. The sensitivities and specificities of this imaging modality can be somewhat variable depending on the stage of the disease but remain in a similar range as detailed above [17, 21, 22]. However, a significant advantage is that this enhanced spatial resolution allows for the tailoring of radiation delivery to target areas of gross disease.

Based on the proven utility of PET, the NCCN recommends PET-CT or CT imaging for newly diagnosed cervical cancer of Stage IB1 or greater [2]. Consequently, it is expected that more patients will be found to have clinically occult PALN involvement, and the management of such patients will become a more common clinical dilemma.

Extended Field Radiotherapy: Treatment of the Para-Aortic Nodal Chain

Elective Irradiation of the Para-Aortic Lymph Node Chain

Prior to the development of imaging modalities to better identify PALN metastases, RTOG 79-20 investigated the use of prophylactic extended field radiation therapy (EFRT) in patients felt to be at high risk for PALN involvement [23, 24]. This included patients with FIGO IB or IIA cervical cancer of at least 4cm in size who were randomized to pelvic radiation or pelvic plus extended field radiation to cover the PALN chain. Traditional cervical cancer radiation fields encompass the whole pelvis with the superior border placed at the interspace between the L4 and L5 vertebral bodies, an anatomical surrogate for the bifurcation of the aorta into the common iliac vessels that is considered the upper extent of the PLN. Forty to 50 Gy in 1.6 to 1.8 Gy daily fractions was delivered to this volume in the standard pelvic field arm. Patients randomized to EFRT underwent similar treatment to the pelvis but had the superior border of the radiation field raised to include the PALN chain. Forty-four to 45 Gy in 1.6 to 1.8 Gy/day fractions was delivered in this manner. In both groups, external beam treatment was followed by intracavitary brachytherapy to provide an additional 30 to 40 Gy prescribed to Point A. No chemotherapy was administered in this trial. Three hundred and sixty seven patients were randomized and an overall survival benefit was demonstrated for extended field irradiation over pelvic radiation for these high risk patients.

Ten year overall survival (OS) was 55% with EFRT and 44% with standard pelvic fields (p=.02). This supports a beneficial role for PAN directed therapy in patients with a high likelihood of harboring occult disease.

The RTOG 90-01 randomized trial then compared the benefit of elective PALN irradiation versus concurrent chemotherapy in those at high risk of PALN involvement (either FIGO IIB-IVA or IB-IIA with tumors > 5cm or PLN involvement; patients with PALN involvement detected by LAG or retroperitoneal surgical exploration were excluded) [25]. Patients were randomized to EFRT versus pelvis RT concurrent with bolus cisplatin and 5-fluorouracil (5-FU) [26]. Forty five Gy in 1.8 Gy per day fractions of external beam RT was delivered to both groups, followed by a brachytherapy boost to a cumulative dose of 85 Gy to point A. At 8 years, outcomes favored the chemoradiotherapy arm, which provided a decrease in locoregional failure (18% v. 35%, p<.0001), and an increase in disease-free survival (61% v. 36%, p<.0001) and overall survival (67% v. 41%, p<.0001). The para-aortic failure rate was similar for the concurrent chemoradiation and EFRT alone arms (9% vs. 4%, respectively, p=.15). Of particular interest, the 8-year non-para-aortic distant failure rate was significantly reduced with the addition of chemotherapy (20% v. 35%, p=.0013) highlighting the systemic effect of bolus cisplatin chemotherapy.

Though it remains possible that the combination of EFRT with concurrent chemotherapy may further improve outcomes, its role has not been evaluated in a randomized trial and combining the two aggressive strategies comes at the cost of considerable toxicity [4, 27]. As such, the general consensus is that prophylactic extended-field chemoradiotherapy with conventional radiation techniques is not recommended. This is especially true with modern imaging that can rule out PALN involvement with greater confidence.

Therapeutic Irradiation of the Para-Aortic Lymph Node Chain (Extended-Field Radiation Therapy Alone)

Given the benefit of elective PALN irradiation, it stands to reason that a similar benefit might be obtained with therapy directed at histologically- or radiographically-positive PALN disease. However, initial efforts with RT alone were met with variable success. A large series from the GOG retrospectively analyzed outcomes of 98 patients enrolled on GOG protocols from 1973 to 1981 [8]. All patients had histologically proven PALN involvement by either staging laparotomy or definitive surgery. Given its retrospective nature, there was significant heterogeneity in patient treatments but typical para-aortic field doses were 44 to 50 Gy, though patients with extensive PALN metastases received as much as 60 Gy. Median survival was 15.2 months in this series and the 3-year overall survival rate was 25%, indicating that a proportion of patients can be cured with para-aortic-directed therapy. Approximately 1/3 of patients experienced pelvic failure, while another 1/3 had distant failure. This highlights the risk of distant progression for patients with PALN involvement, particularly when chemotherapy is not administered. Table 3 summarizes data from several series exploring the treatment of PALN disease with RT alone. It is important to note the limitations of capturing toxicity outcomes with retrospective data and that the reported frequencies may be an underestimation.

Table 3. Selected series of extended-field radiation therapy alone for cervical cancer with involved para-aortic lymph nodes

Study	N	External beam radiation dose/field	Overall Survival	Recurrence Pattern	Grade 3+ gastrointestinal toxicity (acute/late)
Berman [8]	98	40 Gy, plus up to 60 Gy to PA field	3-yr: 25%	Local 48%, distant 52% (as a component of known recurrent sites; 8% of failure sites were unspecified)	NR
Hughes [41]	41	42-51 Gy	5-yr: 29%	NR	NR/5%
Ballon [42]	18	43.2-51.2 Gy	5-yr: 23%	NR	NR
Emami [43] (Tufts University)	29	45-50 Gy	3-yr: 31% NED	38% LF, 17% DF	
Nori [44]	27	44 Gy, plus 6-8Gy boost to PA	5-yr: 29%	NR	22%/NR
Vigliotti [45] (University of Iowa)	43	50.4 Gy	5-yr: 32%	47% pelvic, 53% DM, 26% PA	21%/NR
Grigsby [46] (Washington University of St. Louis)	43	45-50.4 Gy	5-yr: 32%	7% pelvic, 20.9% pelvic & DM, 18.6% DM only (39.5% DM as a component of failure)	NR/4.7%

NR = not reported. PA = para-aortic.

Therapeutic Irradiation of the Para-Aortic Lymph Node Chain with Concurrent Chemotherapy

While it is clear that there exists a small but curable population within this group, enthusiasm for large volume radiation treatments has been tempered by a significant risk of late GI toxicity. This is of particular concern when combining EFRT with concurrent chemotherapy, a treatment shown to dramatically improve survival over radiation alone in locally-advanced cervical cancer [25, 26].

GOG 125 was a phase II study investigating the use of concurrent chemotherapy and EFRT in patients with histologically proven PALN involvement [4]. Eighty-six patients with FIGO stage I-IVA disease were enrolled, and treatment was directed to the PALN chain using an anterio-posterior/posterio-anterior (AP/PA) beam arrangement to a dose of 45 Gy in 1.5 Gy fractions per day. The whole pelvis was treated with a four-field box technique and received 39.6 to 48.6 Gy depending on stage. External beam RT was followed by a brachytherapy boost of 30 to 40 Gy. Concurrent chemotherapy consisted of cisplatin (50mg/m^2) and 5-FU (1000mg/m^2) administered on weeks 1 and 5. The 3-year progression free and overall survival was 34% and 39%, respectively. Recurrence was frequent; 55

patients (64%) recurred and 20.9% were pelvis only, 31.4% had distant disease only, and 10.5% had both distant and pelvic failures. Acute GI toxicity was documented in 18.6% and grade 3+ hematologic in 15.1%. This led to a total treatment time of > 14 weeks in 9 patients (10.5%), a well-known adverse risk factor for disease progression [28, 29].

These results suggest that a subset of patients can experience long-term disease control, though at the cost of increased toxicity. Other prospective studies show similar rates of disease control, but also high rates of acute and late toxicity. RTOG 92-10 was a phase II study delivering 1.2 Gy twice daily to the pelvis and PALN to total doses of 24-48 Gy to the pelvis, 12-36 Gy to parametrium, and 48 Gy to PALN, with a boost to 54-58 Gy to gross PALN metastases, followed by brachytherapy [27]. Cisplatin (75 mg/m2, days 1 and 22) and 5-FU (1000 mg/m2/24 h x 4 days; days 1 and 22) were given for two or three cycles. Though the 4-yr overall survival rate was 29%, and the probability of disease failure at any site was 63% at 3 years, toxicity was significant. Acute chemotherapy-related toxicity from chemotherapy was grade 3 in 48% and grade 4 in 28%. Acute radiotherapy-related toxicity was grade 3 in 21% and grade 4 in 28%. One patient died from acute treatment-related complications. Late grade 3 and 4 toxicity was experienced by 7% and 17%, respectively.

Considerable toxicity was also documented in RTOG 01-16, a small randomized trial, assessing the efficacy of amifostine to reduce the acute toxicity of EFRT with concurrent weekly cisplatin. This study accrued patients with either involved PALN or high common iliac nodes. Unfortunately, amifostine did not reduce the high acute toxicity experienced by patients in both arms, 87% versus 81% of those with and without amifostine (one-sided p = 0.70). Late grade 3-4 toxicity was observed in 20% (3/15) versus 40% (10/25) in those with and without amifostine (one-sided p = 0.08), respectively.

Table 4 is a compilation of selected series of chemo-EFRT for patients with involved PALN, highlighting treatment toxicity.

Intensity-modulated Radiation Therapy with Concurrent Chemotherapy

Despite significant toxicity, chemo-EFRT in patients with involved PALN remains worthwhile given evidence of long-term disease control in a subset of patients and the demonstrated survival benefit of concurrent chemoradiotherapy over radiotherapy alone in the management of pelvic-only locally advanced cervical cancer [25, 26, 30]. As such, efforts have focused at reducing toxicity, primarily by improved conformality of radiation delivery using three-dimensional planning and intensity-modulated radiation therapy (IMRT). Such modern techniques allow the targeting of high radiation doses towards tumor with increased sparing of normal tissues [31-34].

But the use of IMRT in patients with intact cervices is not without controversy. Primarily, the ability of IMRT to limit high doses to smaller tissue volumes has been scrutinized due to the risk of inter- and intrafraction cervical motion. Such motion can shift gross disease out of outside of tight IMRT target volumes [35-37]. As such, consensus guidelines for delineating target volumes that account for motion have been developed [38], though the role of IMRT in the definitive treatment of cervical cancer requires further research.

Nonetheless, the feasibility of IMRT to deliver EFRT with concurrent chemotherapy has already been demonstrated [39]. In a retrospective analysis of largely post-operative patients, 13 patients with gynecological malignancies who required treatment of the PALN region received EFRT using IMRT. Forty-five Gy in 1.8 Gy per day fractions was delivered, followed by a 9 Gy boost for gross nodal disease. Twelve patients received concurrent chemotherapy. Acute toxicity was limited; grade 3+ hematologic toxicity was observed in 3 patients and grade 3+ GI toxicity in 1 patient. No patients required a treatment break due to excessive toxicity. The 1 year rate of local control was 90% and 6 of 8 documented failures were outside of the treatment field. IMRT was successful in decreasing dose to the small bowel, kidneys, and rectum with an accordingly low rate of late toxicity – only one observed small bowel obstruction and one patient with significant lower extremity edema.

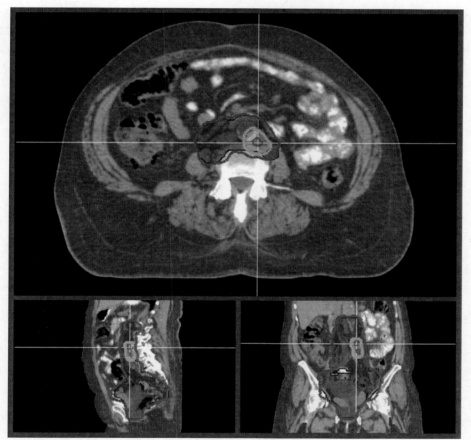

Thick red line = 42.75 Gy isodose line; thick orange line = 52.25 Gy isodose line; blue = gross disease and elective nodal target volume; green = involved para-aortic lymph node.

Figure 1. Representative computed tomography images displaying prescription isodose lines for an intensity modulated radiotherapy (IMRT) plan treating the whole pelvis and para-aortic nodes to 45 Gy and a simultaneous integrated boost to 55 Gy to an involved para-aortic lymph node.

A similar experience from the University of Pittsburgh detailed the results of 36 patients treated in the definitive setting with extended field radiation and concurrent chemotherapy using an IMRT technique [3]. Patients were stage IB2 to IVA, and 19 were lymph node positive. Of these patients, 10 also had involvement of the PALN chain. Chemotherapy consisted of 6 cycles of weekly cisplatin at $40mg/m^2$. A volume encompassing the cervix, uterus, parametria, presacral space and 4cm of adjacent vagina, as well as the pelvic and PANs up to the T12/L1 interspace was generated. This volume received 45 Gy in 1.8 Gy per day fractions. Additionally, all involved lymph nodes received either a sequential or simultaneous integrated boost to deliver an additional 10 to 15 Gy. Parametrial boosts were interdigitated with treatment as needed for a cumulative dose of 50.4 to 59.4 Gy. Brachytherapy was administered in 5 fractions of 5 Gy using an HDR technique. Treatment was well tolerated with 12 (33%) of patients experiencing grade 3 acute toxicity, while no patients experienced grade 4 toxicity. Hematologic effects were the most common adverse effect of therapy (n=10) and 5 patients did require a treatment break, although the overall median treatment time was acceptable at 56 days. Only 1 patient experienced grade 3 GI toxicity. With a median follow up of 18 months, 2 year estimates of local control (80%), disease free survival (51%) and overall survival (65%) have been published. Late toxicity has been rare with one documented small bowel obstruction and one sigmoid stenosis. This compares favorably with the 12% rate of late grade 3 toxicity observed in the extended field irradiation only arm of RTOG 90-01. For the 10 patients with known PALN involvement prior to treatment, 5 remain without evidence of disease, while the other 5 have developed systemic recurrences.

Future Directions

The above study is important as it demonstrates that effective therapy with limited toxicity can be directed at PALN metastases. Unfortunately, despite reasonable locoregional control, distant recurrences remain the predominant pattern of failure. Further study will be needed to define the optimal doses and RT target volumes but future efforts should be preferentially geared towards improvement of systemic therapies. Novel applications such as the use of gemcitabine in combination with cisplatin have been undertaken [40].

A large trial randomized 515 patients with IIB to IVA cervical cancer to conventional pelvic RT and concurrent weekly cisplatin ($40mg/m^2$) with or without gemcitabine ($125mg/m^2$) for 6 weeks. Patients randomized to the gemcitabine-containing arm also received 2 cycles of adjuvant chemotherapy consisting of cisplatin ($50mg/m^2$) and gemcitabine ($1000mg/m^2$) on a 3 week schedule. Three-year PFS (74.4% v. 65%, p=.029) and 3-year OS (80% v. 69%, p=.0224) were improved with the addition of concurrent and adjuvant gemcitabine. As local failure was similar between the arms (11% v. 16%, p=.097), the benefit was largely a reduction in distant failures. Given the trial design, it is not clear if this benefit was derived from concurrent gemcitabine or the use of adjuvant chemotherapy. Despite these improved outcomes, enthusiasm for this regimen has been tempered by the substantial toxicities observed; grade 3 or greater acute toxicity was observed in 86% of the patients in the gemcitabine-containing arm as opposed to 46% in the standard cisplatin arm (p<.001).

Table 4. Selected series of extended-field radiation therapy with concurrent chemotherapy for cervical cancer with involved para-aortic lymph nodes

Study	N	External beam radiation dose/field	Concurrent chemotherapy	Overall Survival	Recurrence Pattern	Grade 3+ radiation-related gastrointestinal toxicity (acute/late)
Malfetano [47] (Albany Medical Center)	13	≥50 Gy to pelvis, 45 Gy to PA.	Cisplatin 1mg/kg (60 mg maximum) weekly during radiotherapy	At 48.7 mos, 8/13 alive.	No local-regional failure; 5/5 recurred distantly	NR/0%
Varia [4] (GOG 125)	95	Stage IB/IIB: 39.6 Gy to pelvis, 45 Gy to PA. Stage IIB/IVA: 48.6 Gy to pelvis, 45 Gy to PA.	Cisplatin (50 mg/m² on d1, 29), 5FU (1,000 mg/m²/24 h, d2-5 and 30-33)	3-yr: 39%	Pelvic alone 20.9%, DM alone 31.4%, pelvic and DM 10.5%	18.6%/14%
Grigsby [27] (RTOG 92-10)	30	1.2 Gy BID. 24-48 Gy to pelvis, 12-36 Gy parametrial boost, 48 Gy to PA.	Cisplatin (75 mg/m² on d1, 22, 43), 5FU (1,000 mg/m²/24 h, d1-4 on d1, 22, 43) for 2 or 3 cycles.	4-yr: 29%	3-yr LRF 50%, 3-yr DF 63%	33%/20% (17% late grade 4 toxicity; 1 patient died of acute toxicity.)
Sood [48]	44	45 Gy to pelvis and PA; median 54 Gy boost to parametria if involved	Cisplatin (20 mg/m²/day) for 5 days for first and fourth week of external beam	5 of 44 died at median 22 mos follow-up	Actuarial 2-yr LF 8%, 2-yr DF 5%	25%/2.3%
Chung [49] (Sun Yat-Sen Cancer Center, Taiwan)	63	45 Gy to pelvis and PA; gross disease boost to 50.4 Gy; parametrial boost to 59.4 Gy.	Bolus cisplatin (50-80 mg/m², week 1 and 5 during external beam.	5-yr: 77%	3% LRF alone, 8% DM alone, 8% LRF plus DM.	2%/6%

Table 4. (Continued)

Study	N	External beam radiation dose/field	Concurrent chemotherapy	Overall Survival	Recurrence Pattern	Grade 3+ radiation-related gastrointestinal toxicity (acute/late)
Kim [50] (Alsan Medical Center and University of Ulsan, Korea)	33	Stage ≤IIB: 41.4 Gy to pelvis. Stage ≥IIIA: 50.4 Gy to pelvis. 36 Gy to PA (using AP-PA) and 9 Gy PA boost using 3DCRT.	Variable; included monthly 5FU (1,000 mg/m²/d) plus cisplatin (20 mg/m2/d), weekly cisplatin (30 mg/m2), paclitaxel (135 mg/m2/d) plus cisplatin (75 mg/m2/d) at 3-week intervals, and paclitaxel (135 mg/m2/d) plus carboplatin (area under the curve, 5) at 3-week intervals.	5-yr: 47%	In-field 4/16, outside field 6/16, persistent disease 6/16	9%/12%
Small [51, 52] (RTOG 0116; accrued patients with positive PA or high common iliac nodes)	41	45 Gy to pelvic and PA; positive high common iliac or PA nodes boosted to 54-59.6 Gy; involved parametrium and/or pelvic nodes boosted 60 Gy.	Cisplatin 40 mg/m², weekly during external beam and once with brachytherapy. 15 patients randomized to receive amifostine 500 mg per fraction of radiotherapy.	2-yr: 55.2% (all patients)	12.5% LRF, 62.5% persistent disease, 25% DF (patterns of failure not reported for patients receiving amifostine)	With amifostine:[¥] 33%/13% Without amifostine:[¥] 38%/24%

NR = not reported. PA = para-aortic. 5FU = 5-fluorouracil. LRF = local-regional failure. DM = distant metastases. DF = distant failure. 3DCRT = 3-dimensional conformal radiotherapy.

[¥] Toxicity reported as combined chemotherapy and radiotherapy toxicity; amifostine did not significantly reduce acute or late toxicity in this study.

Toxicity was largely due to neutropenia (grade 3 in 45%) and diarrhea (grade 3 in 17.7%). Additionally, there were more therapy discontinuations and 2 deaths that were felt to be treatment-related.

Perhaps this toxicity profile could be limited by the more conformal radiation delivery allowed by IMRT with care taken to limit treatment of the bone marrow and bowel. A trial that combines this technique with gemcitabine chemotherapy, either concurrently or adjuvantly, certainly seems reasonable. This could be of particular importance in patients with PALN involvement that require larger radiation volumes and who are also at an increased risk of distant failure.

References

[1]   Benedet J. L., Bender H., Jones H., 3rd, Ngan H. Y., Pecorelli S. FIGO staging classifications and clinical practice guidelines in the management of gynecologic cancers. FIGO Committee on Gynecologic Oncology. *Int J Gynaecol Obstet.* Aug 2000;70(2):209-262.

[2]   NCCN Clinical Practice Guidelines in Oncology (NCCN Guidelines): *Cervical Cancer.* Version 2.2013.

[3]   Beriwal S., Gan G. N., Heron D. E. et al. Early clinical outcome with concurrent chemotherapy and extended-field, intensity-modulated radiotherapy for cervical cancer. *Int J Radiat Oncol Biol Phys.* May 1 2007;68(1):166-171.

[4]   Varia M. A., Bundy B. N., Deppe G. et al. Cervical carcinoma metastatic to para-aortic nodes: extended field radiation therapy with concomitant 5-fluorouracil and cisplatin chemotherapy: a Gynecologic Oncology Group study. *Int J Radiat Oncol Biol Phys.* Dec 1 1998;42(5):1015-1023.

[5]   Bader A. A., Winter R., Haas J., Tamussino K. F. Where to look for the sentinel lymph node in cervical cancer. *Am J Obstet Gynecol.* Dec 2007;197(6):678 e671-677.

[6]   Lagasse L. D., Creasman W. T., Shingleton H. M., Ford J. H., Blessing J. A. Results and complications of operative staging in cervical cancer: experience of the Gynecologic Oncology Group. *Gynecol Oncol.* Feb 1980;9(1):90-98.

[7]   Stehman F. B., Bundy B. N., di Saia P. J., Keys H. M., Larson J. E., Fowler W. C. Carcinoma of the cervix treated with radiation therapy. I. A multi-variate analysis of prognostic variables in the Gynecologic Oncology Group. *Cancer.* Jun 1 1991;67(11): 2776-2785.

[8]   Berman M. L., Keys H., Creasman W., DiSaia P., Bundy B., Blessing J. Survival and patterns of recurrence in cervical cancer metastatic to periaortic lymph nodes (a Gynecologic Oncology Group study). *Gynecol Oncol.* Sep 1984;19(1):8-16.

[9]   Brill A. I., Nezhat F., Nezhat C. H., Nezhat C. The incidence of adhesions after prior laparotomy: a laparoscopic appraisal. *Obstet Gynecol.* Feb 1995;85(2):269-272.

[10] Possover M., Krause N., Kuhne-Heid R., Schneider A. Value of laparoscopic evaluation of paraaortic and pelvic lymph nodes for treatment of cervical cancer. *Am J Obstet Gynecol.* Apr 1998;178(4):806-810.

[11] Heller P. B., Maletano J. H., Bundy B. N., Barnhill D. R., Okagaki T. Clinical-pathologic study of stage IIB, III, and IVA carcinoma of the cervix: extended diagnostic

evaluation for paraaortic node metastasis--a Gynecologic Oncology Group study. *Gynecol Oncol.* Sep 1990;38(3):425-430.

[12] Bipat S., Glas A. S., van der Velden J., Zwinderman A. H., Bossuyt P. M., Stoker J. Computed tomography and magnetic resonance imaging in staging of uterine cervical carcinoma: a systematic review. *Gynecol Oncol.* Oct 2003;91(1):59-66.

[13] Scheidler J., Hricak H., Yu K. K., Subak L., Segal M. R. Radiological evaluation of lymph node metastases in patients with cervical cancer. A meta-analysis. *JAMA.* Oct 1 1997;278(13):1096-1101.

[14] van Vliet E. P., Heijenbrok-Kal M. H., Hunink M. G., Kuipers E. J., Siersema P. D. Staging investigations for oesophageal cancer: a meta-analysis. *Br J Cancer.* Feb 12 2008;98(3):547-557.

[15] Flamen P., Lerut A., van Cutsem E. et al. Utility of positron emission tomography for the staging of patients with potentially operable esophageal carcinoma. *J Clin Oncol.* Sep 15 2000;18(18):3202-3210.

[16] van Loon J., de Ruysscher D., Wanders R. et al. Selective nodal irradiation on basis of (18)FDG-PET scans in limited-disease small-cell lung cancer: a prospective study. *Int J Radiat Oncol Biol Phys.* Jun 1 2010;77(2):329-336.

[17] Kidd E. A., Siegel B. A., Dehdashti F., Grigsby P. W. Pelvic lymph node F-18 fluorodeoxyglucose uptake as a prognostic biomarker in newly diagnosed patients with locally advanced cervical cancer. *Cancer.* Mar 15 2010;116(6):1469-1475.

[18] Kunos C., Radivoyevitch T., Abdul-Karim F. W., Faulhaber P. 18F-Fluoro-2-Deoxy-d-Glucose Positron Emission Tomography Standard Uptake Value Ratio as an Indicator of Cervical Cancer Chemoradiation Therapeutic Response. *Int J Gynecol Cancer.* Aug 2011;21(6):1117-1123.

[19] Rose P. G., Adler L. P., Rodriguez M., Faulhaber P. F., Abdul-Karim F. W., Miraldi F. Positron emission tomography for evaluating para-aortic nodal metastasis in locally advanced cervical cancer before surgical staging: a surgicopathologic study. *J Clin Oncol.* Jan 1999;17(1):41-45.

[20] Grigsby P. W., Siegel B. A., Dehdashti F. Lymph node staging by positron emission tomography in patients with carcinoma of the cervix. *J Clin Oncol.* Sep 1 2001;19(17): 3745-3749.

[21] Wright J. D., Dehdashti F., Herzog T. J. et al. Preoperative lymph node staging of early-stage cervical carcinoma by [18F]-fluoro-2-deoxy-D-glucose-positron emission tomography. *Cancer.* Dec 1 2005;104(11):2484-2491.

[22] Sironi S., Buda A., Picchio M. et al. Lymph node metastasis in patients with clinical early-stage cervical cancer: detection with integrated FDG PET/CT. *Radiology.* Jan 2006;238(1):272-279.

[23] Rotman M., Choi K., Guse C., Marcial V., Hornback N., John M. Prophylactic irradiation of the para-aortic lymph node chain in stage IIB and bulky stage IB carcinoma of the cervix, initial treatment results of RTOG 7920. *Int J Radiat Oncol Biol Phys.* Sep 1990;19(3):513-521.

[24] Rotman M., Pajak T. F., Choi K. et al. Prophylactic extended-field irradiation of para-aortic lymph nodes in stages IIB and bulky IB and IIA cervical carcinomas. Ten-year treatment results of RTOG 79-20. *JAMA.* Aug 2 1995;274(5):387-393.

[25] Eifel P. J., Winter K., Morris M. et al. Pelvic irradiation with concurrent chemotherapy versus pelvic and para-aortic irradiation for high-risk cervical cancer: an update of radiation therapy oncology group trial (RTOG) 90-01. *J Clin Oncol.* Mar 1 2004; 22(5): 872-880.

[26] Morris M., Eifel P. J., Lu J. et al. Pelvic radiation with concurrent chemotherapy compared with pelvic and para-aortic radiation for high-risk cervical cancer. *N Engl J Med.* Apr 15 1999;340(15):1137-1143.

[27] Grigsby P. W., Heydon K., Mutch D. G., Kim R. Y., Eifel P. Long-term follow-up of RTOG 92-10: cervical cancer with positive para-aortic lymph nodes. *Int J Radiat Oncol Biol Phys.* Nov 15 2001;51(4):982-987.

[28] Fyles A., Keane T. J., Barton M., Simm J. The effect of treatment duration in the local control of cervix cancer. *Radiother Oncol.* Dec 1992;25(4):273-279.

[29] Perez C. A., Grigsby P. W., Castro-Vita H., Lockett M. A. Carcinoma of the uterine cervix. I. Impact of prolongation of overall treatment time and timing of brachytherapy on outcome of radiation therapy. *Int J Radiat Oncol Biol Phys.* Jul 30 1995;32(5):1275-1288.

[30] Keys H. M., Bundy B. N., Stehman F. B. et al. Cisplatin, radiation, and adjuvant hysterectomy compared with radiation and adjuvant hysterectomy for bulky stage IB cervical carcinoma. *N Engl J Med.* Apr 15 1999;340(15):1154-1161.

[31] Mundt A. J., Roeske J. C., Lujan A. E. et al. Initial clinical experience with intensity-modulated whole-pelvis radiation therapy in women with gynecologic malignancies. *Gynecol Oncol.* Sep 2001;82(3):456-463.

[32] Brixey C. J., Roeske J. C., Lujan A. E., Yamada S. D., Rotmensch J., Mundt A. J. Impact of intensity-modulated radiotherapy on acute hematologic toxicity in women with gynecologic malignancies. *Int J Radiat Oncol Biol Phys.* Dec 1 2002;54(5):1388-1396.

[33] Mell L. K., Tiryaki H., Ahn K. H., Mundt A. J., Roeske J. C., Aydogan B. Dosimetric comparison of bone marrow-sparing intensity-modulated radiotherapy versus conventional techniques for treatment of cervical cancer. *Int J Radiat Oncol Biol Phys.* Aug 1 2008;71(5):1504-1510.

[34] Hasselle M. D., Rose B. S., Kochanski J. D. et al. Clinical outcomes of intensity-modulated pelvic radiation therapy for carcinoma of the cervix. *Int J Radiat Oncol Biol Phys.* Aug 1 2011;80(5):1436-1445.

[35] Buchali A., Koswig S., Dinges S. et al. Impact of the filling status of the bladder and rectum on their integral dose distribution and the movement of the uterus in the treatment planning of gynaecological cancer. *Radiother Oncol.* Jul 1999;52(1):29-34.

[36] Chan P., Dinniwell R., Haider M. A. et al. Inter- and intrafractional tumor and organ movement in patients with cervical cancer undergoing radiotherapy: a cinematic-MRI point-of-interest study. *Int J Radiat Oncol Biol Phys.* Apr 1 2008;70(5):1507-1515.

[37] van de Bunt L., Jurgenliemk-Schulz I. M., de Kort G. A., Roesink J. M., Tersteeg R. J., van der Heide U. A. Motion and deformation of the target volumes during IMRT for cervical cancer: what margins do we need? *Radiother Oncol.* Aug 2008;88(2):233-240.

[38] Lim K., Small W., Jr., Portelance L. et al. Consensus guidelines for delineation of clinical target volume for intensity-modulated pelvic radiotherapy for the definitive treatment of cervix cancer. *Int J Radiat Oncol Biol Phys.* Feb 1 2011;79(2):348-355.

[39] Salama J. K., Mundt A. J., Roeske J., Mehta N. Preliminary outcome and toxicity report of extended-field, intensity-modulated radiation therapy for gynecologic malignancies. *Int J Radiat Oncol Biol Phys.* Jul 15 2006;65(4):1170-1176.

[40] Duenas-Gonzalez A., Zarba J. J., Patel F. et al. Phase III, open-label, randomized study comparing concurrent gemcitabine plus cisplatin and radiation followed by adjuvant gemcitabine and cisplatin versus concurrent cisplatin and radiation in patients with stage IIB to IVA carcinoma of the cervix. *J Clin Oncol.* May 1 2011;29(13):1678-1685.

[41] Hughes R. R., Brewington K. C., Hanjani P. et al. Extended field irradiation for cervical cancer based on surgical staging. *Gynecol Oncol.* Apr 1980;9(2):153-161.

[42] Ballon S. C., Berman M. L., Lagasse L. D., Petrilli E. S., Castaldo T. W. Survival after extraperitoneal pelvic and paraaortic lymphadenectomy and radiation therapy in cervical carcinoma. *Obstet Gynecol.* Jan 1981;57(1):90-95.

[43] Emami B., Watring W. G., Tak W., Anderson B., Piro A. J. Para-aortic lymph node radiation in advanced cervical cancer. *Int J Radiat Oncol Biol Phys.* Sep 1980;6(9):1237-1241.

[44] Nori D., Valentine E., Hilaris B. S. The role of paraaortic node irradiation in the treatment of cancer of the cervix. *Int J Radiat Oncol Biol Phys.* Aug 1985;11(8):1469-1473.

[45] Vigliotti A. P., Wen B. C., Hussey D. H. et al. Extended field irradiation for carcinoma of the uterine cervix with positive periaortic nodes. *Int J Radiat Oncol Biol Phys.* 1992;23(3):501-509.

[46] Grigsby P. W., Perez C. A., Chao K. S., Herzog T., Mutch D. G., Rader J. Radiation therapy for carcinoma of the cervix with biopsy-proven positive para-aortic lymph nodes. *Int J Radiat Oncol Biol Phys.* Mar 1 2001;49(3):733-738.

[47] Malfetano J. H., Keys H. Aggressive multimodality treatment for cervical cancer with paraaortic lymph node metastases. *Gynecol Oncol.* Jul 1991;42(1):44-47.

[48] Sood B. M., Gorla G. R., Garg M. et al. Extended-field radiotherapy and high-dose-rate brachytherapy in carcinoma of the uterine cervix: clinical experience with and without concomitant chemotherapy. *Cancer.* Apr 1 2003;97(7):1781-1788.

[49] Chung Y. L., Jian J. J., Cheng S. H. et al. Extended-field radiotherapy and high-dose-rate brachytherapy with concurrent and adjuvant cisplatin-based chemotherapy for locally advanced cervical cancer: a phase I/II study. *Gynecol Oncol.* Apr 2005;97(1):126-135.

[50] Kim Y. S., Kim J. H., Ahn S. D. et al. High-dose extended-field irradiation and high-dose-rate brachytherapy with concurrent chemotherapy for cervical cancer with positive para-aortic lymph nodes. *Int J Radiat Oncol Biol Phys.* Aug 1 2009;74(5):1522-1528.

[51] Small W., Jr., Winter K., Levenback C. et al. Extended-field irradiation and intracavitary brachytherapy combined with cisplatin chemotherapy for cervical cancer with positive para-aortic or high common iliac lymph nodes: results of ARM 1 of RTOG 0116. *Int J Radiat Oncol Biol Phys.* Jul 15 2007;68(4):1081-1087.

[52] Small W., Jr., Winter K., Levenback C. et al. Extended-field irradiation and intracavitary brachytherapy combined with cisplatin and amifostine for cervical cancer with positive para-aortic or high common iliac lymph nodes: results of arm II of Radiation Therapy Oncology Group (RTOG) 0116. *Int J Gynecol Cancer.* Oct 2011; 21(7):1266-1275.

In: Cervical Cancer
Editor: Laurie Elit

ISBN: 978-1-62948-062-6
© 2013 Nova Science Publishers, Inc.

Chapter XII

Targeted Therapeutic Management of Locally Advanced, Recurrent and Metastatic Cervical Cancer

Craig J. Mulhall[1] and Jermaine I. G. Coward[1,2,3,]
[1]Mater Adult Hospital, Department of Medical Oncology, Raymond Terrace, Brisbane, Australia
[2] Inflammation & Cancer Therapeutics Group, Mater Research, Translational Research Institute, Woolloongabba, Brisbane, Australia
[3]School of Medicine, University of Queensland, St Lucia, Brisbane, Australia

Abstract

In the sphere of gynaecological malignancies, the chemotherapeutic management of advanced cervical cancer is exceptionally challenging. Significantly, the slow pace in the evolution of novel targeted therapies in treating this disease partly explains why it remains third only to breast and ovarian cancer in terms of female cancer mortality worldwide. Over the course of the past decade, only small increments in overall and progression-free survival using combination chemotherapy has been witnessed, with the doublet of platinum-agents plus paclitaxel becoming established as the optimal first-line regimen. However the median overall survival still remains desperately poor ranging between 9-18 months.

With the recent explosion of adjunctive molecular targeted agents alongside chemotherapy, there has been significant scope for their inclusion into the treatment paradigms for locally advanced, recurrent and metastatic cervical cancer. Considerable impacts have been made by scrutinising the way in which signal transduction pathways can be modulated to improve survival in this setting. Specifically, bevacizumab and other agents targeting vascular endothelial growth factor (VEGF) have returned promising results, prompting a plethora of early-phase trials. Other areas of burgeoning interest include inhibition of epithelial growth factor receptor (EGFR), platelet-derived growth factor (PDGF), mammalian target of rapamycin (mTOR), histone deacetylase (HDAC), cyclooxygenase (COX), insulin growth factor receptor (IGFR) and activators of AMP kinase (AMPK).

Currently, these areas represent exciting new frontiers in advanced cervical cancer management, having already proven a substantial benefit in other numerous tumour types. Though they are yet to make the leap from publication to clinical practice, targeted therapies undoubtedly point the way forward. This chapter aims to outline the current evidence to support their swift introduction in this grave disease, drawing on literature from *in vitro* and *in vivo* studies and also highlights the possible reasons for the paucity of clinical trials focused on the incorporation of agents that have shown efficacy in other gynaecological tumours.

Keywords: Cervical cancer, targeted therapy, chemotherapy, cisplatin, VEGF, EGFR, mTOR, IGFR family, HDAC inhibitors, COX inhibitors

Introduction

Within the current era of targeted therapies, the treatment of advanced cervical cancer (CC) still poses a host of difficult questions that remain unanswered. Despite long established screening programmes, it still remains the third highest cause of female cancer related mortality worldwide with 274,000 deaths per annum [1]. Chemoradiation remains the standard of care for locally advanced disease (i.e. Stage IB-IIIB). However, up until relatively recently, there had previously been an absence of international concordance with respect to the chemotherapeutic management of metastatic disease (Stage IV). Over the past 30 years, numerous studies have investigated the merits of single-agent versus combination therapy; most being predominated by platinum-containing regimens. Initial reports of the efficacy of platinum monotherapy emerged in 1981, with Thigpen et al. demonstrating a 38% objective response rate (ORR) in a Phase II trial with 34 patients with either advanced or recurrent cervical SCC [2]. This was closely followed by the Bonomi study (GOG 43) which established the dose of cisplatin at 50 mg/m^2 in patients treated for recurrent CC [3]. Since then, other monotherapeutic approaches in these settings with paclitaxel [4], topotecan [5], vinorelbine [6], gemcitabine [7] and ifosfamide [8] have been investigated and yielded responses just below 20%. Initial combinatorial approaches alongside cisplatin failed to show survival advantages over single agent platinum and were inevitably more toxic [9, 10]. However, recent seminal studies have confirmed the superiority of combinatorial therapy with a backbone of platinum-based treatment. The first of these was the GOG 169 trial, which compared cisplatin and paclitaxel with cisplatin alone. Although significant improvement in ORR (36% vs 19%; p=0.002) and progression free survival (PFS) (4.8 vs 2.8 months; p<0.001) was evident, this did not translate to overall survival (OS) (8.8 vs 9.7 months) [11]. This naturally led to the development of subsequent trials using cisplatin combined with other drugs showing activity as single agents in CC. The triple-arm GOG 179 study compared cisplatin with cisplatin/topotecan and methotrexate, vinblastine, doxorubicin and cisplatin (MVAC); the latter regimen discontinued due to unacceptable toxicity [12]. However, cisplatin/topotecan demonstrated significant advantages over cisplatin for ORR (27% vs 13%; p=0.004), PFS (4.6 vs 2.9 months; p=0.014) and, for the first time with for a platinum doublet, OS (9.4 and 6.5 months; p = 0.017) [12]. Notably, the ORR for cisplatin monotherapy in both of these sequential studies was less than previously reported. This fuelled the initiation of the landmark Phase III GOG 204 study, which aimed to establish the most effective regimen by comparing the successful doublets used in the aforementioned GOG169 and 179 studies with cisplatin/gemcitabine and cisplatin/vinorelbine [13]. Based on the non-statistically significant advantages over all other treatments in ORR, PFS and OS, cisplatin and paclitaxel highlighted a new 'gold standard' for managing advanced CC. However, learning lessons from other gynaecological malignancies such as epithelial ovarian cancer (EOC), many clinicians had intuitively substituted cisplatin for carboplatin in this doublet in view of the non-inferiority seen with response rates, survival and more favourable toxicity profile [14]. Such intuition has proven valid, with the 2012 JCOG 505 study confirming similar PFS and OS rates for cisplatin/paclitaxel and carboplatin/paclitaxel in patients with recurrent CC [15]; hence paving the way for a new standard with the latter regime. However, subsequent analysis revealed a caveat; whereby patients who were platinum naive had a significantly better OS with cisplatin/paclitaxel [15].

Although these important studies have provided some clarity on the best choice of combination chemotherapy, it must be stressed that the median OS rates are still dismal at approximately 18 months at best [15]. Hence, there is an urge to develop strategies to enhance response and prolong survival for advanced CC and recent attempts have been made through the introduction of targeted therapies. This chapter exhaustively summarises the pre-clinical data on the effects of inhibiting chief effectors of tumour promotion in CC with an additional update on the clinical trials with novel agents (Table 1) for locally advanced, recurrent and metastatic disease.

Table 1. Key targeted therapy trials in locally advanced, recurrent and metastatic CC

Author	Study phase: Targeted therapy regimen	No. Evaluable patients	ORR (%)	PFS (months)	SD rate (%)	OS (months)
Wright et al. 2006 [36]	Retrospective: Bevacizumab + 5FU or capecitabine Patients pre-treated with platinum	6	33	N/A	33	5.1
Goncalves et al. 2008 [70]	Phase II: Gefitinib $2^{nd}/3^{rd}$ line monotherapy	28	0	1.23	20	3.57
Monk et al. 2009 [37]	Phase II: Bevacizumab $2^{nd}/3^{rd}$ line monotherapy	46	10.9	3.4	23.9	7.29

Table 1. (Continued)

Author	Study phase: Targeted therapy regimen	No. Evaluable patients	ORR (%)	PFS (months)	SD rate (%)	OS (months)
Kurtz et al. 2009 [68]	Phase II: Cetuximab + Cisplatin/topotecan Stopped early (due to toxicity)	44	32	5.73	32	7.33
Schilder et al. 2009 [71]	Phase II: Erlotinib monotherapy	28	0	1.87	16	4.96
Mackay et al. 2010 [46]	Phase II: Sunitinib monotherapy	19	0	3.5	84	N/A
Monk et al. 2010 [44]	Phase II: Pazopanib Lapatinib Pazopanib + lapatinib (combination arm discontinued)	 74 78 78	 9 5 N/A	 4.5 4.27 N/A	 43 44 N/A	 12.4 11.0 N/A
Farley et al. 2011 [67]	Phase II: Cetuximab + cisplatin	69	11.59	3.91	N/A	8.77
Santin et al. 2011[66]	Phase II: Cetuximab monotherapy	35	0	1.97	31.4	6.7
Tinker et al. 2013 [72]	Phase II: Temsirolimus monotherapy	37	3	3.52	57.6	N/A
Tewari et al. 2013 [41]	Phase III: Bevacizumab + cisplatin/paclitaxel or cisplatin/topotecan	450	N/A	N/A	N/A	N/A

Angiogenic Targeted Therapy

Angiogenic pathways have long been under the spotlight as a therapeutic target in a number of malignancies. The widespread interest and relative success of this strategy has been attributed to the critical role of angiogenesis in tumour progression. This process involves the expansion of existing blood vessels and is characterised by endothelial tip spouting and insertion of interstitial tissue columns into the lumen of these vessels (i.e. intussusception) [16, 17]. The hallmarks of this 'sprouting phase' are tumour vessel dilatation, increased permeability and leaking due to the effects of vascular endothelial growth factor (VEGF). VEGF, a 45kDa glycoprotein, was the first vascular-specific growth factor to be characterised and is widely accepted to be the essential driver for vasculogenesis [18]. It consists of a family of five structurally related molecules; namely VEGF-A,-B,-C, -D & placental growth factor (PlGF) and signals through three receptor tyrosine kinases namely VEGFR-1 (Flt-1), VEGFR-2 (KDR/Flk-1) and VEGFR-3 (Flt-4) [19]. Most of the aforementioned properties of VEGF are mediated through VEGFR-2 and conversely VEGFR-1 exhibits antagonistic effects by blunting signalling through VEGFR-2 [18]. Furthermore, although VEGFR-1 has a higher affinity for VEGF than VEGFR-2, it only possesses a weak capacity for signal transduction [19, 20].

The influence of hypoxia on VEGF induction is particularly highlighted by the intimate relationship between the Von Hippel Lindau (VHL) tumour suppressor gene and hypoxia inducible factor-1α (HIF-1α). Under normoxic conditions, VHL induces the hydroxylation and subsequent ubiquitin mediated degradation of HIF-1α which in turn modulates the expression of VEGF mRNA [21, 22]. Conversely, under hypoxic conditions, this process is reversed and hence promotes angiogenesis. More specifically, in malignancies such as renal cell carcinomas characterised by VHL mutations, HIF-1α is constitutively activated [23] and aberrant angiogenesis is a prominent feature.

Certainly, with respect to cervical cancer, VEGF appears to have a prominent aetiological role. The HPV 16 E6 and E7 oncoproteins which promote HPV replication also behave as inactivators of the tumour suppressor genes, p53 and Rb. HPV (16 and 18) E6 is known to induce angiogenesis by up-regulating VEGF transcription in a p53-independant fashion [24, 25] . Furthermore HPV 18 E6 and E7 shRNA in HeLa (human CC) cells can decrease VEGF expression in addition to increasing apoptosis and diminishing cell proliferation, invasion and adhesion. All such effects were also observed with shVEGF transfection of these cells [26]

Using cervical biopsy specimens, Guidi et al. demonstrated significantly increased microvascular density (MVD) and VEGF mRNA expression are apparent in high grade CIN and invasive CC in comparison with low grade CIN or benign cervical tissue [27]. It has also been suggested that VEGF may facilitate early invasive disease as high mRNA levels are particularly evident in stage I and II [28]. Furthermore, it has been implied that enhanced VEGF expression facilitates the development of aggressive phenotypes as higher expression has been witnessed in squamous subtypes in comparison to adenocarcinomas which have more favourable outcomes [29]. Moreover, VEGF overexpression is associated with poor prognosis by virtue of correlations with increased tumour size, lymphovascular invasion and risk of nodal metastasis [30-33]. Another putative angiogenic target in CC relates to platelet derived growth factor (PDGF) signalling [34, 35], which has been shown to support tumour growth and progression; processes that are abrogated by PDGF receptor (PDGFR) blockade

[34]. All aforementioned examples have set the platform for the introduction of anti-angiogenic therapies which currently represent the most promising targeted therapeutic strategy for either locally advanced or metastatic CC.

Bevacizumab

Bevacizumab is a humanised monoclonal antibody which targets VEGF-A, effectively preventing activation of VEGFR2 and the previously mentioned signalling pathway. Extensive trials involving an array of tumour types have cemented the role of bevacizumab in the medical oncologist's arsenal. In recent years, the case for bevacizumab in the treatment of metastatic cervical cancer has been compelling. As early as 2006, Wright et al. presented the retrospective analysis of a cohort of six patients, all of whom had been heavily pre-treated, who were given combination therapy including bevacizumab [36]. Two-thirds of the patients demonstrated a clinical benefit, with one complete response (CR) (17%) and one partial response (PR) (17%) documented. The treatment was well-tolerated, in spite of 5-fluorouracil-based protocols being employed, rather than the preferred platinum-taxane doublet. One case of grade 4 toxicity, in the form of neutropenic sepsis was reported. The median time to progression, amongst those who had demonstrated a clinical benefit, was 4.3 months [36].

This preliminary analysis prompted a cascade of Phase II trials focused on bevacizumab, in both the locally-advanced and metastatic setting. Monk et al. published the Gynaecological Oncology Group (GOG) Study on the efficacy of bevacizumab monotherapy, in the context of recurrent squamous cell carcinoma (SCC) of the cervix [37]. 46 patients, of performance status ≤ 2, were treated with bevacizumab 15mg/kg intravenously every 3 weeks, until disease progression or unacceptable toxicity. Progression free survival (PFS) was selected as the primary end-point and assessed at 6 months. In the absence of concurrent chemotherapy, the encouraging results of this trial showed a median PFS of 3.40 months, and median overall survival (OS) of 7.29 months, almost one quarter of patients survived progression-free for at least 6 months on bevacizumab alone (23.9%; 2-sided 90% CI 14%-37%). The most significant toxicity, was grade 3 hypertension (n=7; 15.2%). This study served to highlight the value of anti-angiogenesis in the second- and third-line settings.

The natural progression has been to combine bevacizumab with first-line chemotherapy in order to determine whether this enhances anti-tumour activity. To this end, a recently completed phase II non-randomised efficacy study examined the efficacy of bevacizumab combined with topotecan and cisplatin (GSK 107278). Aiming at a primary end-point of PFS > 6 months, the results of this study are eagerly anticipated and will undoubtedly prompt further studies of bevacizumab combined with other currently recommended first-line doublets. Drawing parallels with the recent success witnessed with the GOG218 and ICON7 studies [38, 39] in epithelial ovarian cancer (EOC), there is certainly scope to study bevacizumab combined with platinum and paclitaxel doublets [13, 15]. Similarly, a recent phase II study has tested the feasibility of combining bevacizumab with chemoradiotherapy and has shown a reasonable safety profile in treatment-naive patients with stage IB-IIIB disease [40]. Yet, for all these studies, there are no data confirming overall survival advantages above and beyond standard chemotherapy.

To this end, drawing bevacizumab into the phase-III arena has proven to be a much-warranted next step. GOG 240 (ClinicalTrials.gov identifier: NCT00803062) is the first such study and the interim analysis of this 2x2 factorial trial were presented at the American Society of Clinical Oncology meeting; June 2013 [41]. Patients with stage IVB, recurrent or persistent CC received paclitaxel in combination with either cisplatin or topetecan and were further randomised to treatment with or without bevacizumab (15mg/kg). With a median follow up of 20.8 months, the results confirmed median PFS of 8.2 and 5.9 months (HR 0.67; 95% CI [0.54, 0.82]; p = 0.0002) and OS of 17 and 13.3 months (HR 0.71; 97.6%, CI [0.54, 0.94]; p=0.0035) for bevacizumab and non-bevacizumab regimes respectively [41]. The significant survival advantages were also reflected in the superior response rates witnessed with bevacizumab over chemotherapy alone (48% vs 36%; p=0.00807). Of further interest, greater than 70% of patients had prior platinum-based therapy and interestingly, paclitaxel and toptecan was neither inferior or superior to paclitaxel and cisplatin [41]. Nevertheless, the addition of bevacizumab conferred improved OS for both regimens. As expected, adverse events relating to thromboembolic phenomena and fistula were more prevalent in the bevacizumab arm, however the incidence was less than 10% [41]. Although these results have yet to mature, the aforementioned results are indeed exciting and, to date, represent the only evidence demonstrating a significant OS advantage for targeted therapy in advanced CC.

Angiogenic Tyrosine Kinase Inhibitors

Following closely behind the encouraging trials of bevacizumab, the VEGFR-specific and multi-targeted tyrosine kinase inhibitors (TKIs) have been a logical progression for the anti-angiogenic approach. The focus of some early preclinical interest in TKI research with CC has been growth factor receptor-bound protein 10 (GRB10). GRB10 is an adaptor protein known to interact with numerous receptor tyrosine kinases, including those associated with VEGFR, PDGF, epithelial growth factor (EGF) and insulin-like growth factor-1 (IGF-1) receptors [42]. Okino et al. confirmed GRB10 mRNA over-expression in 80% of primary SCC samples and observed significant growth inhibition *in vitro* with GRB10 siRNA [42]. In lieu of such effects, TKIs targeting multiple pathways have garnered growing attention in clinical trials.

Pazopanib is a small-molecule 'multikinase' inhibitor with affinity for VEGFR-1, -2, -3, PDGFR and c-KIT tyrosine kinases. It has come into the realm of gynaecological malignancies following success in other tumour streams, most predominantly renal cell carcinoma [43]. A triple-arm, open-label, phase II trial by Monk et al. has shed light on the efficacy of pazopanib in the treatment of metastatic cervical cancer [44]. 152 patients were randomised in a 1:1:1 ratio to pazopanib 800mg once daily (n=74), lapatinib 1500mg once daily (n=78) or combination therapy (one of two regimens: pazopanib 400mg/lapatinib 1000mg or pazopanib 800mg/lapatinib 1500mg), with the primary end-point of PFS. At the point of interim analysis, the combination arm was discontinued, due to crossing the futility boundary compared to either monotherapy arm. Additionally, there were a greater number of significant adverse events (SAEs) in the combination group, with two fatal haemorrhages and one unexplained death. Upon continuing both monotherapy arms, pazopanib demonstrated an improved PFS (HR 0.66, 90%CI 0.48-0.91, p = 0.013) against lapatinib [44]. The secondary end-point of OS was also improved, with median OS being 50.7 weeks (39.1 weeks for lapatinib). The predominating SAE of either grade 3 or 4 was diarrhoea, which occurred in 12% of patients in the pazopanib monotherapy arm [44]. Due to the absence of a standard treatment arm (i.e. platinum-doublet chemotherapy), the true impact of pazopanib in this setting is difficult to establish fully from this study. Yet, there are encouraging aspects which should prompt further trials into its use; namely, its oral delivery mechanism, clear anti-neoplastic activity and low incidence of high-grade toxicities [45].

Other angiogenic TKIs have been represented in the novel therapeutic pipeline for CC over the past few years. Sunitinib is multikinase inhibitor which shares the same targets as pazopanib in addition to Flt3, RET and CSF1R. However, a phase II trial with sunitinib in the second-line setting has returned dissatisfying results, with moderate toxicities (including a higher than anticipated rate of fistula formation) overshadowing a very modest mean PFS of 3.5 months, and no objective response [46]. Cediranib is a multikinase inhibitor with activity against VEGFR and PDGFR. The CIRCCa or Cediranib in Recurrent Cervical Cancer (ClinicalTrials.gov identifier NCT01229930) study is a randomised placebo-controlled phase II trial exploring the use of this agent in combination with carboplatin and paclitaxel. The primary end-point is PFS, with a targeted increase of 50% compared to the placebo arm. Secondary end-points include response, toxicity and quality of life (QOL). The study is currently closed to recruitment and awaiting publication.

Despite mixed outcomes in the existing trials, there is much scope for further scrutiny of angiogenic pathways in CC pathogenesis and treatment. The approach of multikinase inhibition, in the context of halting angiogenesis, remains an attractive and under-investigated prospect. In addition, a resurrection of older antiangiogenic agents such as TNP-470 (fumagillin analogue) which has previously shown significant clinical promise [47-49], certainly requires further investigation.

Epidermal Growth Factor Receptor Family Inhibitors

The epidermal growth factor receptor (EGFR) family consists of four structurally-related tyrosine kinase cell surface receptors which include ErbB-1/EGFR, ErbB2/HER-2/neu, ErbB-3 and ErbB-4 [50-52]. The extracellular domain of EGFR binds to a host of ligands (including epidermal growth factor (EGF), transforming growth factor- α, (TGF-α), amphiregulin) resulting in tyrosine kinase activation and subsequent phosphorylation of two main signalling pathways; Ras-Raf-MEK-ERK and PI3-Akt-mTOR, all of which promote cell proliferation, motility, metastatic spread, chemoresistance and angiogenesis [51].

EGFR overexpression, deregulation and mutations have been identified as a driving force associated with numerous malignancies. With respect to CC, EGFR expression appears to be highly variable, ranging between 6% to 90% [52]. Furthermore, there appear to be specific patterns of EGFR family expression according to subtype, whereby stronger correlations are associated with EGFR and SCC as opposed to adenocarcinomas which are more associated with HER2-neu [53]. As downstream signal transduction mediates a number of tumourigenic processes, it follows that EGFR expression influences survival and treatment outcomes in CC. Indeed, there are several reports to support EGFR over-expression as an independent prognostic marker in the context of poor response to chemo-radiation and inferior survival rates [52-56]. This observation also extends to surgical outcomes in CC. For example, in a study of 136 patients undergoing radical surgery for stage I and II cervical cancer, 54% were found to have moderate or strong expression of EGFR. Moreover, such expression was associated with reduced disease-free survival (DFS) and OS [57]. Although some other studies have failed to show any such relationship [58-60], there is sufficient evidence to support the introduction of targeted EGFR therapies in CC.

Cetuximab

Cetuximab is a chimeric monoclonal antibody which binds with higher affinity to the EGFR extracellular domain compared with the endogenous ligands; EGF and TGF-α [61]. This binding induces EGFR downregulation and modulation of downstream signalling; potentially inhibiting cell proliferation and anti-apoptotic effects [62]. Cetuximab has perhaps demonstrated its' greatest success in augmenting the efficacy of chemotherapy in the treatment of colorectal cancer and head and neck SCC [63, 64]. Amongst a panel of human CC cell lines *in vitro*, cetuximab can effectively internalise EGFR [65]. However, from a translational perspective, results have unfortunately varied between modest to disappointing. In 2011, Santin et al. conducted a phase II study investigating cetuximab monotherapy, with an induction dose of 400mg/m^2 followed by 250mg/m^2 weekly, until disease progression or unacceptable toxicity [66]. PFS was selected as the primary end-point. Five of thirty-five patients demonstrated a PFS beyond 6 months (14.3%; 90% CI 5.8% - 30%). These patients notably all showed squamous cell histology, suggesting that perhaps this subgroup make the most suitable candidates for investigating adjunctive treatment with cetuximab. In spite of this finding, the study yielded no clinical responses. Further attempts at coupling cetuximab with topotecan and cisplatin have also garnered dissatisfying results, showing limited activity and ORR, as well as prohibitive rates of morbidity and mortality [67, 68].

A further attempt at producing a competitive inhibitor of ligand binding to EGFR with the humanised monoclonal antibody; matuzumab, met with initial phase II success which was offset by gastrointestinal, haematologic and dermatologic toxicities [69]. However, production of this drug was ceased in 2008.

Lapatinib

Lapatinib is a dual inhibitor of EGFR and HER2, with its most established role in breast cancers refractory to trastuzumab, anthracycline and taxane chemotherapy. As previously discussed, Monk et al. studied the utility of lapatinib monotherapy, and in combination with pazopanib for cervical cancer with no significant success seen [44].

EGFR Tyrosine Kinase Inhibitors

Erlotinib

As with VEGFR, inhibition of EGFR autophosphorylation and downstream signal transduction is also feasible by targeting the receptor tyrosine kinase. The small molecule reversible TKIs, erlotinib and gefitinib, have risen to prominence as well-tolerated oral agents, with appreciable activity in an array of tumour types.

Over the past decade, erlotinib has developed an established role in adenocarcinoma of the lung, as well as some upper gastrointestinal tumours. The evidence is also mounting in favour of its use in locally advanced CC. At a clinical level, combined therapy with chemoradiation and erlotinib is certainly feasible. In patients with IIB and IIIB CC, Nogueira-Rodrigues et al. used escalating doses of erlotinib (50-150mg), with cisplatin and radiotherapy (external beam followed by brachytherapy). The regimen with the maximal dose of 150mg was well tolerated. Using a similar protocol, Ferreira et al. presented phase II data on 37' treatment-naive patients also with stage IIB to IIIB cervical cancer [73]. Out of 23 evaluable patients, 21 patients (91.3%, 95%CI 70.5% - 98.5%) presented with CR; which compares favourably to the historical CR rates of 38%-75% achieved with standard chemoradiotherapy [73]. A further two patients (8.7%) demonstrated PR, over a median treatment duration of 77 days (range 64 – 106 days). Notably, during a median follow-up period of 9 months (range 3 – 25), none of the evaluable patients progressed. Grade 3 toxicities included diarrhoea (3 patients, 12%), skin rash (5 patients, 20%) and one patient presented with grade 4 hepatotoxicity [73]. In summary, the addition of erlotinib showed a favourable response rate, with a toxicity profile consistent with clinical experience of TKI usage. Given such results, the adjunctive use of erlotinib to chemotherapy in locally advanced disease merits ongoing investigation.

However, in the metastatic setting, there is still much work to be done. In 2009, Schilder et al. presented a phase II trial of erlotinib monotherapy in recurrent SCC of the cervix. Unfortunately, there were no objective responses and only one patient experienced a PFS of 6 months or more [71]. Clearly attention must now focus on combining erlotinib with standard chemotherapy regimens; however this has yet to be adequately assessed.

Gefitinib

Like erlotinib, gefitinib has gained substantial prominence in the landscape of clinical management for non-small cell lung cancer (NSCLC) [74]. By contrast, data exploring its use in treating CC are sparse. A recent French multi-centre phase-II study by Goncalves et al. investigated gefitinib as a second- or third-line management strategy in recurrent locoregional or metastatic disease [70]. A cohort of 28 patients was prescribed 500mg/day of gefitinib, with the objective of correlating outcomes to the degree of EGFR expression. Although there were no objective responses, and no identifiable correlation between EGFR expression levels and outcome, six patients (20%) had demonstrable stable disease. This interesting finding indicates that our understanding of cervical cancer biology warrants further development. Hopefully, with data correlated from larger cohorts, this may be realised in the near future.

Activators of AMP Kinase

5' AMP-activated protein kinase (AMP-K) is a serine/threonine kinase which is a critical sensor for cellular energy homeostasis [75]. It is a linchpin for numerous metabolic processes, including glycolysis and fatty acid oxidation; and as such, is linked to chronic diseases such as obesity and diabetes mellitus [76]. From an oncological perspective, AMP-K has a pivotal role in blocking the functions of mTOR, with downstream inhibition of protein synthesis and cell growth. It is also known to potentiate the effect of p53, promoting cell cycle arrest in G_1-S [77]. Furthermore, there is a suggested link between AMP-K and the inhibition of glucose-activated gene expression, though details of this mechanism are not completely understood [78].

Compelling evidence has surfaced since the mid-2000s with regard to harnessing the effects of AMP-K in cancer treatment. To date, such publications exist in the sphere of pre-clinical studies, including both *in vitro* and *in vivo* work using pharmacological activators of AMP-K; AICAR and A23187. With specific regard to cervical cancer, Yu et al. demonstrated *in vitro* that co-treatment with AICAR and A23187 was able to enhance anti-proliferative effects, and inhibit cell growth, in CC cells [79].

To date, the AMP-K story is continuing to emerge. Kwan et al. have recently attempted to shed new light on our understanding of the mechanism for AMP-K-driven tumour suppression, utilising both *in vivo* and *in vitro* techniques [80]. The focus of this work has been DVL3, a cell proliferation regulating protein which is upregulated in CC. This study identifies a reduction in DVL3 protein levels as the means by which AMP-K activation impairs cervical cancer cell growth [80]. Whether this new knowledge can contribute to anti-cancer therapy or as a surrogate marker of treatment efficacy is yet to be determined. Nevertheless, AMP-K activation provides another way forward in the challenge to find suitable CC targets.

Insulin-Like Growth Factor (IGF) System Inhibition

The insulin-like growth factor (IGF) system has integral roles in numerous physiological and pathological processes. It consists of three ligands (IGF-1, IGF-2 and insulin) and their respective cell surface receptors (IGF-1R, IGF-2R, IR); all of which share a structural and functional homology [81-83]. Their interaction initiates a surge of downstream signalling events predominantly via Ras-Raf-MAPK and PI3K-Akt transduction pathways which facilitate tumourigenesis by promoting cellular proliferation, angiogenesis, invasion, metastatic potential and inhibiting apoptosis. Such signalling is regulated by six IGF-binding proteins (IGFBP-1 to -6) which are associated with IGFBP proteases and receptors (IGFBP-R) [83, 84]. The mode of regulation is complex in that all IGFBPs can inhibit IGF activity but select IGFBPs (i.e. IGFBP-1, -3 & -5) can enhance IGF functioning. In turn, the ratios of IGFs and IFGBPs influence the extent of either normal or pathological cellular proliferation [84, 85].

Predictably, the IGF system has been highlighted as a putative therapeutic target in several malignancies which is exemplified by several recent Phase I/II trials conducted with anti-IR/IGFR inhibitors in this setting [86]. With respect to CC, there is certainly convincing evidence to support the introduction of this approach in managing this disease. Interestingly, in a study of 98 gynaecological tumours, Hirano et al. observed variable IGFBP and high IGFR-1 mRNA expression in all 32 cervical cancer specimens; implicating the importance of the IGF system in tumour growth [87]. There is also a wealth of preclinical data to support this perception. Steller et al. were the first to report overexpression of IGF-1R in primary cervical cancer cell lines in comparison with normal cervical cells [88]. In addition, mitogenic effects exerted by epidermal growth factor (EGF) could be effectively abrogated by using antisense oligonucleotide to IGF-2 [88]. IGFR-1 also contributes to the proliferative potential of CC by enhancing KCl cotransport ((KCC); a key regulator of cell volume and epithelial cell transport) [89] and facilitates invasion through interactions with $\alpha v \beta 3$ integrin signalling [90].

Steller et al. have also inferred a distinct role for IGFR-1 in the aetiology of CC via its intimate relationship with HPV. Using fibroblast cells with an IGFR-1 gene disruption stably transfected with HPV 16 E6 and E7, they observed that IGFR-1 and E6 were required for E7 transformation. Furthermore, this was potentially mediated through cell survival pathways supporting inhibition of apoptosis [91]. A subsequent report has consolidated the links between the IGF system, HPV and tumourigenesis; whereby IGFR-1 expression is elevated in CINIII and invasive carcinomas and IGFR-1 phosphorylation increases in accordance with disease progression [92]. This group also hypothesised that the upregulation of IGFR-1 was as a consequence of HPV E6 mediated p53 deregulation [92].

However, there are conflicting reports with respect to the role of the IGF system as a prognostic factor in CC. Huang et al. have noted high grade IGFR-1 expression and elevated preoperative squamous cell carcinoma antigen as independent predictors of death and recurrence; and in combination both could aid stratification of patients with higher risk of death [93]. Similarly, higher serum levels of IGF-2 are evident in patients with CIN and invasive carcinoma in comparison with healthy controls and returned to normal with successful therapeutic intervention [94]. Conversely, Serrano et al. have shown significantly lower IGF-2 levels in patients with invasive disease compared to control cases [95]. These opposing observations are also reflected in IGF-1 concentrations and IGF-1:IGFBP3 ratios with reports of either low levels found in CC patients [96] or higher levels found in CIN with no significant association with invasive disease [97]. Adding to the complexity, Schaffer et al. noted an inverse correlation between IGF-1 and high grade CIN in young women [98]; however an explanation for this inferred protective effect has yet to be elucidated.

Nevertheless, high IGFR-1 certainly portends poor therapeutic response and significantly shorter disease free and overall survival in patients undergoing chemoradiation for locally advanced disease [99]. From a clinical perspective, these findings would support targeting of the IGF system alongside chemotherapy in the metastatic setting as a means to prolong response. To date, only a single clinical trial has encompassed this strategy in advanced CC. Molife et al. conducted a Phase Ib study with the IGFR-1 monoclonal antibody, Figitumumab, in combination with docetaxel for patients with advanced solid tumours [100]. The combination appeared to be well tolerated and 12 out of 46 patients had a best response of stable disease (SD); one of which included a case of advanced CC with a modest stabilisation period of 7 months [100]. Although this result is encouraging, clearly a larger study is required to explore the true efficacy of this regime in this setting. Furthermore, in view of the emerging evidence relating to resistance to IGFR-1 inhibition through compensatory signalling via IR [101], it would appear logical to adopt synchronous targeting of IGFRs (e.g. with dual IGFR-1/IR inhibitors such as OSI-906) for future clinical trials.

Mammalian Target of Rapamycin (mTOR) Inhibitors

In parallel with other gynaecological malignancies, targeting the Akt/PI3K signal transduction pathway has also stimulated a degree of interest in CC. Yet again, despite the preclinical efficacy witnessed, this has yet to be substantially translated into clinical trials. This particular pathway has diverse biological roles ranging from regulation of cell proliferation, transcription, survival and apoptosis. These processes are mediated by a number of downstream effectors, which appears to be dominated by Akt activation of mTOR; a serine/threonine protein kinase which consists of a Rictor- containing complex of two proteins (mTORC1 and mTORC2). Additionally, PI3K signalling is tightly modulated by the tumour suppressor gene, PTEN, which inhibits phosphorylation of plasma membrane phospholipids critically involved in Akt activation. As aberrations in this pathway are frequently observed within the tumour microenvironment, it serves as an attractive therapeutic target in numerous tumour types. Using immunohistochemistry to analyse markers of mTOR pathway expression, Feng et al. reported significantly higher expression of cytoplasmic p-mTOR (Ser2448) and nuclear p-p70S6K (Thr389) in both high grade CIN and invasive SCC compared to normal cervical epithelium [102]. Furthermore, elevated pmTOR expression has also been shown to predict poor survival and response to neoadjuvant platinum-based chemotherapy in patients with advanced CC [103]. Interestingly, the interaction between mTOR and the translator inhibitor 4E-BP1 has been shown to maintain high levels of the HPV E7 oncoprotein, an effect that can be abrogated in CaSki cell lines *in vitro* by mTOR inhibition with rapamycin [104]. More recently, Ji et al. witnessed cell cycle inhibition and induction of apoptosis through mTOR inhibition either via rapamycin or using siRNA knockdown [105]. Similarly, Li et al. have reported that *in vitro* overexpression of the micro RNA (miRNA), mir-218, which is frequently reduced in CC [106, 107], cells can inhibit tumour growth and enhance cisplatin sensitivity by downregulating mTOR [107].

Published translational studies with mTOR inhibitors thus far have been limited to two small studies. An initial Phase I study by Temkin et al. using a weekly regimen of temsirolimus and topetecan in 15 patients with gynaecological malignancies; 2 with recurrent CC (108). The main dose limiting effect was myelosuppression and no specific information relating to the CC cases was documented [108]. More recently, Tinker et al. have published the results of a phase II study with weekly temsirolimus monotherapy in 37 patients with recurrent, unresectable, locally advanced or metastatic CC [72]. Amongst the evaluable patients, they observed 1 PR (3.0%) and 19 SD (57.6%) with a median duration of 6.5 months. The 6-month PFS rate was modest at 28% and toxicity profile was acceptable in alignment with many other temsirolimus studies [72].

With respect to everolimus, a trial investigating its efficacy in recurrent/metastatic disease has recently been suspended due to poor patient accrual (ClinicalTrials.gov identifier NCT00967928). However, patients with locally advanced CC are currently being recruited in a Phase I study (PHOENIX 1; ClinicalTrials.gov identifier NCT01217177) focusing on varying doses of everolimus in combination with chemoradiation.

Cyclooxygenase Inhibitors

Cancer related inflammation has long been established as a key aetiological factor in the development of lower genital tract cancers [109]. Specifically, cervical inflammation is associated with both high grade CIN and invasive CC [110-113]. In addition high concentrations of proinflammatory cytokines (e.g. IL-6, IL-8 and TNF-α) are associated with persistent HPV infection [114]. Hence, targeting inflammatory mediators would appear an intuitive strategy in this disease and, from a translational perspective, most of the research in this field has revolved around inhibiting cyclooxygenases (COXs). The principal role of COXs is to catalyse the conversion of arachidonic acid to prostaglandin H2, a process that serves as a key regulatory step in inflammation. These enzymes exist as two isoforms; COX-1 which is constitutively expressed by a variety of cells and mediates the housekeeping functions of prostaglandins, and COX-2 which is induced by inflammatory cytokines [115]. Seemingly, elevated COX-1 and COX-2 expression have been reported in CC. Indeed Sales et al. not only confirmed enhanced COX-1 activity in both squamous and adenocarcinomas of the cervix, but also reported up-regulation of COX-2 by COX-1; an effect that was impeded by dual COX inhibition with indomethacin and not via selective COX-2 inhibition with NS-398 [116]. Furthermore, Kulkarni et al. confirmed COX-2 expression in both CIN and CC as opposed to normal cervical tissue and demonstrated significant induction of COX-2 activity by EGF, which is also commonly overexpressed in CC [117]. Moreover, COX-2 overexpression is associated with increased metastatic/invasive potential and poor prognosis in this disease [118-120].

Numerous publications have consolidated the concept of prostaglandin-related radioprotection of tumours through enhanced cell survival following radiation, repair of DNA damage and reduced sensitivity to radiation induced apoptosis [121]. This has stimulated further exploration into the potential of role COX inhibitors in reversing this phenomenon in CC. The first report relating to this focused on the effect of oxyphenbutazone; a prostoglandin antagonist, which significantly improved survival when combined with radiotherapy for CC patients compared with radiotherapy alone. The authors hypothesised that such benefits were secondary to prostaglandin inhibition causing tumour growth regression [122]. Further reports have confirmed effective *in vitro* radiosensitisation with celecoxib by downregulation of both COX-2 and VEGF-C [123]. In addition, Xia et al. observed that radiation resistance induced by activation of the PI3K/Akt/COX-2 pathway could be effectively reversed in a synergistic fashion in HeLa cells treated combinatorially with RT, celecoxib and the PI3K inhibitor, LY294002 [124].

Similarly, COX inhibition also has profound effects on blunting chemoresistance in CC. Ogino et al. demonstrated indomethacin treatment of SKG and HKUS cell lines *in vitro* enhanced the cytoxicity of 5-FU and cisplatin by increasing their intracellular uptake. However, indomethacin alone failed to exhibit any cytotoxic effects [125]. As chemoresistance is often facilitated by upregulation of pro-survival genes, it is interesting to note that celecoxib has been shown to effectively increase apoptosis in HeLa cells *in vitro* by inducing caspase-3 and suppressing expression of the anti-apoptotic protein, survivin, at both the mRNA and protein level [126]. Furthermore, an earlier study by Kim et al. suggested that these enhanced apoptotic effects could occur independently from COX inhibition and mediated via upregulation of caspases 8 and 9 and through increased activity of the inflammatory transcription factor, NF-κB [127].

The clinical application of concurrent COX inhibition with chemoradiation in CC has been investigated in two recent studies. Herrera et al. conducted a prospective Phase I/II trial evaluating toxicity and efficacy of celecoxib (400mg b.d.) administered to 31 patients 2 weeks before and during chemoradiation [128]. Although early toxicities were deemed tolerable, unexpected higher frequencies of late complications (e.g. fistula formation) were observed. Moreover, no significant improvement in response in comparison to chemoradiation alone was demonstrated [128]. Another Phase II study has confirmed unacceptably high rates of acute toxicities with celecoxib combined with chemotherapy, pelvic radiation and brachytherapy [129]. In view of the adverse events witnessed in these trials, there appears to be justifiable reticence in further exploring these particular treatment algorithms. Nevertheless, in view of the inferences from preclinical data, this should not preclude the development of future trials with celecoxib and chemotherapy in the metastatic setting.

Histone Deacetylase (HDAC) & DNA Methylation Inhibitors

Perhaps one of the most exciting novel therapeutics on the horizon is embodied by the emergence of histone deacetylase (HDAC) inhibitors. Histone proteins are key chromatin components and their N-terminus post-translational modification through acetylation to form a "histone code" is critical to silencing tumour suppressor gene transcription [130, 131]. Specifically, in relation to CC, HPV E6 oncoprotein targets p53 for proteosomal degradation [132] and E7 also functions through indirect binding with HDAC1 and HDAC 2 [133]. Over the past 5 years, a plethora of studies have shown *in vitro* and *in vivo* activity of different classes of HDAC inhibitors in experimental CC models. Vorinostat (Suberoylanilide Bishydroxamine; SAHA) is a hydroxamic acid inhibitor which has been shown to have a favourable toxicity profile *in vivo* [131]. In view of the tumorigenic effects of HPV mediated through p53 downregulation and co-option with HDACs, Lin et al. aimed to exploit these mechanisms and confirmed that combinatorial therapy with Vorinostat and the proteasome inhibitor, bortezomib (Velcade) resulted in synergistic killing in HPV-positive C33A, HeLa and HT3 CC cell lines. Furthermore, this effect was not evident in HPV-negative cells [134]. The butyrate classes of HDAC inhibitors (e.g. sodium butyrate, phenylbutyrate) have also been shown to mediate anti-tumour activity in CC by facilitating extrinsic cell death, inducing G1/S growth arrest, abrogating cdk2 function and up-regulating the cyclin-dependent kinase inhibitors, p21 and p27 [131, 135, 136]. Similarly, treatment of HeLa cells *in vitro* with the novel HDAC inhibitor, BML-210, has been shown to inhibit cell growth, induce apoptosis and significantly increase p21 levels [137]. In addition, Trichostatin A (TSA) has been shown to enhance radiosensitivity in HeLa cell lines under hypoxic conditions through dowregulation of HIF-1α and VEGF [138].

As with all other targeted therapies for metastatic CC, the clinical application of these drugs has currently been limited to small Phase I and II trials. Valproic acid, an anticonvulsant drug with significant *in vitro* HDAC inhibitory effects [139, 140], has been studied within in a Phase I study [141], with twelve newly diagnosed patients with CC treated with oral magnesium valproate (30-50mg for 5 days). The authors observed decreased tumour deacetylase activity in 8 patients (80%) alongside histone hyperacetylation and significant differences in pre- and post-treatment HDAC activity [141]. Entinostat, a synthetic benzamine derivative, is another HDAC inhibitor which exerts anti-neoplastic activity through upregulating p21 and impeding cell proliferation [131]. Ryan et al. conducted a Phase I trial with entinostat in 31 patients with advanced/refractory malignancies. The single patient with CC gained reasonable clinical benefit with disease stabilisation lasting 10 months [142].

The interest in epigenetic targeted therapy also extends to inhibitors of DNA methylation with drugs such as hydralazine; which are also able to reactivate tumour suppressor gene expression [49]. Moreover, a recent study in advanced CC has investigated the efficacy of combinatorial treatment with hydralazine, magnesium valproate and radiotherapy in newly diagnosed stage IIIB disease [143]. Although well tolerated, the suboptimal delivery of brachytherapy limited a true assessment of therapeutic efficacy [143]. A randomised phase III study using a combination of hydralazine and valproate with standard cisplatin/topetecan compared with cisplatin/topetecan plus placebo has been registered with ClinicalTrials.gov (ClinicalTrials.gov identifier NCT00532818, last updated March 2009); however recent verification of this study is ominously absent.

Conclusion

To further the case for deeper exploration using these targeted agents in metastatic cervical cancer, lessons could be learnt by taking a brief foray into the evidence involving their use in other advanced gynaecological tumour types. Although it could be argued that the biological disparity between CC and other gynaecological cancers should preclude any direct comparisons regarding the utilisation of novel drugs, the similarities in their current chemotherapeutic management proves otherwise. For example, platinum-taxane doublets have long been heralded as the cornerstone for treating advanced CC, EOC and endometrial cancer; the latter for either progestin resistant or progesterone receptor negative subtypes. Furthermore, although the multiple episodes of platinum rechallenge adopted in EOC are seldom seen in CC, patients relapsing years after completing chemoradiation, can be expected to respond reasonably to platinum-based palliative chemotherapy.

Interestingly, there appear to be distinct patterns of success shared amongst the gynaecological malignancies with certain targeted therapies. Undoubtedly, the most successful approach has been with targeting angiogenesis. Phase III trials employing bevacizumab in EOC have implicated a role for both primary and maintenance therapy, with some promise in advancing PFS beyond 14 months in the GOG-0218 and ICON7 trials [38, 39]. Similar studies, supporting the activity of combinatorial regimes with chemotherapy and bevacizumab in both platinum-sensitive (OCEANS) [144] and platinum-resistant/recurrent ovarian cancer (AURELIA) [145] have also provided room for optimism in a disease where only minimal increments in OS have been evident over the past 15 years. Similarly, a phase II trial with bevacizumab monotherapy against recurrent endometrial cancer, has exhibited good tolerance and activity, with PFS beyond 6 months in 40.4% of patients [146]. Outside of PARP and PI3K inhibitors for EOC and EC respectively, these trials currently represent the most promising strategy in prolonging chemotherapeutic response and survival rates. In parallel with these observations, amongst all the targeted therapy studies pertaining to CC, this approach has manifested the most success, as lucidly exemplified by the survival advantages in the GOG240 study; which at the time of writing, represents the only Phase III molecularly targeted study in advanced/metastatic CC [41].

In relation to the study of anti-angiogenic tyrosine kinase inhibitors in other advanced gynaecological cancers, a wealth of study data are on the horizon. Pazopanib, and cediranib are both the subject of numerous phase III clinical trials in these diseases. Pazopanib is under scrutiny as maintenance therapy following first line combination chemotherapy for women with epithelial ovarian, fallopian tube and primary peritoneal carcinoma (OVAR 16/VEG110655). In addition, for recurrent EOC, monotherapy has a favourable toxicity profile and promising activity in the context of a phase II trial (147). Similarly, for metastatic CC encouraging results have been seen with single agent therapy in another Monk study [44] and hence there is an urge to expedite further trials with pazopinib in combination with platinum-based chemotherapy in this setting. Cediranib is under the spotlight in platinum sensitive EOC with the ICON6 study, a triple-armed, placebo-controlled trial which has recently closed to recruitment (Clinicaltrials.gov identifier: NCT00532194). This also parallels with the CIRCCa study in CC, as detailed earlier in this chapter.

With regards to EGFR family targeted agents, response rates using these drugs in EOC are particularly poor despite the abundance of EGFR expression (148-151). Again, the latter results are also witnessed with small studies in advanced CC and the failure has been attributable to the paucity of EGFR mutations in these tumour types [52, 152-154]. Despite a clear preclinical rationale for targeting the PI3K/Akt/mTOR signalling axis in CC [105], this has only resulted in two small studies using temsirolimus, with the most recent showing some promise with modest rates of disease stabilisation [72]. However, there remains a distinct lag in progress relative to the success seen with numerous studies using PI3K/mTOR inhibitors in endometrial cancer [155].

The question remains; despite substantial preclinical evidence supporting the introduction of molecular targeted therapies in gynaecological cancer, why has advanced cervical cancer fared the worst in this exciting era of translational oncology? Why have the first interim results of the Phase III GOG 240 study been presented nearly a decade after those from the ICON7 & GOG218 trials in EOC? Clearly, the relatively fewer presentations of advanced CC in comparison to EOC and endometrial cancer have prohibited progress in this field as this would inevitably result in poor trial accrual. Furthermore, although just under 300,000 patients worldwide succumb to this disease per annum [1], most of these will be in developing countries where the infrastructure for clinical trials may not align with centres in the more affluent developed world. The situation may also be compounded by the advent of Gardasil®, which has possibly instilled a significant degree of reluctance amongst the pharmaceutical industry to substantially invest in phase II/III clinical trials for this disease. However, as the true effects of Gardasil® will not be realised for several years, such nihilism is unwarranted and there is still a pressing need to improve OS in such patients whose clinical outcomes remain bleak. Hence there is a call for collaborative groups such as ICON and GOG to develop dynamic studies in this field. Moreover, such trials should attempt to exploit the use of neoadjuvant therapy, whereby genomic analysis from pre- and post-treatment biopsies can elucidate predictive biomarkers and ultimately assist appropriate stratification of patients likely to gain benefit from novel targeted therapy in combination with chemotherapy or chemoradiation.

Another possible contributing factor to this gap is the lack of some potentially targetable activating mutations, such as HER2 and BRCA1/2, which may add to the armament of treatments available for trial in ovarian and uterine malignancies respectively. Although the situation with PARP inhibition for high grade EOC is exciting, epic failures with EGFR/HER2 inhibition due to the relative lack of activating mutations in these receptors appears to have placed the nail in the coffin with this approach. Hence attention has turned towards targeting the supporting tumour microenvironment. This chapter has highlighted some of the proven success with COX inhibition and may serve as a platform for targeting other inflammatory mediators such as IL-6; an established tumour promoter in CC [109] and whose inhibition has shown clinical efficacy in EOC [156].

Undoubtedly, obtaining adequate financial support is paramount to the swift progress of translational research. The priority must now rest with collaborative groups in developing robustly designed clinical trials based on the promising pre-clinical and clinical data previously described in both locally advanced and metastatic settings. In this regard, window of opportunity trials, whereby patients receive novel therapies prior to standard treatment, may serve as the way forward. Such attempts to refresh current treatment algorithms must be adopted in order to appreciate both the true efficacy and survival impact of targeted agents in advanced cervical cancer.

References

[1]   Parkin D.M., Bray F., Ferlay J., Pisani P., Global cancer statistics, 2002. *CA Cancer J. Clin.*, 2005;55: 74-108.

[2]   Thigpen T., Shingleton H., Homesley H., Lagasse L., Blessing J., Cis-platinum in treatment of advanced or recurrent squamous cell carcinoma of the cervix: a phase II study of the Gynecologic Oncology Group. *Cancer,* 1981; 48: 899-903.

[3]   Bonomi P., Blessing J.A., Stehman F.B., DiSaia P.J., Walton L., Major F.J., Randomized trial of three cisplatin dose schedules in squamous-cell carcinoma of the cervix: a Gynecologic Oncology Group study. *J. Clin. Oncol.,* 1985; 3: 1079-1085.

[4]   McGuire W.P., Blessing J.A., Moore D., Lentz S.S., Photopulos G., Paclitaxel has moderate activity in squamous cervix cancer. A Gynecologic Oncology Group study. *J. Clin. Oncol.,* 1996; 14: 792-795.

[5]   Fiorica J.V., Blessing J.A., Puneky L.V. et al., A Phase II evaluation of weekly topotecan as a single agent second line therapy in persistent or recurrent carcinoma of the cervix: a Gynecologic Oncology Group study. *Gynecol. Oncol.,* 2009; 115: 285-289.

[6]   Muggia F.M., Blessing J.A., Waggoner S. et al., Evaluation of vinorelbine in persistent or recurrent nonsquamous carcinoma of the cervix: a Gynecologic Oncology Group Study. *Gynecol. Oncol.,* 2005; 96: 108-111.

[7]   Schilder R.J., Blessing J., Cohn D.E., Evaluation of gemcitabine in previously treated patients with non-squamous cell carcinoma of the cervix: a phase II study of the Gynecologic Oncology Group. *Gynecol. Oncol.,* 2005; 96: 103-107.

[8] Sutton G.P., Blessing J.A., Adcock L., Webster K.D., DeEulis T., Phase II study of ifosfamide and mesna in patients with previously-treated carcinoma of the cervix. A Gynecologic Oncology Group study. *Invest New Drugs,* 1989; 7: 341-343.

[9] Alberts D.S., Kronmal R., Baker L.H. et al., Phase II randomized trial of cisplatin chemotherapy regimens in the treatment of recurrent or metastatic squamous cell cancer of the cervix: a Southwest Oncology Group Study. *J. Clin. Oncol.,* 1987; 5: 1791-1795.

[10] Omura G.A., Blessing J.A., Vaccarello L. et al., Randomized trial of cisplatin versus cisplatin plus mitolactol versus cisplatin plus ifosfamide in advanced squamous carcinoma of the cervix: a Gynecologic Oncology Group study. *J. Clin. Oncol.,* 1997; 15: 165-171.

[11] Moore D.H., Blessing J.A., McQuellon R.P. et al., Phase III study of cisplatin with or without paclitaxel in stage IVB, recurrent, or persistent squamous cell carcinoma of the cervix: a gynecologic oncology group study. *J. Clin. Oncol.,* 2004; 22: 3113-3119.

[12] Long H.J., 3rd, Bundy B.N., Grendys E.C., Jr. et al., Randomized phase III trial of cisplatin with or without topotecan in carcinoma of the uterine cervix: a Gynecologic Oncology Group Study. *J. Clin. Oncol.,* 2005; 23: 4626-4633.

[13] Monk B.J., Sill M.W., McMeekin D.S. et al., Phase III trial of four cisplatin-containing doublet combinations in stage IVB, recurrent, or persistent cervical carcinoma: a Gynecologic Oncology Group study. *J. Clin. Oncol.,* 2009; 27: 4649-4655.

[14] Neijt J.P., Engelholm S.A., Tuxen M.K. et al., Exploratory phase III study of paclitaxel and cisplatin versus paclitaxel and carboplatin in advanced ovarian cancer. *J. Clin. Oncol.,* 2000; 18: 3084-3092.

[15] Kitagawa R., Katsumata N., Shibata T. et al., A randomized, phase III trial of paclitaxel plus carboplatin (TC) versus paclitaxel plus cisplatin (TP) in stage IVb, persistent or recurrent cervical cancer: Japan Clinical Oncology Group study (JCOG0505). *J. Clin. Oncol., 2012*; 30 (suppl; abstr 5006).

[16] Carmeliet P., Jain R.K., Angiogenesis in cancer and other diseases. *Nature,* 2000; 407: 249-257.

[17] Patan S., Munn L.L., Jain R.K., Intussusceptive microvascular growth in a human colon adenocarcinoma xenograft: a novel mechanism of tumor angiogenesis. *Microvasc. Res.,* 1996; 51: 260-272.

[18] Ferrara N., Gerber H.P., LeCouter J., The biology of VEGF and its receptors. *Nat. Med.,* 2003; 9: 669-676.

[19] Kerbel R.S., Tumor angiogenesis. *N. Engl. J. Med.,* 2008; 358: 2039-2049.

[20] Shibuya M., Claesson-Welsh L., Signal transduction by VEGF receptors in regulation of angiogenesis and lymphangiogenesis. *Exp. Cell Res.,* 2006; 312: 549-560.

[21] Mole D.R., Maxwell P.H., Pugh C.W., Ratcliffe P.J., Regulation of HIF by the von Hippel-Lindau tumour suppressor: implications for cellular oxygen sensing. *IUBMB Life, 2001*; 52: 43-47.

[22] Maxwell P.H., Ratcliffe P.J., Oxygen sensors and angiogenesis. *Semin. Cell Dev. Biol.,* 2002; 13: 29-37.

[23] Maxwell P.H., Wiesener M.S., Chang G.W. et al., The tumour suppressor protein VHL targets hypoxia-inducible factors for oxygen-dependent proteolysis. *Nature,* 1999; 399: 271-275.

[24] Clere N., Bermont L., Fauconnet S. et al., The human papillomavirus type 18 E6 oncoprotein induces Vascular Endothelial Growth Factor 121 (VEGF121) transcription from the promoter through a p53-independent mechanism. *Exp. Cell Res.,* 2007; 313: 3239-3250.

[25] Lopez-Ocejo O., Viloria-Petit A., Bequet-Romero M., Mukhopadhyay D., Rak J., Kerbel R.S., Oncogenes and tumor angiogenesis: the HPV-16 E6 oncoprotein activates the vascular endothelial growth factor (VEGF) gene promoter in a p53 independent manner. *Oncogene,* 2000; 19: 4611-4620.

[26] Chen L., Wu Y.Y., Liu P. et al., Down-regulation of HPV18 E6, E7, or VEGF expression attenuates malignant biological behavior of human cervical cancer cells. *Med. Oncol.,* 2011; 28 Suppl 1: S528-539.

[27] Guidi A.J., Abu-Jawdeh G., Berse B. et al., Vascular permeability factor (vascular endothelial growth factor) expression and angiogenesis in cervical neoplasia. *J. Natl. Cancer Inst.,* 1995; 87: 1237-1245.

[28] Kodama J., Seki N., Tokumo K. et al., Vascular endothelial growth factor is implicated in early invasion in cervical cancer. *Eur. J. Cancer,* 1999; 35: 485-489.

[29] Santin A.D., Hermonat P.L., Ravaggi A., Pecorelli S., Cannon M.J., Parham G.P., Secretion of vascular endothelial growth factor in adenocarcinoma and squamous cell carcinoma of the uterine cervix. *Obstet. Gynecol.,* 1999; 94: 78-82.

[30] Cheng W.F., Chen C.A., Lee C.N., Chen T.M., Hsieh F.J., Hsieh C.Y., Vascular endothelial growth factor in cervical carcinoma. *Obstet. Gynecol.,* 1999; 93: 761-765.

[31] Cheng W.F., Chen C.A., Lee C.N., Wei L.H., Hsieh F.J., Hsieh C.Y., Vascular endothelial growth factor and prognosis of cervical carcinoma. *Obstet. Gynecol.,* 2000; 96: 721-726.

[32] Loncaster J.A., Cooper R.A., Logue J.P., Davidson S.E., Hunter R.D., West C.M., Vascular endothelial growth factor (VEGF) expression is a prognostic factor for radiotherapy outcome in advanced carcinoma of the cervix. *Br. J. Cancer,* 2000; 83: 620-625.

[33] Delli Carpini J., Karam A.K., Montgomery L., Vascular endothelial growth factor and its relationship to the prognosis and treatment of breast, ovarian, and cervical cancer. *Angiogenesis,* 2010; 13: 43-58.

[34] Pietras K., Pahler J., Bergers G., Hanahan D., Functions of paracrine PDGF signaling in the proangiogenic tumor stroma revealed by pharmacological targeting. *PLoS Med.,* 2008; 5: e19.

[35] Murata T., Mizushima H., Chinen I. et al., HB-EGF and PDGF mediate reciprocal interactions of carcinoma cells with cancer-associated fibroblasts to support progression of uterine cervical cancers. *Cancer Res.,* 2011; 71: 6633-6642.

[36] Wright J.D., Viviano D., Powell M.A. et al., Bevacizumab combination therapy in heavily pretreated, recurrent cervical cancer. *Gynecol. Oncol.,* 2006; 103: 489-493.

[37] Monk B.J., Sill M.W., Burger R.A., Gray H.J., Buekers T.E., Roman L.D., Phase II trial of bevacizumab in the treatment of persistent or recurrent squamous cell carcinoma of the cervix: a gynecologic oncology group study. *J. Clin. Oncol.,* 2009; 27: 1069-1074.

[38] Burger R.A., Brady M.F., Bookman M.A. et al., Incorporation of bevacizumab in the primary treatment of ovarian cancer. *N. Engl. J. Med.,* 2011; 365: 2473-2483.

[39] Perren T.J., Swart A.M., Pfisterer J. et al., A phase 3 trial of bevacizumab in ovarian cancer. *N. Engl. J. Med.*, 2011; 365: 2484-2496.

[40] Schefter T.E., Winter K., Kwon J.S. et al., A phase II study of bevacizumab in combination with definitive radiotherapy and cisplatin chemotherapy in untreated patients with locally advanced cervical carcinoma: preliminary results of RTOG 0417. *Int. J. Radiat. Oncol. Biol. Phys.*, 2012; 83: 1179-1184.

[41] Tewari K.S., Sill M., Long H.J. et al., Incorporation of bevacizumab in the treatment of recurrent and metastatic cervical cancer: A phase III randomized trial of the Gynecologic Oncology Group. *J. Clin. Oncol.*, 2013; 31: 2013 (suppl; abstr 3).

[42] Okino K., Konishi H., Doi D. et al., Up-regulation of growth factor receptor-bound protein 10 in cervical squamous cell carcinoma. *Oncol. Rep.*, 2005; 13: 1069-1074.

[43] Escudier B.J., Porta C., Bono P. et al., Patient preference between pazopanib (Paz) and sunitinib (Sun): Results of a randomized double-blind, placebo-controlled, cross-over study in patients with metastatic renal cell carcinoma (mRCC)—PISCES study, NCT 01064310. *J. Clin. Oncol.*, 2012;30(18)suppl (June 20 Supplement) CRA4502.

[44] Monk B.J., Mas Lopez L., Zarba J.J. et al., Phase II, open-label study of pazopanib or lapatinib monotherapy compared with pazopanib plus lapatinib combination therapy in patients with advanced and recurrent cervical cancer. *J. Clin. Oncol.*, 2010; 28: 3562-3569.

[45] Kim K., Ryu S.Y., Major clinical research advances in gynecologic cancer 2009. *J. Gynecol. Oncol.*, 2009; 20: 203-209.

[46] Mackay H.J., Tinker A., Winquist E. et al., A phase II study of sunitinib in patients with locally advanced or metastatic cervical carcinoma: NCIC CTG Trial IND.184. *Gynecol. Oncol.*, 2010; 116: 163-167.

[47] Kudelka A.P., Levy T., Verschraegen C.F. et al., A phase I study of TNP-470 administered to patients with advanced squamous cell cancer of the cervix. *Clin. Cancer Res.*, 1997; 3: 1501-1505.

[48] Kudelka A.P., Verschraegen C.F., Loyer E., Complete remission of metastatic cervical cancer with the angiogenesis inhibitor TNP-470. *N. Engl. J. Med.*, 1998; 338: 991-992.

[49] Zagouri F., Sergentanis T.N., Chrysikos D., Filipits M., Bartsch R., Molecularly targeted therapies in cervical cancer. A systematic review. *Gynecol. Oncol.*, 2012; 126: 291-303.

[50] Yarden Y., Sliwkowski M.X., Untangling the ErbB signalling network. *Nat. Rev. Mol. Cell Biol.*, 2001; 2: 127-137.

[51] Herbst R.S., Review of epidermal growth factor receptor biology. *Int. J. Radiat. Oncol. Biol. Phys.*, 2004; 59: 21-26.

[52] Gadducci A., Guerrieri M.E., Greco C., Tissue biomarkers as prognostic variables of cervical cancer. *Crit. Rev. Oncol. Hematol.*, 2013; 86: 104-129.

[53] Lee W.I., Bacchni P., Bertoni F., Maeng Y.H., Park Y.K., Quantitative assessment of HER2/neu expression by real-time PCR and fluorescent in situ hybridization analysis in low-grade osteosarcoma. *Oncol. Rep.*, 2004; 12: 125-128.

[54] Noordhuis M.G., Eijsink J.J., Ten Hoor K.A. et al., Expression of epidermal growth factor receptor (EGFR) and activated EGFR predict poor response to (chemo)radiation and survival in cervical cancer. *Clin. Cancer Res.*, 2009; 15: 7389-7397.

[55] Kim Y.T., Park S.W., Kim J.W., Correlation between expression of EGFR and the prognosis of patients with cervical carcinoma. *Gynecol. Oncol.*, 2002; 87: 84-89.

[56] Perez-Regadera J., Sanchez-Munoz A., De-la-Cruz J. et al., Impact of epidermal growth factor receptor expression on disease-free survival and rate of pelvic relapse in patients with advanced cancer of the cervix treated with chemoradiotherapy. *Am. J. Clin. Oncol.,* 2011; 34: 395-400.

[57] Kersemaekers A.M., Fleuren G.J., Kenter G.G. et al., Oncogene alterations in carcinomas of the uterine cervix: overexpression of the epidermal growth factor receptor is associated with poor prognosis. *Clin. Cancer Res.,* 1999; 5: 577-586.

[58] Scambia G., Ferrandina G., Distefano M., D'Agostino G., Benedetti-Panici P., Mancuso S., Epidermal growth factor receptor (EGFR) is not related to the prognosis of cervical cancer. *Cancer Lett.,* 1998; 123: 135-139.

[59] Ngan H.Y., Cheung A.N., Liu S.S., Cheng D.K., Ng T.Y., Wong L.C., Abnormal expression of epidermal growth factor receptor and c-erbB2 in squamous cell carcinoma of the cervix: correlation with human papillomavirus and prognosis. *Tumour. Biol.,* 2001; 22: 176-183.

[60] Yamashita H., Murakami N., Asari T., Okuma K., Ohtomo K., Nakagawa K., Correlation among six biologic factors (p53, p21(WAF1), MIB-1, EGFR, HER2, and Bcl-2) and clinical outcomes after curative chemoradiation therapy in squamous cell cervical cancer. *Int. J. Radiat. Oncol. Biol. Phys.,* 2009; 74: 1165-1172.

[61] Goldstein N.I., Prewett M., Zuklys K., Rockwell P., Mendelsohn J., Biological efficacy of a chimeric antibody to the epidermal growth factor receptor in a human tumor xenograft model. *Clin. Cancer Res.,* 1995; 1: 1311-1318.

[62] Fan Z., Lu Y., Wu X., Mendelsohn J., Antibody-induced epidermal growth factor receptor dimerization mediates inhibition of autocrine proliferation of A431 squamous carcinoma cells. *J. Biol. Chem.,* 1994; 269: 27595-27602.

[63] Cohen M.H., Chen H., Shord S. et al., Approval summary: cetuximab in combination with Cisplatin or Carboplatin and 5-Fluorouracil for the first-line treatment of patients with recurrent locoregional or metastatic squamous cell head and neck cancer. *Oncologist,* 2013; 18: 460-466.

[64] Jonker D.J., O'Callaghan C.J., Karapetis C.S. et al., Cetuximab for the treatment of colorectal cancer. *N. Engl. J. Med.,* 2007; 357: 2040-2048.

[65] Eiblmaier M., Meyer L.A., Watson M.A., Fracasso P.M., Pike L.J., Anderson C.J., Correlating EGFR expression with receptor-binding properties and internalization of 64Cu-DOTA-cetuximab in 5 cervical cancer cell lines. *J. Nucl. Med.,* 2008; 49: 1472-1479.

[66] Santin A.D., Sill M.W., McMeekin D.S. et al., Phase II trial of cetuximab in the treatment of persistent or recurrent squamous or non-squamous cell carcinoma of the cervix: a Gynecologic Oncology Group study. *Gynecol. Oncol.,* 2011; 122: 495-500.

[67] Farley J., Sill M.W., Birrer M. et al., Phase II study of cisplatin plus cetuximab in advanced, recurrent, and previously treated cancers of the cervix and evaluation of epidermal growth factor receptor immunohistochemical expression: a Gynecologic Oncology Group study. *Gynecol. Oncol.,* 2011; 121: 303-308.

[68] Kurtz J.E., Hardy-Bessard A.C., Deslandres M. et al., Cetuximab, topotecan and cisplatin for the treatment of advanced cervical cancer: A phase II GINECO trial. *Gynecol. Oncol.,* 2009; 113: 16-20.

[69] Blohmer J., Gore M., Kuemmel S. et al., Phase II study to determine the response rate, pharmacokinetics (PK), pharmacodynamics (PD), safety and tolerability of treatment with the humanised anti-epidermal growth factor receptor (EGFR) monoclonal antibody EMD 72000 (matuzumab) in patients with recurrent cervical cancer. . *J. Clin. Oncol.,* 2005 ASCO Annual Meeting Proceedings 2005; 23 (16S)

[70] Goncalves A., Fabbro M., Lhomme C. et al., A phase II trial to evaluate gefitinib as second- or third-line treatment in patients with recurring locoregionally advanced or metastatic cervical cancer. *Gynecol. Oncol.,* 2008; 108: 42-46.

[71] Schilder R.J., Sill M.W., Lee Y.C., Mannel R., A phase II trial of erlotinib in recurrent squamous cell carcinoma of the cervix: a Gynecologic Oncology Group Study. *Int. J. Gynecol. Cancer,* 2009; 19: 929-933.

[72] Tinker A.V., Ellard S., Welch S. et al., Phase II study of temsirolimus (CCI-779) in women with recurrent, unresectable, locally advanced or metastatic carcinoma of the cervix. A trial of the NCIC Clinical Trials Group (NCIC CTG IND 199). *Gynecol. Oncol.,* 2013.

[73] Ferreira C.G., Erlich F., Carmo C.C. et al., Erlotinib (E) combined with cisplatin (C) and radiotherapy (RT) for patients with locally-advanced squamous cell cervical cancer: a phase II trial. *J. Clin. Oncol.,* 2008;26(15S) (May 20 Supplement): 5511.

[74] Cufer T., Ovcaricek T., O'Brien M.E., Systemic therapy of advanced non-small cell lung cancer: major-developments of the last 5-years. *Eur. J. Cancer,* 2013; 49: 1216-1225.

[75] Hardie D.G., AMP-activated/SNF1 protein kinases: conserved guardians of cellular energy. *Nat. Rev. Mol. Cell Biol.,* 2007; 8: 774-785.

[76] Luo Z., Saha A.K., Xiang X., Ruderman N.B., AMPK, the metabolic syndrome and cancer. *Trends Pharmacol. Sci.,* 2005; 26: 69-76.

[77] Fay J.R., Steele V., Crowell J.A., Energy homeostasis and cancer prevention: the AMP-activated protein kinase. *Cancer Prev. Res. (Phila),* 2009; 2: 301-309.

[78] Woods A., Azzout-Marniche D., Foretz M. et al., Characterization of the role of AMP-activated protein kinase in the regulation of glucose-activated gene expression using constitutively active and dominant negative forms of the kinase. *Mol. Cell Biol.,* 2000; 20: 6704-6711.

[79] Yu S.Y., Chan D.W., Liu V.W., Ngan H.Y., Inhibition of cervical cancer cell growth through activation of upstream kinases of AMP-activated protein kinase. *Tumour. Biol.,* 2009; 30: 80-85.

[80] Kwan H.T., Chan D.W., Cai P.C. et al., AMPK activators suppress cervical cancer cell growth through inhibition of DVL3 mediated Wnt/beta-catenin signaling activity. *PLoS One,* 2013; 8: e53597.

[81] Werner H., Weinstein D., Bentov I., Similarities and differences between insulin and IGF-I: structures, receptors, and signalling pathways. *Arch. Physiol. Biochem.,* 2008; 114: 17-22.

[82] Furstenberger G., Senn H.J., Insulin-like growth factors and cancer. *Lancet Oncol.,* 2002; 3: 298-302.

[83] Bruchim I., Werner H., Targeting IGF-1 signaling pathways in gynecologic malignancies. *Expert. Opin. Ther. Targets,* 2013; 17: 307-320.

[84] Serrano M., Umaña-Pérez A., Garay-Baquero D.J., Sánchez-Gómez M., New Biomarkers for Cervical Cancer – Perspectives from the IGF System. In Rajamanickam R. ed. Topics on Cervical Cancer With an Advocacy for Prevention. InTech, 2012; 215-236.

[85] Mohan S., Baylink D.J., IGF-binding proteins are multifunctional and act via IGF-dependent and -independent mechanisms. *J. Endocrinol.*, 2002; 175: 19-31.

[86] Seccareccia E., Brodt P., The role of the insulin-like growth factor-I receptor in malignancy: an update. *Growth Horm. IGF Res.*, 2012; 22: 193-199.

[87] Hirano S., Ito N., Takahashi S., Tamaya T., Clinical implications of insulin-like growth factors through the presence of their binding proteins and receptors expressed in gynecological cancers. *Eur. J. Gynaecol. Oncol.*, 2004; 25: 187-191.

[88] Steller M.A., Delgado C.H., Bartels C.J., Woodworth C.D., Zou Z., Overexpression of the insulin-like growth factor-1 receptor and autocrine stimulation in human cervical cancer cells. *Cancer Res.*, 1996; 56: 1761-1765.

[89] Shen M.R., Lin A.C., Hsu Y.M. et al., Insulin-like growth factor 1 stimulates KCl cotransport, which is necessary for invasion and proliferation of cervical cancer and ovarian cancer cells. *J. Biol. Chem.*, 2004; 279: 40017-40025.

[90] Shen M.R., Hsu Y.M., Hsu K.F., Chen Y.F., Tang M.J., Chou C.Y., Insulin-like growth factor 1 is a potent stimulator of cervical cancer cell invasiveness and proliferation that is modulated by alphavbeta3 integrin signaling. *Carcinogenesis*, 2006; 27: 962-971.

[91] Steller M.A., Zou Z., Schiller J.T., Baserga R., Transformation by human papillomavirus 16 E6 and E7: role of the insulin-like growth factor 1 receptor. *Cancer Res.*, 1996; 56: 5087-5091.

[92] Kuramoto H., Hongo A., Liu Y.X. et al., Immunohistochemical evaluation of insulin-like growth factor I receptor status in cervical cancer specimens. *Acta. Med. Okayama*, 2008; 62: 251-259.

[93] Huang Y.F., Shen M.R., Hsu K.F., Cheng Y.M., Chou C.Y., Clinical implications of insulin-like growth factor 1 system in early-stage cervical cancer. *Br. J. Cancer*, 2008; 99: 1096-1102.

[94] Mathur S.P., Mathur R.S., Underwood P.B., Kohler M.F., Creasman W.T., Circulating levels of insulin-like growth factor-II and IGF-binding protein 3 in cervical cancer. *Gynecol. Oncol.*, 2003; 91: 486-493.

[95] Serrano M.L., Sanchez-Gomez M., Bravo M.M., Cervical scrapes levels of insulin-like growth factor-II and insulin-like growth factor binding protein 3 in women with squamous intraepithelial lesions and cervical cancer. *Horm. Metab. Res.*, 2010; 42: 977-981.

[96] Serrano M.L., Romero A., Cendales R., Sanchez-Gomez M., Bravo M.M., Serum levels of insulin-like growth factor-I and -II and insulin-like growth factor binding protein 3 in women with squamous intraepithelial lesions and cervical cancer. *Biomedica*, 2006; 26: 258-268.

[97] Lee S.W., Lee S.Y., Lee S.R., Ju W., Kim S.C., Plasma levels of insulin-like growth factor-1 and insulin-like growth factor binding protein-3 in women with cervical neoplasia. *J. Gynecol. Oncol.*, 2010; 21: 174-180.

[98] Schaffer A., Koushik A., Trottier H. et al., Insulin-like growth factor-I and risk of high-grade cervical intraepithelial neoplasia. *Cancer Epidemiol. Biomarkers Prev.*, 2007; 16: 716-722.

[99] Lloret M., Lara P.C., Bordon E. et al., IGF-1R expression in localized cervical carcinoma patients treated by radiochemotherapy. *Gynecol. Oncol.,* 2007, 106, 8-11.

[100] Molife L.R., Fong P.C., Paccagnella L. et al., The insulin-like growth factor-I receptor inhibitor figitumumab (CP-751,871) in combination with docetaxel in patients with advanced solid tumours: results of a phase Ib dose-escalation, open-label study. *Br. J. Cancer,* 2010; 103: 332-339.

[101] Buck E., Gokhale P.C., Koujak S. et al., Compensatory insulin receptor (IR) activation on inhibition of insulin-like growth factor-1 receptor (IGF-1R): rationale for cotargeting IGF-1R and IR in cancer. *Mol. Cancer Ther.,* 2010; 9: 2652-2664.

[102] Feng W., Duan X., Liu J., Xiao J., Brown R.E., Morphoproteomic evidence of constitutively activated and overexpressed mTOR pathway in cervical squamous carcinoma and high grade squamous intraepithelial lesions. *Int. J. Clin. Exp. Pathol.,* 2009; 2: 249-260.

[103] Faried L.S., Faried A., Kanuma T. et al., Predictive and prognostic role of activated mammalian target of rapamycin in cervical cancer treated with cisplatin-based neoadjuvant chemotherapy. *Oncol. Rep.,* 2006; 16: 57-63.

[104] Oh K.J., Kalinina A., Park N.H., Bagchi S., Deregulation of eIF4E: 4E-BP1 in differentiated human papillomavirus-containing cells leads to high levels of expression of the E7 oncoprotein. *J. Virol.,* 2006; 80: 7079-7088.

[105] Ji J., Zheng P.S., Activation of mTOR signaling pathway contributes to survival of cervical cancer cells. *Gynecol. Oncol.,* 2010; 117: 103-108.

[106] Zhou X., Chen X., Hu L. et al., Polymorphisms involved in the miR-218-LAMB3 pathway and susceptibility of cervical cancer, a case-control study in Chinese women. *Gynecol. Oncol.,* 2010; 117: 287-290.

[107] Li J., Ping Z., Ning H., MiR-218 Impairs Tumor Growth and Increases Chemo-Sensitivity to Cisplatin in Cervical Cancer. *Int. J. Mol. Sci.,* 2012; 13: 16053-16064.

[108] Temkin S.M., Yamada S.D., Fleming G.F., A phase I study of weekly temsirolimus and topotecan in the treatment of advanced and/or recurrent gynecologic malignancies. *Gynecol. Oncol.,* 2010; 117: 473-476.

[109] Coward J.I., Kulbe H., The role of interleukin-6 in gynaecological malignancies. *Cytokine Growth Factor Rev.,* 2012; 23: 333-342.

[110] Castle P.E., Hillier S.L., Rabe L.K. et al., An association of cervical inflammation with high-grade cervical neoplasia in women infected with oncogenic human papillomavirus (HPV). *Cancer Epidemiol. Biomarkers Prev.,* 2001; 10: 1021-1027.

[111] Schwebke J.R., Zajackowski M.E., Effect of concurrent lower genital tract infections on cervical cancer screening. *Genitourin. Med.,* 1997; 73: 383-386.

[112] Jones C.J., Brinton L.A., Hamman R.F. et al., Risk factors for in situ cervical cancer: results from a case-control study. *Cancer Res.,* 1990; 50: 3657-3662.

[113] Brinton L.A., Hamman R.F., Huggins G.R. et al., Sexual and reproductive risk factors for invasive squamous cell cervical cancer. *J. Natl. Cancer Inst.,* 1987; 79: 23-30.

[114] Kemp T.J., Hildesheim A., Garcia-Pineres A. et al., Elevated systemic levels of inflammatory cytokines in older women with persistent cervical human papillomavirus infection. *Cancer Epidemiol. Biomarkers Prev.,* 2010; 19: 1954-1959.

[115] O'Banion M.K., Winn V.D., Young D.A., cDNA cloning and functional activity of a glucocorticoid-regulated inflammatory cyclooxygenase. *Proc. Natl. Acad. Sci. USA,* 1992; 89: 4888-4892.

[116] Sales K.J., Katz A.A., Howard B., Soeters R.P., Millar R.P., Jabbour H.N., Cyclooxygenase-1 is up-regulated in cervical carcinomas: autocrine/paracrine regulation of cyclooxygenase-2, prostaglandin e receptors, and angiogenic factors by cyclooxygenase-1. *Cancer Res.,* 2002; 62: 424-432.

[117] Kulkarni S., Rader J.S., Zhang F. et al., Cyclooxygenase-2 is overexpressed in human cervical cancer. *Clin. Cancer Res.,* 2001; 7: 429-434.

[118] Ryu H.S., Chang K.H., Yang H.W., Kim M.S., Kwon H.C., Oh K.S., High cyclooxygenase-2 expression in stage IB cervical cancer with lymph node metastasis or parametrial invasion. *Gynecol. Oncol.,* 2000; 76: 320-325.

[119] Gaffney D.K., Holden J., Davis M., Zempolich K., Murphy K.J., Dodson M., Elevated cyclooxygenase-2 expression correlates with diminished survival in carcinoma of the cervix treated with radiotherapy. *International Journal of Radiation Oncology Biology Physics,* 2001; 49: 1213-1217.

[120] Kim H.J., Wu H.G., Park I.A., Ha S.W., High cyclooxygenase-2 expression is related with distant metastasis in cervical cancer treated with radiotherapy. *Int. J. Radiat. Oncol. Biol. Phys.,* 2003; 55: 16-20.

[121] Nakata E., Mason K.A., Hunter N. et al., Potentiation of tumor response to radiation or chemoradiation by selective cyclooxygenase-2 enzyme inhibitors. *Int. J. Radiat. Oncol. Biol. Phys.,* 2004; 58: 369-375.

[122] Weppelmann B., Monkemeier D., The influence of prostaglandin antagonists on radiation therapy of carcinoma of the cervix. *Gynecol. Oncol.,* 1984; 17: 196-199.

[123] Wang A.H., Tian X.Y., Yu J.J., Mi J.Q., Liu H., Wang R.F., Celecoxib radiosensitizes the human cervical cancer HeLa cell line via a mechanism dependent on reduced cyclo-oxygenase-2 and vascular endothelial growth factor C expression. *J. Int. Med. Res.,* 2012; 40: 56-66.

[124] Xia S., Zhao Y., Yu S., Zhang M., Activated PI3K/Akt/COX-2 pathway induces resistance to radiation in human cervical cancer HeLa cells. *Cancer Biother Radiopharm.,* 2010; 25: 317-323.

[125] Ogino M., Minoura S., Indomethacin increases the cytotoxicity of cis-platinum and 5-fluorouracil in the human uterine cervical cancer cell lines SKG-2 and HKUS by increasing the intracellular uptake of the agents. *Int. J. Clin. Oncol.,* 2001; 6: 84-89.

[126] Fukada K., Takahashi-Yanaga F., Sakoguchi-Okada N. et al., Celecoxib induces apoptosis by inhibiting the expression of survivin in HeLa cells. *Biochem. Biophys. Res. Commun.,* 2007; 357: 1166-1171.

[127] Kim S.H., Song S.H., Kim S.G. et al., Celecoxib induces apoptosis in cervical cancer cells independent of cyclooxygenase using NF-kappaB as a possible target. *J. Cancer Res. Clin. Oncol.,* 2004; 130: 551-560.

[128] Herrera F.G., Chan P., Doll C. et al., A prospective phase I-II trial of the cyclooxygenase-2 inhibitor celecoxib in patients with carcinoma of the cervix with biomarker assessment of the tumor microenvironment. *Int. J. Radiat. Oncol. Biol. Phys.,* 2007; 67: 97-103.

[129] Gaffney D.K., Winter K., Dicker A.P. et al., A Phase II study of acute toxicity for Celebrex (celecoxib) and chemoradiation in patients with locally advanced cervical cancer: primary endpoint analysis of RTOG 0128. *Int. J. Radiat. Oncol. Biol. Phys.,* 2007; 67: 104-109.

[130] Strahl B.D., Allis C.D., The language of covalent histone modifications. *Nature,* 2000; 403: 41-45.

[131] Takai N., Kira N., Ishii T., Nishida M., Nasu K., Narahara H., Novel chemotherapy using histone deacetylase inhibitors in cervical cancer. *Asian. Pac. J. Cancer Prev.,* 2011; 12: 575-580.

[132] Werness B.A., Levine A.J., Howley P.M., Association of human papillomavirus types 16 and 18 E6 proteins with p53. *Science,* 1990; 248: 76-79.

[133] Brehm A., Nielsen S.J., Miska E.A. et al., The E7 oncoprotein associates with Mi2 and histone deacetylase activity to promote cell growth. *EMBO J.,* 1999; 18: 2449-2458.

[134] Lin Z., Bazzaro M., Wang M.C., Chan K.C., Peng S., Roden R.B., Combination of proteasome and HDAC inhibitors for uterine cervical cancer treatment. *Clin. Cancer Res.,* 2009; 15: 570-577.

[135] Darvas K., Rosenberger S., Brenner D. et al., Histone deacetylase inhibitor-induced sensitization to TNFalpha/TRAIL-mediated apoptosis in cervical carcinoma cells is dependent on HPV oncogene expression. *Int. J. Cancer,* 2010; 127: 1384-1392.

[136] Finzer P., Kuntzen C., Soto U., zur Hausen H., Rosl F., Inhibitors of histone deacetylase arrest cell cycle and induce apoptosis in cervical carcinoma cells circumventing human papillomavirus oncogene expression. *Oncogene, 2001*; 20: 4768-4776.

[137] Borutinskaite V.V., Magnusson K.E., Navakauskiene R., Histone deacetylase inhibitor BML-210 induces growth inhibition and apoptosis and regulates HDAC and DAPC complex expression levels in cervical cancer cells. *Mol. Biol. Rep.,* 2012; 39: 10179-10186.

[138] Yu J., Mi J., Wang Y., Wang A., Tian X., Regulation of radiosensitivity by HDAC inhibitor trichostatin A in the human cervical carcinoma cell line Hela. *Eur. J. Gynaecol. Oncol.,* 2012; 33: 285-290.

[139] Blaheta R.A., Nau H., Michaelis M., Cinatl J., Jr., Valproate and valproate-analogues: potent tools to fight against cancer. *Curr. Med. Chem.,* 2002; 9: 1417-1433.

[140] Phiel C.J., Zhang F., Huang E.Y., Guenther M.G., Lazar M.A., Klein P.S., Histone deacetylase is a direct target of valproic acid, a potent anticonvulsant, mood stabilizer, and teratogen. *J. Biol. Chem.,* 2001; 276: 36734-36741.

[141] Chavez-Blanco A., Segura-Pacheco B., Perez-Cardenas E. et al., Histone acetylation and histone deacetylase activity of magnesium valproate in tumor and peripheral blood of patients with cervical cancer. A phase I study. *Mol. Cancer,* 2005; 4: 22.

[142] Ryan Q.C., Headlee D., Acharya M. et al., Phase I and pharmacokinetic study of MS-275, a histone deacetylase inhibitor, in patients with advanced and refractory solid tumors or lymphoma. *J. Clin. Oncol.,* 2005; 23: 3912-3922.

[143] Candelaria M., Cetina L., Perez-Cardenas E. et al., Epigenetic therapy and cisplatin chemoradiation in FIGO stage IIIB cervical cancer. *Eur. J. Gynaecol. Oncol.,* 2010; 31: 386-391.

[144] Aghajanian C., Blank S.V., Goff B.A. et al., OCEANS: a randomized, double-blind, placebo-controlled phase III trial of chemotherapy with or without bevacizumab in patients with platinum-sensitive recurrent epithelial ovarian, primary peritoneal, or fallopian tube cancer. *J. Clin. Oncol.,* 2012; 30: 2039-2045.

[145] Pujade-Lauraine E., Hilpert F., Weber B. et al., AURELIA: A randomized phase III trial evaluating bevacizumab (BEV) plus chemotherapy (CT) for platinum (PT)-resistant recurrent ovarian cancer (OC). . *J. Clin. Oncol.,* 2012;30(18S) (June 20 Supplement): LBA5002.

[146] Aghajanian C., Sill M.W., Darcy K.M. et al., Phase II trial of bevacizumab in recurrent or persistent endometrial cancer: a Gynecologic Oncology Group study. *J. Clin. Oncol.,* 2011; 29: 2259-2265.

[147] Friedlander M., Hancock K.C., Rischin D. et al., A Phase II, open-label study evaluating pazopanib in patients with recurrent ovarian cancer. *Gynecol. Oncol.,* 2010; 119: 32-37.

[148] Bookman M.A., Darcy K.M., Clarke-Pearson D., Boothby R.A., Horowitz I.R., Evaluation of monoclonal humanized anti-HER2 antibody, trastuzumab, in patients with recurrent or refractory ovarian or primary peritoneal carcinoma with overexpression of HER2: a phase II trial of the Gynecologic Oncology Group. *J. Clin. Oncol.,* 2003; 21: 283-290.

[149] Secord A.A., Blessing J.A., Armstrong D.K. et al., Phase II trial of cetuximab and carboplatin in relapsed platinum-sensitive ovarian cancer and evaluation of epidermal growth factor receptor expression: a Gynecologic Oncology Group study. *Gynecol. Oncol.,* 2008; 108: 493-499.

[150] Murphy M., Stordal B., Erlotinib or gefitinib for the treatment of relapsed platinum pretreated non-small cell lung cancer and ovarian cancer: a systematic review. *Drug Resist. Updat.,* 2011; 14: 177-190.

[151] Vergote I., Joly F., Katsaros D. et al., Randomized Phase III study of erlotinib versus observation in patients with no evidence of disease progression after first-line platin-based chemotherapy for ovarian carcinoma: a GCIG and EORTC–GCG study. *J. Clin. Oncol.,* 2012; 30(Suppl.): Abstract LBA5000.

[152] Lassus H., Sihto H., Leminen A. et al., Gene amplification, mutation, and protein expression of EGFR and mutations of ERBB2 in serous ovarian carcinoma. *J. Mol. Med. (Berl),* 2006; 84: 671-681.

[153] Arias-Pulido H., Joste N., Chavez A. et al., Absence of epidermal growth factor receptor mutations in cervical cancer. *Int. J. Gynecol. Cancer,* 2008; 18: 749-754.

[154] Steffensen K.D., Waldstrom M., Olsen D.A. et al., Mutant epidermal growth factor receptor in benign, borderline, and malignant ovarian tumors. *Clin. Cancer Res.,* 2008; 14: 3278-3282.

[155] Slomovitz B.M., Coleman R.L., The PI3K/AKT/mTOR pathway as a therapeutic target in endometrial cancer. *Clin. Cancer Res.,* 2012; 18: 5856-5864.

[156] Coward J., Kulbe H., Chakravarty P. et al., Interleukin-6 as a therapeutic target in human ovarian cancer. *Clin. Cancer Res.,* 2011; 17: 6083-6096.

In: Cervical Cancer
Editor: Laurie Elit

ISBN: 978-1-62948-062-6
© 2013 Nova Science Publishers, Inc.

Chapter XIII

Screening and Treatment of Cervical Cancer in Pregnancy

Jonathan R. Foote, MD and Jennifer Young Pierce, MD
Medical University of South Carolina, Charleston, SC, US

Abstract

A diagnosis of cancer or precancer of the cervix in pregnancy poses major challenges for a woman and her family. Can she continue her pregnancy? What are her options for treatment? Fortunately the majority of cases present at an early stage, and overall survival remains the same as for the non-pregnant patient. Eighty-three percent of cases present with Stage I disease, while 10% present with Stage II disease. Five-year survival rates for stage IA disease are >95%, with five-year survival rates for Stage IB ranging from 76% to 95%. The incidence of cervical cancer in pregnancy is low, 1-10 per 10,000 pregnancies. However, this number is likely to increase as women continue to delay their childbearing years. The stakes are high for these women, which makes the discussion of management options imperative. This chapter will review the most up to date recommendations for cervical cancer screening, diagnosis, and treatment in pregnancy. Cervical cancer in pregnancy demands a multi-disciplinary approach including the patient, her obstetrician, a maternal fetal medicine specialist, and a gynecologic oncologist. Patient education and empathy should lead the discussion of management, and a patient's wishes will ultimately guide her plan.

Keywords: Cervical Cancer, Pregnancy

Introduction

Cervical cancer in pregnancy occurs 1-10/10,000 pregnancies, depending on inclusion criteria. In the United States this number may continue to rise as women delay childbearing and as reproductive technology improves. Although cervical cancer in pregnancy is infrequent, the stakes are high and discussion of management is imperative. The diagnosis of cervical cancer in pregnancy must be considered on a case-to-case basis. Each case should involve a multi-disciplinary team in coordination with the patient and the patient's family. This chapter will review the current cervical screening guidelines and colposcopic guidelines in pregnancy, as well explore the most up to date recommendations for cervical cancer treatment in pregnancy.

Section 1: Screening and Pre-Invasive Disease

1.1. Screening

In the United States, 2-7% of women will have an abnormal pap smear during pregnancy. [1, 2, 3] Cervical cancer screening in pregnancy should follow national guidelines recommended by the American Cancer Society, the American Society for Colposcopy and Cervical Pathology (ASCCP), and the American Society of Clinical Pathology. [4] Pap smear testing has been demonstrated to be as accurate in pregnancy as in the non-pregnant patient. [3] Table 1 lists the current national guidelines that were recently endorsed by the American Congress of Obstetricians and Gynecologists (ACOG) in Practice Bulletin 131. Most women during pregnancy will fall between 21-35 years of age, although advanced maternal age (AMA) is being encountered more often as women delay pregnancy and as assisted reproductive technology improves. Prior to 21 years of age, no screening should be performed regardless of pregnancy. As well, pregnancy is not an indication to perform screening. If a woman is up-to-date on screening guidelines, repeat testing is not recommended at the start of pregnancy. Further, repeating screening post-partum is not recommended.

1.2. Abnormal Cervical Cytology Algorithms in Pregnancy

The ASCCP updated management algorithms for cervical cytology in April 2013. ACOG and the American Cancer Society have endorsed the new ASCCP guidelines. Cervical cytology algorithms should continue to be followed in pregnancy, although most colposcopic recommendations can be deferred until after pregnancy. Cervical cancer screening in pregnancy has the purpose of diagnosing cancer, and subsequently providing appropriate treatment counseling. Cytology results that predicate colposcopy during pregnancy include atypical glandular cells (AGC), atypical squamous cells – cannot rule out high grade (ASC-H), and high-grade squamous lesions (HSIL). Low-grade squamous lesions (LSIL) can be managed with colposcopy during pregnancy or deferred until at least 6 weeks postpartum.

Economos et al. demonstrated that almost all colposcopic examinations are adequate by 20 weeks of gestation secondary to cervical eversion. [5] Failure to collect biopsies is associated with missing diagnosis of cancer and delayed treatment options. [6] Cervical biopsies during colposcopy have not been associated with increased risk of bleeding or loss of pregnancy, and providers should counsel their patients to this effect. [5] However, most experts recommend a biopsy only if there is a concern for invasive cancer. Endocervical curettage (ECC) and endometrial biopsy (EMB) are always contraindicated during pregnancy and should not be performed in any situation. One retrospective study reported on ECC performed in 33 pregnant patients with a diagnosis of CIS (carcinoma in situ). Ninety-seven percent delivered at term without any significant increase in maternal or neonatal morbidity. [7] However, ECC remains "unacceptable" in pregnancy. [8] Routine diagnostic excisional procedures are no longer part of ASCCP cytology guidelines, and have always been contraindicated in pregnancy. An excisional procedure should be considered if there is a possibility of cancer and that diagnosis would alter the outcome of the pregnancy. These situations will be discussed in more detail below.

Table 1. Screening Methods for Cervical Cancer: Joint Recommendations of the American Cancer Society, the American Society for Colposcopy and Cervical Pathology, and the American Society for Clinical Pathology [4]

Population	Recommended Screening Method	Comment
Women younger than 21 years	No screening	
Women aged 21–29 years	Cytology alone every 3 years	
Women aged 30–65 years	Human papillomavirus and cytology co-testing (preferred) every 5 years Cytology alone (acceptable) every 3 years	Screening by HPV testing alone is not recommended
Women older than 65 years	No screening is necessary after adequate negative prior screening results	Women with a history of CIN 2, CIN 3 or adenocarcinoma in situ should continue routine age-based screening for at least 20 years
Women who underwent total hysterectomy	No screening is necessary	Applies to women without a cervix and without a history of CIN 2, CIN 3, adenocarcinoma in situ, or cancer in the past 20 years
Women vaccinated against HPV	Follow age-specific recommendations (same as unvaccinated women)	

Abbreviations: CIN indicates cervical intraepithelial neoplasia; HPV, human papillomavirus.
Modified from Saslow, D., Solomon, D., Lawson, H. W., Killackey, M., Kulasingam, S. L., Cain, J., et al. American Cancer Society, American Society for Colposcopy and Cervical Pathology, and American Society for Clinical Pathology screening guidelines for the prevention and early detection of cervical cancer.

1.2.1. Atypical Glandular Cells

A diagnosis of atypical glandular cells is frequently associated with a high grade or cancerous lesion in the nonpregnant patient. However, in pregnant patients, the possibility of a benign finding is more likely. The Arias-Stella reaction in pregnancy can be misinterpreted as glandular atypia. [1, 9] In 1954, Javier Arias-Stella first described a reaction of gestational endometrium characterized by hyper-secretory glands with architectural complexity and nuclear enlargement. [10] Cytological features characteristic of this reaction are also associated with endocervical adenocarcinoma and poorly differentiated squamous cell carcinoma. Arias-Stella reaction was found in 9% of hysterectomy specimens close to gestation and should not be mistaken for malignancy during pregnancy. [1] Kim et al. reviewed 21 patients with AGC during pregnancy, which lead to the diagnosis of carcinoma in situ (CIS) in only one patient. [11]

The ASCCP published new guidelines in 2013, which advocate the evaluation of AGC in pregnancy with colposcopy. ECC and EMB are still contraindicated. Careful visual inspection with acetic acid should be performed with biopsies done if a lesion is identified. Repeat colposcopy can be performed each trimester if the clinical exam is concerning. [4] Conization procedure should be considered in those patients with an exam, repeat pap, or biopsy concerning for invasive cancer. This should be limited to the second trimester and again should only be considered in which the results of the biopsy would change the outcome of the pregnancy.

1.2.2. High-Grade Squamous Lesions

The ASCCP continues to recommend colposcopy during pregnancy for HSIL. Seventy to 80% of HSIL patients will have high-grade disease (CIN 2/3) at time of cervical biopsy. [1] Murta et al. reported on 53 patients with HSIL managed conservatively, demonstrating that 75% of patients had persistent high-grade disease after pregnancy. However, of utmost importance, no patients progressed to invasive disease. [12] Vlahos et al. reported on 78 patients with HSIL, demonstrating no progression to invasive disease. [13] It remains imperative to perform colposcopy in this subset of patients, but it is reassuring that overt cancer in pregnancy is unlikely.

1.3. Cervical Intraepithelial Neoplasia

Cervical intraepithelial neoplasia can present as CIN 1, CIN 2, and CIN 3. In March of 2012, the College of American Pathologists and the ASCCP convened a consensus conference entitled the Lower Anogenital Squamous Terminology (LAST) Project. This project may eventually change our terminology of intraepithelial neoplasia into "low-grade" squamous intraepithelial lesion and "high-grade" squamous intraepithelial lesion (SIL). This terminology would mirror current cytology reports. "Low-grade" SIL correlates with CIN1 disease and "high-grade" SIL correlates with CIN 2 and CIN 3 disease. The LAST Project also addresses the use of p16 tissue immuno-staining to help delineate intraepithelial disease into "high-grade" and benign "low-grade" disease. [14] Positive p16 staining is associated with high-risk disease, and likely represents CIN 3 disease. CIN 2 as a category is hard to identify by pathologists, but p16 testing has helped to delineate these lesions into low grade vs. high grade. [15]

Depending on clinical suspicion, CIN 2 and CIN 3 cervical biopsies can be followed by repeat colposcopy at most every 12 weeks during pregnancy or can be followed up at least 6 weeks postpartum. [4] Colposcopy should be performed by a seasoned provider who is familiar with colposcopy in pregnancy. CIN 1 on biopsy can be re-evaluated postpartum with repeat cytology and colposcopy. [4] The ASCCP recommends cervical conization "when the diagnosis of microinvasive/invasive cancer would change the outcome of the pregnancy or the mode of delivery." [4] Treatment of CIN disease during pregnancy is associated with significant perinatal morbidity, including hemorrhage, preterm birth, etc. It is also associated with incomplete excision, resulting in persistence of CIN and recurrent disease. [16] If invasive cancer is not present or suspected, CIN 2/3 can be managed conservatively with repeat colposcopy at least 6 weeks postpartum and treatment based on the findings of the postpartum colposcopy.

1.4. Conization Procedures in Pregnancy

There are many options for treatment of cervical dysplasia including a loop electrocautery excisional procedure (LEEP), cold knife conization (CKC), and cryotherapy ablation. We recommend an excisional procedure in all patients with high-grade dysplasia on pap or biopsy given the need for pathologic confirmation. Many patients can have concurrent microinvasive cancer or adenocarcinoma in situ and these lesions may be missed on cryotherapy. However, there are specific considerations for excisional procedures in pregnancy. In regards to loop electro-cautery excisional procedure (LEEP), Hunter reviewed a number of studies demonstrating LEEP in pregnancy can be considered "with a reasonable degree of maternal safety." [16, 17] Mitsuhashi et al. demonstrated that LEEP performed in the first trimester in 9 patients did not result in any miscarriages, premature delivery, or excessive bleeding. In contrast, Robinson et al. published data on 20 women who underwent LEEP between 8 to 34 weeks gestation. In women greater than 27 weeks gestation, there was significantly increased morbidity, including need for blood transfusions, preterm birth, and intrauterine fetal demise. [16] Given the increased risk with LEEP and insufficient comparison to the traditional CKC, most providers do not feel comfortable performing this procedure. Subsequently, for most purposes, the LEEP is contraindicated in pregnancy.

The safety of cold knife conization in pregnancy has varied in the literature. There is an increased amount of bleeding in 5-15% of pregnant patients. The rate of miscarriage occurred in 15-33% of patients and at least 50% of women undergoing CKC or LEEP in pregnancy had recurrent CIN following antepartum conization. [16] As well, 30-57% of conizations during pregnancy will have dysplasia or microinvasion at the margins. For this reason, CKC should not be considered therapeutic in pregnancy and should only be used for diagnostic purposes. [18] If an excisional procedure is warranted, the coin biopsy should be considered an alternative to typical conization. [18] A coin biopsy is similar to CKC, but excises only a shallow portion of the cervix. It also uses the placement of six hemostatic sutures placed on the cervix near the cervico-vaginal interface. These sutures reduce the blood flow to the cervix and help evert the transformation zone. This procedure should be performed only in the operative room under appropriate anesthesia with appropriate blood products available in preparation for possible complications. As well, any of the aforementioned procedures should be limited to pre-viable pregnancies, preferably in the second trimester.

As discussed earlier, progression of high-grade disease (CIN 2/3) or pre-invasive disease to invasive cancer during gestation is rare. Treatment of CIN and CIS in pregnancy should be delayed until at least 6 weeks postpartum, unless invasive cancer is suspected. If invasive cancer is suspected, and this would change treatment options in pregnancy, a coin biopsy should be performed for diagnosis. The ASCCP recommends conization "when the diagnosis of microinvasive/invasive cancer would change the outcome of the pregnancy or the mode of delivery." [4]

Section 2: Cervical Cancer in Pregnancy

Each case of cervical cancer in pregnancy presents a unique and special circumstance. There is a great deal of emotion, family, personal beliefs, religious beliefs, cultural beliefs and stigma that each patient brings to the table. Each patient should receive counseling involving a maternal fetal medicine (MFM) specialist, a gynecology oncologist, and their primary obstetrician. For some women, termination of pregnancy may be desired, while for some, termination of pregnancy is not even a choice. A review of the literature demonstrates that delaying treatment until postpartum does not increase risk of disease progression or overall survival. Ishioka reported on treatment delay up to 19 weeks with no change in tumor growth or staging. [28] Duggan et al. reported on 8 patients who delayed treatment for up to 212 days with no evidence of recurrence at a median follow-up of 23 months. [19] Women who choose to delay treatment must have close surveillance of their tumor during pregnancy. If there is evidence of progression on exam, delaying treatment is no longer recommended. Currently there is no evidence to suggest that serial MRI scans in pregnancy are warranted. Disease surveillance should be clinically assessed by a gynecologic oncologist by pelvic exam and colposcopy at least once per trimester.

2.1. Assessment and Staging

Cervical cancer frequently presents in early stages when it is often curable. Eighty-three percent of cases present with Stage I disease. Five-year survival rates for stage IA disease are >95%, with five-year survival rates for Stage IB ranging from 76% to 95%. Only 7% of women present with advanced stage cervical cancer. The diagnosis of invasive cancer in pregnancy should lead to further evaluation, exploring for the presence of lymphadenopathy, metastatic disease, and possible hydronephrosis. Chest radiography (CXR) should be performed to explore the presence of pulmonary metastatic disease. Typically, computed tomography (CT) scans have been used in the past and have minimal risk in pregnancy. [20] However, multiple CT scans should be avoided and should be used with caution in early gestation. Magnetic resonance imaging (MRI) does not subject the fetus to ionizing radiation and can be used in place of CT scan for initial evaluation. MRI has a reported high negative predictive value for predicting invasion into the parametria, vagina, and pelvic lymph nodes, 95%, 96%, and 93%, respectively. [21, 22] Few studies have explored MRI in pregnancy, but there is growing amount of evidence to support MRI helping to characterize tumor size, tumor location, depth of invasion, and parametrial invasion and adenopathy. [23] Positron emission tomography (PET) may be beneficial in cervical cancer, but given unknown effects of radioactive isotopes used, this imaging modality is contraindicated in pregnancy.

2.1.1. Fetal Assessment

Fetal assessment in the presence of cervical cancer should follow normal guidelines. Accurate assessment of fetal gestation age is important in any pregnancy. Detailed anatomy scans and first trimester screening or quad screening should be offered to all pregnant females. Discussion of possible screening for aneuploidy and/or neural tube defects should be routine in these women. The fetus is part of the patient and fetal assessment will play a large role in the management of cervical cancer in pregnancy.

2.2. Early Cervical Cancers

Most cervical cancer presents as Stage I disease. Treatment options in Stage I disease will vary regarding classification. The International Federation of Gynecology and Obstetrics (FIGO) and the Society of Gynecologic Oncologists agreed in the revised FIGO staging of cervical cancer to divide stage IA into IA1 and IA2, as can be seen in Table 2. Stage IA1 can be considered micro-invasive disease with depth of invasion less than 3mm and horizontal spread less than 7mm. Discussion regarding management of Stage I disease varies regarding status of invasion, and each stage will be discussed separately. Figure 1 displays a flow chart outlining basic treatment guidelines and principles.

Table 2. FIGO Cervical Cancer Staging

Stage	Description
I	Carcinoma is strictly confined to the cervix
IA1	*Stromal invasion ≤ 3mm in depth with extension ≤ 7mm*
IA2	*Stromal invasion > 3mm and ≤ 7mm*
IB1	*Clinically visible lesion ≤ 4cm in greatest dimension*
IB2	*Clinically visible lesion > 4cm in greatest dimension*
II	Cervical carcinoma invades beyond the uterus, but no to the pelvic wall or the lower third of the vagina
IIA1	*No parametrial invasion, clinically visible lesion ≤ 4cm in greatest dimension*
II2	*No parametrial invasion, clinically visible lesion > 4cm in greatest dimension*
IIB	*Obvious parametrial invasion*
III	Tumor extends to the pelvic wall, involves the lower third of the vagina, or causes hydronephrosis or impaired kidney function
IIIA	*Tumor involves the lower third of the vagina, with no extension to the pelvic wall*
IIIB	*Extension to the pelvic wall, hydronephrosis, or impaired kidney function*
IV	Carcinoma extends beyond the true pelvis or has involved the mucosa of the bladder or rectum (biopsy proven)
IVA	*Spread to adjacent organs, such as bladder or rectum*
IVB	*Spread to distant organs, such as liver, lung, bones, lymph nodes*

2.2.1. Stage IA1

In the non-pregnant patient, definitive treatment consists of conization with negative margins followed by extra-fascial hysterectomy in those patients who have completed child-bearing. Less than 1% of stage IA1 cervical cancer has positive lymph nodes, and lymph node dissection is not routinely performed or recommended. Review of the literature, demonstrates that delaying conservative treatment until at least 6 weeks postpartum is safe for women who desire to continue with their pregnancy.

In relation to delivery, vaginal delivery is preferred for fertility preservation and conservative management. Normal labor guidelines should be followed, and cesarean section performed only if obstetrically indicated. However, if patient desires definitive treatment and has completed childbearing, a routine cesarean hysterectomy can be performed at the time of delivery, although vaginal delivery with minimally invasive hysterectomy postpartum provides less surgical risk to the patient.

Treatment postpartum should always consist of excisional conization to confirm absence of more advanced disease (if not already performed). In 2004, Diakomanolis et al. reported on 90 patients undergoing CO2 laser conization in microinvasive disease. After a mean follow-up of 54 months, they found no recurrence of high-grade or invasive lesions. [24] In 1999, Okamoto et al. reported on 198 patients with microinvasive disease that underwent laser conization and demonstrated no recurrences. [25] Conservative management is safe in stage IA1 cervical cancer and should be offered to patients desiring to maintain their fertility. Delaying treatment until postpartum is the treatment of choice in these women. There is no increased risk of disease growth or change in stage. [19, 28] Hysterectomy is recommended after completion of childbearing.

In women who desire termination of pregnancy and have completed childbearing, termination of the pregnancy prior to surgery or hysterectomy with fetus in utero are both options. A conization should still be performed prior to hysterectomy to confirm diagnosis of microinvasive cancer which can only be assured by conization with negative margins. Larger or more deeply invasive lesions need further evaluation and possibly more radical surgery.

2.2.2. Stage IA2, IB1

FIGO staging of Stage IA2 is confined to the cervix with no more than 3-5mm depth of invasion and less than 7mm horizontal spread. Stage IB1 is defined as a clinically visible lesion less than 4cm in greatest diameter. Providers can consider early stage 1B1 disease (<2cm) to be similar to stage IA2 and can be managed similarly. Counseling is very important in this group of patients as the treatment options are numerous.

Nodal status is important in cervical cancer in regards to overall survival and disease-free survival. The presence of lymph node metastases occurs in 7.8% of patients, warranting the consideration of lymph node dissection in these patients. If lymphovascular space invasion (LVSI) is present, the rate of nodal metastases increases to 15.7%. [26] While MRI and/or CT help to evaluate nodal disease at time of diagnosis, these may not be able to characterize microscopic nodal disease. In 2008, Alouini et al. published data on pelvic lymphadenectomy in pregnancy in 5 women with stage IB1, two women with stage IB2, and one woman with stage IIIA. Each patient underwent pelvic and/or para-aortic lymphadenectomy via laparoscopy. Researchers found no increase in fetal or maternal morbidity. The mean number of lymph nodes collected was 18 and the operation was found to be safe in all 3 trimesters. [27] In women who desire to maintain their pregnancy, or who may be on the fence regarding treatment options and survival data, laparoscopic lymphadenectomy should be considered. A gynecologic oncologist should always be central to these discussions. If the lymph node assessment is negative for metastatic disease, treatment can be delayed until at least 6 weeks postpartum. Vaginal delivery is recommended for women desiring fertility preservation. In 2009, Ishioka et al. reported on 5 patients who delayed treatment for up to 20 weeks. There was no evidence of tumor growth or change in stage during this time. [28]

Definitive treatment outside of pregnancy is radical hysterectomy and pelvic and para-aortic lymphadenectomy. Recent review of the literature raises the question if conization with pelvic lymphadenectomy in low-risk disease is a viable option for treatment. Frumovitz et al.

reported on 125 women in low-risk category defined as any grade tumor, primary tumor size less than 2cm and with the absence of LVSI. None of these 125 women had parametrial involvement. [29] Kinney et al. reported a 0% risk of parametrial spread in early cervical cancer with primary tumor less than 2cm and no evidence of LVSI. [30] Risks of conization in pregnancy are discussed above and should be reviewed with the patient. The decision of conization in pregnancy versus postpartum should be made on a case by case basis with special consideration to the patients desires for the pregnancy and gestational age at diagnosis.

Radical trachelectomy should be considered as an alternative fertility-sparing treatment in the nonpregnant patient. There is a small amount of literature published on the performance of this procedure in pregnancy. Given the lack of change in outcomes for delaying treatment until postpartum, this procedure is not recommended in pregnancy. There is an expected increased risk of fetal loss and bleeding. However, the literature continues to report successful case reports of radical trachelectomy outside of pregnancy in fertility sparing surgeries. This option should be limited to those patients with a tumor less than 2 cm and with a squamous or adenocarcinoma histology. High-risk cancers including neuroendocrine and glassy cell cervical carcinomas should be treated with definitive surgery. Shepherd et al. reported on 123 patients who underwent radical vaginal trachelectomy and pelvic lymphadenectomy for fertility sparing treatment. Recurrence risk was 2.7%. Sixty-three women attempted pregnancy following surgery. Over the first 5 years, the conception rate was 52.8%. However, preterm birth was a significant risk at 25%. [31] Nishio et al. also reported on 31 patients undergoing radical abdominal trachelectomy for fertility sparing treatment. Seventy-two percent of patients had infertility problems requiring reproductive technology. Of those who wished to conceive, the fecundity rate was 36.2%. Preterm birth rate less than 32 weeks was 12%, while the majority of patients (65%) delivered between 32-37 weeks. The remainder delivered greater than 37 weeks. [32] If fertility preservation is desired, radical trachelectomy during the postpartum period following delivery is safe and should be offered.

Vaginal delivery is safe in these women and there is no need for early delivery or confirmation of fetal lung maturity. Definitive treatment can be delayed until the postpartum period for patients undergoing vaginal delivery with either fertility-preserving surgery as described above or with definitive radical hysterectomy and pelvic lymphadenectomy. Performance of these surgeries postpartum offers women the option of minimally invasive techniques with associated decrease in risk of postoperative complications, blood loss, and recovery time. There is no increased risk of disease spread during this time. If obstetrical indications predicate a cesarean delivery, a radical cesarean hysterectomy with pelvic lymph node dissection should be considered for women who have completed their childbearing. [32]

If pregnancy and fertility are not desired and the fetus is pre-viable, definitive radical hysterectomy with fetus in utero with pelvic lymphadenectomy is the treatment of choice. Monk et al. demonstrated that there is minimal associated morbidity with a radical hysterectomy following cesarean delivery or with fetus in utero. Average blood loss was 1.4 liters in his subset of patients following cesarean delivery. [33] This procedure is certainly safe and should be performed when definitive management is desired. Disease-free survival at 40 months for radical hysterectomy and lymphadenectomy following cesarean section or when the fetus was in utero was 95%.

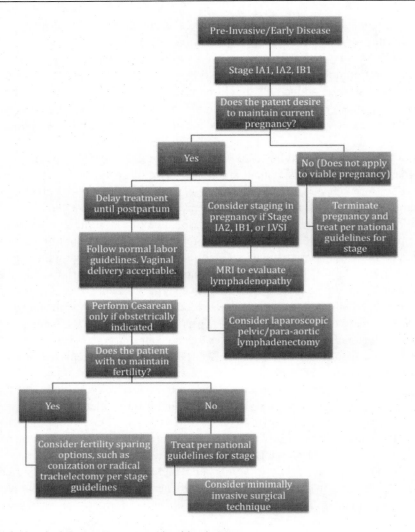

Figure 1. Early Cervical Cancer Treatment Algorithm in Pregnancy.

2.3. Advanced Cervical Cancer

2.3.1. Stage IB2

FIGO staging of stage IB2 cervical cancer consists of clinically visible lesions greater than 4cm in greatest dimension. Stage IB2 should be offered immediate treatment. Immediate treatment does not preclude pregnancy termination. Figure 2 outlines a treatment algorithm for Stage IB2 lesions in pregnancy. If a patient presents late in gestation, fetal lung maturity should be documented and cesarean delivery should be considered. Following delivery, stage IB2 can be treated in the typical fashion with chemotherapy and radiation. If a patient presents early in gestation, peri-viable or previable, a great deal of counseling should be offered. If continuation of the current pregnancy is desired, MRI to evaluate nodal status should be considered.

If there is evidence of nodal disease, overall survival is decreased and immediate treatment should be considered. If the MRI is negative, further consideration can be given to pelvic lymphadenectomy with minimally invasive techniques given risk of microscopic metastatic disease. If the lymph nodes are negative, delaying treatment can be considered. In these women who desire maintaining their current pregnancy, neoadjuvant chemotherapy should be considered and recommended. If continuation of the present pregnancy is not desired, and childbearing is completed, chemotherapy and radiation can be initiated with fetus in utero.

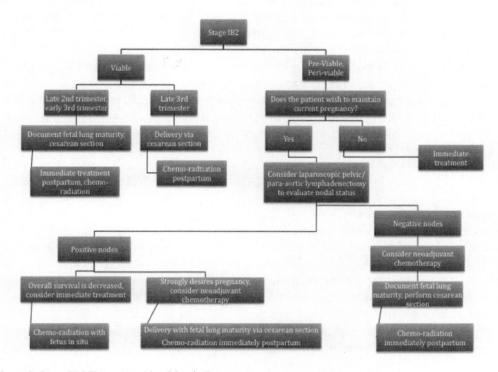

Figure 2. Stage IB2 Treatment Algorithm in Pregnancy.

2.3.2. Special Consideration: Neoadjuvant Chemotherapy

Neoadjuvant chemotherapy is a novel approach to cervical cancer treatment in women desiring to maintain their pregnancy. While neoadjuvant chemotherapy is most germane to stage IB2 cervical cancer, it should be applied to all patients with advanced stage disease who refuse to interrupt their pregnancy at any given gestational age. There are numerous other case reports in the literature in regards to neoadjuvant chemotherapy in stage IB2 and more advanced disease.

Creasman et al. reviewed the literature of cervical cancer patients (IB2, IIA, and IIB) undergoing neoadjuvant chemotherapy in pregnancy. Each regimen included platinum based therapy with cisplatin (50 mg/m^2). Two patients also received vincristine, while a third also received bleomycin. There was considerable disease regression, and in each case of IB2 and IIA, radical hysterectomy was performed at the time of cesarean delivery. One patient was without evidence of recurrence at 2 years. Unfortunately, both stage II patients had lethal recurrences at 5 months and 13 months following delivery. The infants remained healthy during these follow-up periods. There were no ill effects from chemotherapy. [18, 34]

In 2011, Gottschalk reviewed the safety of cisplatin in eight pregnancies with cervical cancer. Each patient underwent conization/biopsy in the second trimester and/or pelvic laparoscopic lymphadenectomy. Each patient received 2-4 cycles of cisplatin and underwent delivery after 31 weeks gestation by cesarean section followed by radical hysterectomy. Cisplatin concentrations in the umbilical cord, amniotic fluid, and breast milk were compared to maternal blood levels. Respectively they measured 31-65%, 13-42%, and 1-10% the concentration in maternal blood. Gottschalk et al. demonstrated cisplatin had decreased levels in fetal circulation and reassured providers and patients that cisplatin is safe. [35] Indeed, normal child growth and development is reported in these case reports, without evidence of hematologic toxicity, ototoxicity, or renal toxicity.

Neoadjuvant chemotherapy should be considered in all patients with stage IB2 or greater who desire to maintain their current pregnancy and would not meet criteria for delivery in the upcoming 4 weeks. In addition to platinum-based regimens, one should consider the addition of paclitaxel for more ideal treatment regimen. Use of paclitaxel in pregnancy in regards to cervical cancer is not well established. However, paclitaxel remains part of the standard of treatment outside of pregnancy and has been proven to be safe in pregnancy in other gynecological cancers. [36]

Often following neoadjuvant chemotherapy, the tumor size shrinks during pregnancy and the patient becomes a candidate for radical surgery including radical hysterectomy and pelvic lymphadenectomy. Important to this discussion is prognosis following surgery. While neoadjuvant chemotherapy may shrink the size of the tumor, the data on neoadjuvant chemotherapy in cervical cancer outside of pregnancy suggests that pre-treatment risk factors in these women are more indicative of overall survival. [39] Risk of recurrence is related to initial size of the tumor, parametrial involvement, and nodal status rather than the size of the tumor and invasion at the time of surgery. Sedlis et al. reports that adjuvant chemo-radiation is beneficial in stage IB disease with preoperative risk factors including depth of stromal invasion, size of the tumor, LVSI, and histology. Overall survival and disease-free time were improved with adjuvant chemo-radiation and should be considered in most patients with Stage IB2 and higher meeting these criteria at diagnosis. [38]

2.3.3. Stage II through IV

While Stage IB2 cervical cancer can be managed conservatively during pregnancy as noted above, some may argue that advanced stage disease should be treated immediately regardless of pregnancy. In the documented literature above, two patients with Stage II disease undergoing neoadjuvant chemotherapy developed a lethal recurrence shortly after completion of pregnancy. [18, 34] Certainly if disease progression occurs in pregnancy, regardless of stage, immediate treatment is warranted. Standard of treatment for advanced cervical cancer outside of pregnancy is pelvic radiation, both external and brachytherapy, in conjunction with chemotherapy. Review of the literature demonstrates that combined chemotherapy and radiation improves overall and disease-free survival. [39] This same regimen should be implemented in pregnant patients, and treatment should be considered immediately regardless of gestational age. If a patient presents between 28-34 weeks gestation, consideration of a steroid course for fetal lung maturity should be considered.

Optimal delivery time is 32-34 weeks gestation. Evidence in non-pregnant patients demonstrates that optimal time to treatment should not be delayed beyond 2-4 weeks. [40, 41] If a patient happens to present greater than 34 weeks gestation, outright delivery and treatment is warranted. If a patient presents in the early second trimester, a discussion regarding peri-viability and risk of cervical cancer progression and treatment options is indicated. If the patient strongly desires to maintain this pregnancy, neoadjuvant chemotherapy and/or premature delivery should be considered and treatment started. If this patient desires outright treatment without preservation of the current pregnancy, treatment should be initiated with fetus in utero. Sood et al. reported on 26 women undergoing radiation in pregnancy, treated with both external beam and intra-cavitary in all 3 trimesters. Planned delay in treatment was offered in late second and early third trimesters prior to initiation of radiotherapy. However, in the first trimester and early second trimester treatment was started immediately. Spontaneous abortion occurred in 20-24 days for patients in the early pregnancy. Complication rate was comparable to the control group of non-pregnant women undergoing the same treatment. [42]

In regards to delivery, vaginal delivery is not recommended in advanced disease. In 2000, Sood et al. reported on 56 women diagnosed with cervical cancer during pregnancy. There was a 14% recurrence rate among patients delivered by cesarean, while there was a 56% recurrence rate among vaginal deliveries. The authors recognize their study did not have significant power to make definitive conclusions, although this data is quite suggestive. [43] Other authors have also reported similar improved survival in patients undergoing cesarean section for advanced stage disease. [44] There are also case reports/series reporting local recurrence at episiotomy sites and perineal laceration sites. [45, 46] The evidence suggests that in advanced stage disease, cesarean delivery is beneficial to overall survival. If the tumor size or disease spread is such that it cannot be removed surgically with negative margins, radical hysterectomy at the time of cesarean section is not recommended. Survival rates are improved if the uterus is left in situ to allow for definitive chemoradiation including brachytherapy in the postpartum period. However, debulking of lymph nodes greater than 2cm in size at the time of cesarean section can be beneficial.

2.4. Prognosis

Overall survival of cervical cancer in pregnancy is similar to survival in non-pregnant patients. Figure 3 represents relative survival ratios of cervical cancer for all histological types based on FIGO staging. [51] In 1970, Creasman et al. reported similar data. Stage I survival was 85% (n=24) in the pregnant patient and 80% (n=371) in the non-pregnant patient. Stage II survival was 60% (n=18) and 70% (n=502) in the pregnant and non-pregnant patient respectively. [48] Zemilickis et al. retrospectively compared 40 women with cervical cancer to 89 non-pregnant women matched for age, stage, and tumor type. Long-term survival over 30 years was similar in both groups. [49] Lee JM et al. reported on 40 patients with early-stage cervical cancer in pregnancy diagnosed between 1995-2003. There was no difference in survival. [50] Clearly early stage cervical cancer can be managed during pregnancy conservatively with similar survival rates as compared to non-pregnant patients. Advanced stage cervical cancer has poor outcomes and immediate treatment is imperative to overall survival.

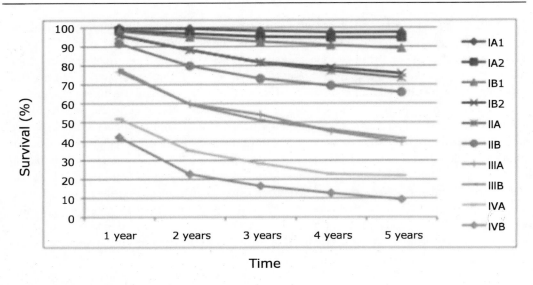

Figure 3. Prognosis of cervical cancer by stage [51].

Conclusion

Cervical cancer in pregnancy demands a multi-disciplinary approach including the patient, her obstetrician, a maternal fetal medicine specialist, and a gynecologic oncologist. Patient education and empathy should lead the discussion of management. Counseling must explore all possible management options and consider each patient as an individual including her desires for this pregnancy and future fertility. While there are many recommendations of treatment, a patient must ultimately decide her treatment plan for herself, her family, and her fetus. As physicians we must help provide education to our patients and establish a medical team that will be able to implement and coordinate the best possible care plan.

References

[1]   Hunter, Mark I.; Monk, Bradley J., Cervical neoplasia in pregnancy. Part 1: screening and management of preinvasive disease. *American Journal of Obstetrics and Gynecology,* July 2008.

[2]   Douvier, S., Flipuzzi, L., Sagot, P. Management of cervical intra-epithelial neoplasm during pregnancy. *Gynecol. Obstet. Fertil.* 2003;31:851-5.

[3]   Morimura, Y., Fujimori, K., Soeda, S., et al. Cervical cytology during pregnancy – comparison with non-pregnant women and management of Pregnant women with abnormal cytology. *Fukushima J. Med. Sci.* 2002;48:27-37.

[4]   Massad, Stewart L., et al. 2012 Updated Consensus Guidelines for the Management of Abnormal Cervical Cancer Screening Tests and Cancer Precursors. *J. of Lower Genital. Tract Disease,* Vol. 17, No 5, 2013, S1-S27.

[5]   Economos, K., Perez Veridiano, N., Delke, I., Collado, M. L., Tancer, M. L. Abnormal cervical cytology in pregnancy: A 17 year experience. *Obstet. Gynecol.* 1993;81:915-8.

[6]   Woodrow, N., Permezel, M. Abnormal cervical cytology in pregnancy: experience of 811 cases. *Aust. N. Z. J. Obstet. Gynaecol.* 1998 May; 38(2):161-5.

[7]   El-Basatawissi, A. Y., Becker, T. M., Dalin, J. R. Effect of cervical carcinoma in situ and its management on pregnancy outcome. *Obstet. Gynecol.* 1999;93:207-12.

[8]   Jain, A. G., Higgins, R. V., Boyle, M. J. Management of low-grade squamous intraepithelial lesions during pregnancy. *Am. J. Obstet. Gynecol.* 1997;177:298-302.

[9]   Kobayashi, T. K., Okamoto, H. Cytopathology of pregnancy-induced cell patterns in cervico vaginal smears. *Am. J. Clin. Pathol.* 2000;114:S6-20.

[10]   Arias-Stella, J. Atypical endometrial changes associated with the presence of chorionic tissue. *Arch. Pathol.* 1954;58:112-128.

[11]   Kim, T. J., Kim, H. S., Park, C. T., et al. Clinical evaluation of follow-up methods and results of atypical glandular cells of undetermined significance (AGUS) detected on cervicovaginal Pap smears. *Gynecol. Oncol.* 1999;73:292-8.

[12]   Murta, E. F., et al. High-grade cervical squamous intraepithelial lesion during pregnancy. *Tumori* 2002;88:246-50.

[13]   Vlahos, G., et al. Conservative management of cervical intraepithelial neoplasia in pregnant women. *Gynecol. Obstet. Invest.* 2002;54:78-81.

[14]   Waxman, Alan G., et al. Revised terminology for cervical histopathology and its implications for management of high-grade squamous intraepithelial lesions of the cervix. *Obstet. Gynecol.* 2012; 120:1465-1471.

[15]   Bergeron, Christine, et al. Conjunctive p16(INK4a) testing significantly increases accuracy in diagnosing high-grade cervical intraepithelial neoplasia. *Am. J. Clin. Pathol.* 2010;133:395-406.

[16]   Robinson, W. R., Webb, S., et al. Management of cervical intraepithelial neoplasia during pregnancy with LOOP excision. *Gynecol. Oncol.* 1997;64:153-5.

[17]   Mitsuhashi, A. et al. Loop electrosurgical excision procedure during first trimester of pregnancy. *Int. J. Gynaecol. Obstet.* 2000;71:237-9.

[18]   DiSaia, P., Creasman, W. eds. *Clinical Gynecologic Oncology.* St Louis (MO): Mosby Inc; 2007.

[19]   Duggan, B., Muderspach, L. I., Roman, L. D., Curtin, J. P., d'Ablaing, G. 3rd, Morrow, C. P., Cervical cancer in pregnancy: Reporting on planned delay in therapy. *Obstet. Gynecol.* 1993;82:598-602.

[20]   Ratnapalan, S., et al. Physicians' perceptions of teratogenic risk associated with radiography and CT during early pregnancy. *AJR Am. J. Roentgenol.* 2004;182:1107-9.

[21]   Choi, H. J., Roh, J. W., Seo, S. S., et al. Comparison of the accuracy of magnetic resonance imaging and positron emission tomography/computed tomography in the pre-surgical detection of lymph node metastases in patients with uterine cervical carcinoma: a prospective study. *Cancer* 2006;106:914-22.

[22]   Choi, S. H., et al. Preoperative magnetic resonance imaging staging uterine cervical carcinoma: Results of prospective study. *J. Comput. Assist. Tomogr.* 2004;28:620-7.

[23]   Nicklas, A. H., Baker, M. E. Imaging strategies in the pregnant cancer patient. *Semin. Oncol.* 2000;27:623-32.

[24] Diakomanolis, E., et al. Laser CO2 conization: a safe mode of treating conservatively microinvasive carcinoma of the uterine cervix. *Eur. J. Obstet. Gynecol. Reprod. Biol.* 2004;113(2):229-33.

[25] Okamoto, Y., et al. Pathological indications for conservative therapy in treating cervical cancer. *Acta Obstet. Cynecol. Scand.* 1999;7818-23.

[26] Benedet, J. L., Anderson, G. H. Stage IA carcinoma of the cervix revisited. *Obstet. Gynecol.* 1996 87;6:1052-59.

[27] Alouini, S., et al. Cervical cancer complicating pregnancy: implications of laparoscopic lymphadenectomy. *Gynecol. Oncol.* 2008 Mar.; 108(3):472-7.

[28] Ishioka, S., et al. Outcomes of planned delivery delay in pregnant patients with invasive gynecologic cancer. *Int. J. Clin. Oncol.* 2009;14:321-325.

[29] Frumovitz, M., et al. Parametrial involvement in radical hysterectomy specimens for women with early stage cervical cancer. *Obstet. Gynecol.* 2009;114:93-9.

[30] Kinney, W. K., Hodge, D. O., et al. Identification of a low-risk subset of patients with stage IB invasive squamous cancer of the cervix possibly suited to less radical surgical treatment. *Gynecol. Oncol.* 1995;57:3-6.

[31] Shepherd, J. H., et al. Radical vaginal trachelectomy as fertility-sparing procedure in women with early-stage cervical cancer – cumulative pregnancy rate in a series of 123 women. *BJOG* 2006;113:719-724.

[32] Nishio, H., et al. Reproductive and obstetric outcomes after radical abdominal trachelectomy for early-stage cervical cancer in a series of 31 pregnancies. *Hum. Reprod.* 2013. Vol. 0:1-6.

[33] Monk, B. J., Montz, F. J.: Invasive cervical cancer complicating intrauterine pregnancy: treatment with radical hysterectomy. *Obstet. Gynecol.* 80:199-203, 1992.

[34] Marana, H. R. C., et al. Chemotherapy in the treatment of locally advanced cervical cancer and pregnancy. *Gynecol. Oncol.* 2001;80:272-274.

[35] Lanowska, M., et al. Addressing concerns about cisplatin application during pregnancy. *J. Perinat. Med.* 2011;39:279-285.

[36] Mendez, L. E., et al. Paclitaxel and carboplatin chemotherapy administered during pregnancy for advanced epithelial ovarian cancer. *Obstet. Gynecol.* 2003;5:1200-2.

[37] Morice, P., et al. Are the outcomes of neoadjuvant chemotherapy for stage IB2 cervical cancer similar in pregnant and nonpregnant patient. *Gynecol. Oncol.* 2012;127;1:257-258.

[38] Sedlis, A., et al. A randomized trial of pelvic radiation versus no further therapy in selected patients with stage IB carcinoma of the cervix after radical hysterectomy and pelvic lymphadenectomy. A Gynecologic Oncology Group Study. *Gynecol. Oncol.* 1999 May;73(2):177-83.

[39] Morris, M., et al. Pelvic radiation with concurrent chemotherapy compared with pelvic and para-aortic radiation for high-risk cervical cancer. *N Engl. J. Med.* 1999;340:1137-43.

[40] Coles, C. E., et al. An audit of delays before and during radical radiotherapy for cervical cancer – effect on tumor cure probability. *Clin. Oncol.* 2003;15:47-54.

[41] Wyatt, R. M., et al. The effects of delays in radiotherapy treatment on tumor control. *Phys. Med. Biol.* 2003;48:139-55.

[42] Sood, A. K., et al. Radiotherapeutic management of cervical carcinoma that complicates pregnancy. *Cancer* 1997, 15;80(6):1073-8.

[43] Sood, A. K., et al. Cervical cancer diagnosed shortly after pregnancy: Prognostic variables and delivery routes. *Obstet. Gynecol.* 2000;95:832-8.

[44] Barber, H. R., Brunschwig, A. Gynecologic cancer complicating pregnancy. *Am. J. Obstet. Gynecol.* 1963;85:156-64.

[45] Cliby, W. A., et al. Cervical cancer complicated by pregnancy: Episiotomy site recurrences following vaginal delivery. *Obstet. Gynecol.* 1994;84:179-82.

[46] Gordon, A. N., et al. Squamous carcinoma of the cervix complicating pregnancy: Recurrence in episiotomy after vaginal delivery. *Obstet. Gynecol.* 1989;73:850-2.

[47] Andrae, B., et al. Screening and cervical cancer cure: population based cohort study. *BMJ* 2012;344:e900.

[48] Creasman, W. T., et al. Carcinoma of the cervix associated with pregnancy. *Obstet. Gynecol.* 1970, 36:495-501.

[49] Zemlickis, D., Lishner, M., et al. Maternal and fetal outcome after invasive cervical cancer in pregnancy. *J. Clin. Oncol.* 1991;9:1956.

[50] Lee, J. M., Lee, K. B., et al. Cervical cancer associated with pregnancy: results of a multicenter retrospective Korean study (KGOG-1006). *Am. J. Obstet. Gynecol.*, 2008; 198(1):92.e1.

[51] Quinn, M. A., Benedet, J. L., et al. Carcinoma of the Cervix uteri. FIGO 26th Annual Report on the Results of Treatment in Gynecological Cancer. *Int. J. Gynaecol. Obstet.* 2006 Nov.;95 Suppl. 1:S43-103.

In: Cervical Cancer
Editor: Laurie Elit

ISBN: 978-1-62948-062-6
© 2013 Nova Science Publishers, Inc.

Chapter XIV

Historical Overview on Cervical Cancer

Ciro Comparetto[1,] and Franco Borruto[2]*

[1]Division of Obstetrics and Gynecology, City Hospital, Azienda USL 4, Prato, Italy
[2]Professor of Obstetrics and Gynecology, Princess Grace Hospital,
Principality of Monaco

Abstract

For a long time, cancer of the cervix has been the most common form of cancer for women, but in recent years the picture has changed dramatically. In developing countries, in fact, this cancer is still the second leading cause of cancer death, because of poor sanitation, while in the West the number of cases and the deaths continue to decline thanks to the introduction of the Papanicolaou (Pap) test. Thanks to this early very effective diagnostic tool, carcinoma of the uterine cervix has a small impact on cancers in women in the Western world while it is much more common in the less industrialized countries. In 2012, almost 500,000 cases of cervical cancer have been recorded in the world. In Europe, the most affected countries are Belarus, Bulgaria, and Hungary. In Italy, every year 3,500 women are affected by cervical cancer, with a national average of one case per 10,000 women, but the chances of dying from this disease are < 1 per 1000. The number of such tumors increases with age. It can occur at any age, although the highest incidence is shown around 40-45 years. Human Papillomavirus (HPV) is the causative agent of cervical cancer. It is recommended to perform a cancer screening at 20 years of age, and to repeat it cyclically. If the Pap test is negative, it may be repeated after three years, but if abnormalities are found, additional exams may be prescribed, such as the search for HPV deoxy-ribonucleic acid (DNA) or colposcopy with biopsy. Once the diagnosis of cervical cancer has been made, other tests may be prescribed such as computed tomography (CT), magnetic resonance imaging (MRI), or positron emission tomography (PET) to accurately determine the extent of the tumor. Gynecological examination under sedation is also rather useful for cancer staging. Other tests are urography, lymphangiography (also called lymphography), bone scintigraphy, intravenous pyelography, and sigmoidoscopy. The choice of treatment for cancer of the

---

* Correspondence concerning this article should be addressed to Ciro Comparetto at Via Castelfidardo, 33-50137 Florence, Italy. Email: cicomp@tin.it.

cervix mainly depends on the stage of disease at the time of diagnosis, but is also based on other criteria such as for example, the general state of health of the patient, her age, and her needs. Often, it is possible also to proceed by combining two or more treatments to achieve maximum effectiveness. Surgery is one of the possible choices and the type of surgery varies depending on the spread of the disease. Radiation therapy is a valid treatment in some cases. A third option for the treatment of cancer of the cervix, however reserved for the advanced or invasive forms, is chemotherapy: different drugs against the tumor are administered intravenously, often combined with each other. The prognosis is good for stage I. We can arrive, however, at a 5% probability of survival at 10 years after diagnosis for stage IV. In recent years, moreover, women have another weapon against HPV, a vaccine towards the two types of HPV responsible for the majority of cervical cancers (HPV 16 and HPV 18). In Italy, the vaccine is now available free to girls of 12 years of age. Numerous studies are underway to evaluate the efficacy of vaccination in adult women with an active sex life and in women who have already been in contact with the virus.

Keywords: Cervical cancer, Human Papillomavirus, prevention, screening, vaccination

Introduction

Carcinoma of the uterine cervix is one of the commonest genital malignancies in women worldwide and the fourth most common neoplasm in women. The mortality from this tumor has dropped with the advent of Papanicolaou (Pap) smears and routine periodic screening, particularly in high-risk populations. Diagnosis and staging includes a careful physical examination, the use of colposcopy, directed biopsy, intravenous urogram, and cystoscopy. Computed tomography (CT) and lymphangiography may be helpful for detection of iliac or para-aortic lymph nodes. Early, noninvasive stages of this disease may be treated with cryosurgery or laser vaporization. Carcinoma in situ (CIS) and microinvasive carcinoma are usually treated with simple hysterectomy for cure [1]. The incidence of invasive carcinoma of the cervix is decreasing in developed countries. This appears to be related to improvements in socioeconomic level and adequate utilization of the Pap smear in the population. Mortality from carcinoma of the cervix has shown a 60% reduction in the last 60 years. Most likely, this is related to the observed reduction in the incidence of the invasive forms of the disease, earlier diagnosis, and improvements in therapy. Optimal therapy of the clinically evident invasive forms of the disease is a combination of external irradiation and intracavitary brachytherapy. Surgery would be of value for specific clinical situations as an adjuvant to irradiation (barrel-shaped types), in post-irradiation recurrences, inadequate brachytherapy, etc. Chemotherapy may provide some palliation to patients with recurrent tumors but does not increase long-term survivorship. The yield in terms of survival and disease-free status in the pelvis is high for the early stages of the disease (approximately 90% 5-year survival and 97% control of pelvic tumor for stage I). Yet, stage IIIB and IV cases show a failure rate of close to 50% or more in the irradiated volume and a high incidence of metastases to the para-aortic nodes and elsewhere [2].

There is a decreased incidence and mortality rate from cervical cancer with well-organized population-based screening programs using cervical smears. Strong evidence exists for a sexually transmitted etiologic agent in cervical cancer. Treatment of occult and early clinically lesions is ideally by a spectrum of surgical procedures which are carefully tailored to the extent of the lesion, but of advanced cancers mainly with radiation therapy and adjuvant surgery and/or chemotherapy in selected cases. Best results for cervical cancer treatment are obtained when treatment facilities are centralized and treatment performed by experienced individuals who individualize therapy or integrate the use of all therapeutic modalities of surgery, radiation, and chemotherapy [3]. Over the last years, the majority of research on the pathology of the cervix has been focused on the Human Papillomavirus (HPV) and its role in the pathogenesis of cervical neoplasia. Several major points emerged from these studies. First, the incidence of latent HPV infection in the general population is greater than previously thought. Up to 31% of a college-aged population has HPV deoxyribonucleic acid (DNA) detected in cervical swabs. Second, in situ hybridization (ISH) to detect HPV has been found to be a useful quality control measure for laboratories diagnosing cervical lesions. Finally, it is now recognized that many different HPV types can infect the cervix and be associated with cervical neoplasia. With regard to treatment, the introduction of loop electrosurgical excision procedures (LEEP) for treating cervical intraepithelial neoplasia (CIN) lesions had a significant impact on the management of cervical disease [4].

The majority of patients with low-stage cervical cancer are cured. Results obtained in the past only in the categorical cancer centers are currently being achieved more broadly. This reflects the work of formally trained gynecologic oncologists often in collaboration with formally trained radiation therapists distributing themselves in a horizontal fashion to more and more university medical centers, teaching hospitals, and quality tertiary hospitals in the private sector. The formalization of training in gynecologic oncology has been pivotal in this development. This group of physicians, working with physicians in other disciplines, has impacted significantly on patient care and has provided many clinical and pathologic studies to better define favorable low-stage cases and poor prognosis cases. The need to explore the use of currently available modalities in a variety of different combinations and to define and develop new techniques to apply to these poor prognosis subsets of disease represent areas of progress and challenge [5-9].

Historical Notes

The death rate from invasive cervical cancer has decreased by 70% since the classic work by Papanicolaou and Traut in 1941 on the use of cytologic evaluation to detect cancer of the uterine cervix in the preinvasive in situ stage, a nearly 100% curable disease. Unfortunately, the survival stage for stage of invasive cervical cancer has remained static over the nearly 5 decades since their report. However, discoveries in the decade of the 1970s of the natural spread of cervical cancer, not only to the known pelvic lymph nodes, but the increasing incidence of para-aortic lymph node metastasis with advanced stages, the higher dose of radiation required to sterilize pelvic lymph node metastasis discovered at the time of radical hysterectomy or for locally advanced cervical cancer treated solely by radiation therapy, and the use of radiation potentiators, such as hydroxyurea, led to the significant reduction in the annual 7,000 deaths from this disease in the decade of the 1990s [10]. The accepted procedure for evaluating women with inflammatory atypia on a Pap smear has changed over the years. Early studies reflected a consensus that inflammatory atypia was normal and required no further evaluation. In the early 1970s, several authors noted a higher-than-expected incidence of CIN and even cervical cancer in these patients. Further work in the late 70s and early 80s demonstrated that up to 79% of patients who had both initial and repeat atypical Pap smears had CIN or worse on biopsy. Those studies were flawed in their methodology. However, recent studies have been sounder methodologically. They clearly showed that 18-56% of initially atypical smears are associated with CIN, HPV, or cervical cancer. Furthermore, they demonstrated an alarmingly high number of false-negative repeat smears. Those studies pointed to a need for a more aggressive approach to the evaluation of inflammatory atypia seen on the initial smear [11].

The etiological role of viruses in various animal cancers is no longer in doubt. Indeed, until recently, virus infections were considered responsible for only a small proportion of the clinical states encountered in humans and the view that viruses could be etiological agents for human malignant tumors was not seriously entertained. With the introduction of more advanced techniques in immunovirology, the role of viruses in clinical syndromes the etiology of which had been obscure became clearer. The Emory University Group first postulated in 1964 an association between Herpes Simplex Virus (HSV) infection and cervical neoplasia, following studies of an infant with neonatal HSV infection and his mother's cervical HSV infection. This postulate was based on the observation that women with genital HSV (HSV type-2 [HSV-2]) infection have a greater frequency of cervical neoplasia than women in the general population. Demographic surveys of cancer of the cervix have established patterns of high risk that strongly suggest that the disease may be transmitted venereally. Similarly, evidence has accumulated to show that HSV-2 is a sexually transmitted disease (STD). It was thus postulated that this virus could be an initiating or promoting carcinogenic factor transmitted to the female during sexual intercourse. Various multicentric approaches, from epidemiological studies to molecular studies, have been employed to substantiate this association. Even though the weight of circumstantial evidence supporting the role of HSV-2 in human carcinoma of the cervix had increased, no definitive "cause-and-effect" association was established between the virus and carcinoma of the cervix. The question arose, therefore, whether or not an etiological association between the virus and the disease could be confirmed. To prove a definitive cause-and-effect relationship, further studies were required, such as the successive demonstration of the involvement of HPV [12]. In the genital tract, the venereal wart (Condyloma acuminatum) has been recognized since ancient times, and known to be a STD. In 1976, two other morphologically distinct HPV lesions were described in the uterine cervix, known currently as a flat and an inverted condyloma. Subsequently, these new HPV lesions were shown to be frequently associated with concomitant CIN and CIS lesions, and occasionally with invasive cervical carcinomas as well. These morphological findings, substantiated by the increasing number of reports of malignant transformation of HPV lesions, as well as data from animal experiments and epidemiological surveys, have lent support to the concept that HPV might be involved in the development of cervical (and other) human squamous cell carcinomas (SCC). Further evidence has been provided by the subsequent discoveries of HPV structural proteins (viral antigens) and HPV type 11 DNA in lesions of CIN, as well as HPV 16 and 18 DNA predominantly in invasive cervical carcinomas. Cervical (and other) HPV lesions have been the subject of intense study utilizing epidemiological, morphological, immunohistochemical, biochemical, and molecular biological methods (recombinant gene technology) to provide further evidence of the suggested causal relationship between HPV and cancer, to explore the natural history of cervical HPV lesions, as well as the factors (immunological, epidemiological, synergistic actions, etc.) which modify it [13, 14].

Therefore, though the existence of disease associated with HPV has been documented for centuries, it has been only within the past four decades that we have recognized the clinical diversity and significant morbidity and mortality associated with HPV infections. The original lack of interest and nonavailability of in vitro culture systems has hampered research. However, with the advent of molecular diagnostic techniques, strong evidence suggests that HPV plays a major role in the development of specific anogenital cancers, including cervical, vaginal, vulvar, penile, and anal. It is this association between anogenital cancers and HPV that may result in treatment guidelines that eventually will eliminate these cancers. Moreover, to the extent that this association has resulted in overdiagnosis and unnecessarily aggressive treatment, new and ongoing research may create more appropriate treatment options [15]. Death rates from cervical cancer have already fallen this century and for patients with invasive cervical cancer five year survival rates are greater than for most solid tumors. Better screening for premalignant changes may further reduce the incidence of invasive cancer: indeed, it has been claimed that the reduction in mortality could be as high as 90%, though estimates of screening efficacy have varied greatly [16-18].

Epidemiology and Etiopathogenesis

The overall incidence of and mortality from cervical cancer has declined in Western countries and in most developing countries. In women under 40 years of age, however, mortality rates are levelling off or increasing in most countries. The earliest and most marked increases in young women occurred in England and Wales, Scotland, Ireland, New Zealand, and Australia. Mortality rates in young women from eastern European countries began to increase later than in the United Kingdom (UK), but the increases are of concern because baseline mortality rates are high in these countries. The reasons for the overall decline in cervical cancer appear to be linked to improvements in the general standard of living. The increases in young women may well be due to the increasing prevalence of HPV infection. Screening for cervical cancer has undoubtedly led to a decline in cervical cancer incidence and mortality in many countries [19]. The epidemiology of cervical cancer presents a number of unique challenges, mainly with respect to disentangling correlated factors and to elucidating biological mechanisms. The available evidence suggests a complex multifactorial etiology, although the relative contributions of risk factors and their interactions remain obscure. Infectious agents have been always strongly suspected, and now conclusively identified. It is unclear whether there are subgroups of women or periods of life that are most susceptible to the action of infectious agents, and the contribution of the "male factor" needs to be defined. Several epidemiologic leads can be pursued through biochemical and molecular techniques. The recent evidence has linked certain HPV types to cervical abnormalities, including cancer, and newly developed probes could be incorporated into epidemiologic studies to evaluate an array of risk factors. Endocrine and metabolic assays have been helpful in clarifying the role of exogenous and possibly endogenous hormones. The effects of cigarette smoking have been further evaluated by studying constituents of tobacco smoke and their metabolites in cervical mucus. Finally, the relationship of diet to cervical cancer has been assessed by examining the levels of micronutrients, trace minerals, and other nutritional indices in body tissues and fluids, as well as through interview data. An understanding of cervical cancer etiology required a better identification of risk factors for precursor lesions as well as factors that enhance their progression to invasive cancer. Through studies that focus on disease stage and time-related events, it has been possible to clarify the multi-stage processes involved in cervical carcinogenesis, and those factors that may inhibit as well as promote transition rates. The protective effects of screening programs deserve further attention, and research into dietary factors may lead in time to nutritional intervention. Investigation by cell type has also been pursued to define the epidemiology of the adenocarcinomas and adenosquamous carcinomas of the cervix. Finally, preventive strategies should be targeted to high-risk populations, especially those of the lower socioeconomic classes and with limited access to medical care. The need for a renewed focus on epidemiology and prevention is emphasized by recent increases in exposure to several postulated risk factors, including sexual promiscuity, oral contraceptives (OC), and smoking [20].

Despite a long history of research into the epidemiology and biology of cervical carcinoma, a definitive statement about its causes has been reached only recently. Although vigorously pursued, an increased risk from OC has not been convincingly demonstrated. Varieties of venereally transmitted organisms appear to be frequent cohabitants with cervical neoplastic cells. HSV-2 has long been the prime suspect in the complex pathogenesis of cervical neoplasia. Clinical findings, biological characteristics of the virus, serological studies and interactions of host cells and viral particles have stimulated the most intensive investigative efforts [21]. The causation of cervical cancer is conveniently discussed by using themes emergent from a great volume of field studies and by using the manner in which this evidence has been exploited in the clinic and laboratory. Epidemiology themes dwell on the strong correlation of disease incidence with sexual behavior of both male and female, sufficient to regard cervical cancer as a type of venereal disease and an equally strong correlation with socioeconomic class. Mortality rises when the male partner resides in the lower social classes. Laboratory and clinical studies have defined the tissue at risk and studies attempted definition of reasons for such risk. The accent in these studies was on a derangement of the cell filament system seen as grades of unusual keratinization. The vast bulk of laboratory studies have been devoted to a definition of the carcinogen. The venereal nature of the epidemiological evidence rendered a transmissible agent as most suspect. Viruses have been a popular subject because of their demonstrable capacity to transform cells in vitro and in vivo. Studies have concentrated on a component of the sperm as carcinogen or co-carcinogen [22].

Risk factors of cervical cancer have been studied in the following aspects:

1) sociodemographic factors including educational level, urbanizational level, socioeconomic status, race, and marriage;
2) sexual activity including age at first marriage, age at first coitus, multiple marriage, multiple sexual partners, broken marriage, unstable sex relationship, syphilis/gonorrhea history, coital frequency, multiple pregnancies, and age at menarche;

3) factors related to husband including circumcision, sperm, smegma, previous wife with cervical cancer, and occupations entailed mobility of husband and periods away from home;

4) psychosocial factors including stressful emotional status, deprived economic background, and discontent home situation;

5) virus including HSV-2 and HPV; and

6) other factors including smoking, barrier and OC [23].

The importance of viruses as oncogenic agents in animals is well established. Recent work suggested that viruses are also etiologically related to some human cancers. Viruses may contribute to the development of human tumors by different mechanisms: indirectly by inducing immunosuppression or by modifying the host cell genome without persistence of viral DNA and directly by inducing oncoproteins or by altering the expression of host cell proteins at the site of viral DNA integration. Human cancers associated with HPV, Hepatitis B and C Virus (HBV and HCV), Epstein-Barr Virus (EBV), and Human T cell Leukemia-lymphoma Virus (HTLV) infections are responsible for approximately 15% of the worldwide cancer incidence. Cancer of the cervix and hepatocellular carcinoma account for about 80% of virus-linked cancers. Because experimental and epidemiologic data imply a causative role for viruses, particularly in cervical and liver cancer, viruses must be thought of as the second most important risk factor for cancer development in humans, exceeded only by tobacco consumption [24]. HSV-2 has long been prime suspect in carcinomas involving the female lower genital tract. In particular, a close association had been found between HSV-2 infection and cervical neoplasia in cytohistopathologic and seroepidemiologic studies. Preliminary results of prospective studies showed further that women with genital herpetic infection were at increased risk of developing cervical neoplasia. Additional studies on animal models, including subhuman primates, and efforts continued in the attempt to confirm the presence of viral genetic material or its expression in human cervical cancer cells [25]. After four decades of investigation, the proposed etiological link between HSV-2 and human carcinoma of the cervix remained unproved. The initial sero-epidemiological studies, which were of a retrospective nature, were in favor of the etiological relationship, whereas the more recent prospective studies suggested that HSV infection is a co-variable. The detection of HSV genes and their products in tumor tissues has been plagued by problems of cross reactivity, but the most recent results indicate that while HSV-2 DNA can be detected in a small proportion of cancer tissues, HSV proteins or tumor antigens probably do not persist in the tumors. The same situation applies with respect to in vitro transformation. Although HSV, and isolated DNA fragments from the viral genome, can transform tissue culture cells (mainly of rodent origin) and under some conditions can cause cervical abnormalities (including cancer) in experimental animals, in no instance need the viral genes be maintained in the transformed cells. A number of mechanisms, including viral mutagenesis, have been proposed to explain this unusual feature, but the relevance of this work to the induction of human cervical carcinoma by HSV-2 in vivo has been difficult to prove [26]. Human Cytomegalovirus (CMV) is another sexually transmitted virus which has also been implicated in both cervical cancer and its precancerous state, CIN [27].

Evidence of a biologically significant association between subclinical HPV infection and cervical neoplasia rose the question of whether this was a causal relationship. HPV infection of metaplastic epithelium in the cervical transformation zone is relatively common, producing latent infection in susceptible persons. The epidemiological characteristics of subclinical HPV infection and cervical cancer are essentially identical and there was a strong clinico-pathological association between condylomas and anogenital carcinoma. Tissue culture cells have been transformed from a normal to a neoplastic phenotype by animal papillomaviruses, and there are data reporting upon the successful identification of HPV genomic sequences in tumor cells. Subclinical HPV infection commonly coexists with foci of CIN. Areas of apparent transition are seen, and these two lesions are linked by a discernible spectrum of morphologic change. Such circumstantial evidence gave biological plausibility to the suggestion that HPV is a cervical carcinogen. It was postulated that cervical neoplasia arises by progression from benign viral hyperplasia, through varying stages of koilocytotic atypia with associated dysplasia, to unremarkable CIS. Invasion was presumed to reflect the emergence of an aggressive heteroploid clone, an age-related decline in host immune surveillance, or an interaction of both factors [28]. With the recent development of new analytic methods, notably the DNA hybridization technique, many benign and malignant gynecologic tumors including CIS, verrucous carcinoma, and invasive carcinomas of the vulva, the vagina, and the cervix have been found to be associated with HPV infection. Benign warts and multiple neoplasms frequently appear synchronously or metachronously in a single patient, and thus present as the genital neoplasm-papilloma syndrome (GENPS) [29]. Current data implicating an etiological role of HPV infections in precancer lesions (intraepithelial neoplasia) and SCC of both the genital tract and other sites (oral cavity, larynx, skin, esophagus, nasal cavity, and bronchus) can be summarized as follows:

1) HPV involvement in both benign benign and malignant genital squamous cell lesions has been demonstrated by morphological, immunohistochemical, and DNA hybridization techniques;
2) HPV infections in the genital tract are STD and associated with the same risk factors as development of cervical carcinoma;
3) the natural history of cervical HPV lesions is equivalent to that of CIN, i.e. they are potentially progressive to CIS;
4) latent HPV infections exist in the genital tract of both sexes;
5) animal models exist, where papillomaviruses induce malignant transformation;
6) HPV induces transformation of human squamous epithelium in vivo (nude mouse renal subcapsule assay);
7) malignant transformation of HPV lesions seems to depend on virus type and the physical state of its DNA, i.e. whether or not integrated in the host cell DNA;
8) malignant transformation most probably requires synergistic actions between HPV and chemical or physical carcinogens or other infectious agents;
9) genetic disposition (at least in animals) significantly contributes to malignant transformation; and
10) immunological defence mechanisms of the host probably are capable of modifying the course of HPV infection.

Many details of the molecular mechanisms remain to be clarified, however. No applicable model systems exist to elucidate these issues, or the mechanisms leading to the progression to invasive cancer. Improved tissue culture systems for in vitro differentiation of keratinocytes helped in elucidating the biology of HPV and their interaction with cell division and differentiation [30, 31]. Thus, HPV has emerged over the past decades as the sexually transmitted etiological factor in cervical cancer. Although it appeared that HPV types 16 and 18 were associated with a higher risk of advanced cervical neoplasia, most of the evidence came from studies that did not satisfy basic epidemiological requirements, and were therefore difficult to interpret. The most significant problems were the small sample size, potentially biased selection of study subjects, the difficulties in cytologically distinguishing precancerous lesions from HPV infection of the cervix, the unknown specificity and sensitivity of the various hybridization methods for determining HPV infection status, and the statistical analyses and presentation of results [32].

In both the United States of America (USA) and the UK, condylomata acuminata is the most commonly diagnosed viral STD. The highest incidence is among females 20-24 years of age. The results of six studies to examine the prevalence of HPV suggest a rate of 1-13%, with a positive association to the prevalence of CIN in that population. It is estimated that genital HPV infection has 10% prevalence among men and women in the USA 15-49 years of age: 1% have condylomata, 2% have lesions visible only by magnification with the colposcope or hand lens, and 7% have clinically inapparent infections. HPV types 6 and 11 tend to cause condylomata and low-grade epithelial cell atypia, while types 16, 18, and 31 have been found in higher-grade intraepithelial neoplasia and invasive cervical cancers. Current evidence suggests a latency between acquisition of genital HPV infection and the development of cervical malignancy. From an epidemiological point of view, the current research literature lacks evidence of careful selection and definition of study populations, consistent quality control of clinical and laboratory methods, and thorough statistical analyses [33]. In vitro transformation studies indicate that these viruses can transform primary mammalian cells in co-operation with Ha-ras. This may mean that these viruses have at least a c-myc like activity that is consistent with their ability on their own to immortalize primary keratinocytes. The fact that HPV 6 can also transform mammalian cells, at a low frequency, in co-operation with Ha-ras, indicates the need to use appropriate cells and systems that will elucidate differences in virus-cell interactions between benign HPV types 6 and 11 and the viruses associated with severe disease 16 and 18 [34]. Epidemiological studies on the association between HPV and cervical cancer using HPV DNA hybridization methods to assess the presence of viral markers have yielded compelling evidence that HPV has a causal role in the disease: the association is strong, consistent, and specific to a limited number of viral types. A dose-response relationship has been reported between increasing estimated viral load and risk of cervical cancer. Indirect evidence suggests that HPV DNA detected in cancer cells is a good marker of HPV infection occurring before cancer development. An increased risk for progression to more advanced CIN lesions has been reported among HPV 16/18-positive women as compared to women with other HPV types or to women without any viral DNA [35].

The question of whether HPV infection causes, or at least contributes to, the development of cervical carcinoma has been a topic of much scrutiny and controversy over the past years. The sexual mode of transmission of genital HPV and detection of viral DNA in cervical tumors suggest a causal role at some stage during malignant progression. To some extent, it seems that the epidemiological data accumulated so far have served to confuse as much as to clarify the issue, and the distribution of genital HPV in the general population appears to be more complex than originally anticipated. However, experimental systems that have been used to study HPV, in particular recent studies utilizing human genital epithelial cells, have provided strong evidence that certain HPV types can cause premalignant changes in these cells. The development of cervical cancer is a multistage process, and HPV infection alone is clearly not sufficient for full malignant transformation. Nevertheless, identification and control of HPV infection may be of critical importance in the diagnosis and treatment of this disease [36]. In fact, although morbidity rates have declined in the past several decades because of wide-scale screening, the disease remains an important public health problem. Recently, important epidemiological incoherences have been found with respect to the sexual transmission route of HPV infection in the causal pathway of cervical cancer. HPV infection rates in asymptomatic women do not seem to be related to sexual behavior, and if analyzed simultaneously, sexual behavior and HPV infection seem to be independent predictors of cervical cancer risk. If confirmed by further research, these findings could signify that there may be alternative etiologic mechanisms for cervical cancer. Since some researchers have recently proposed public health action because of the acceptance of HPV infection as a necessary cause of cervical cancer, it is imperative that the aforementioned incoherences be immediately resolved by further research [37]. Measurement errors have been an important concern in studies of HPV and anogenital cancers. Misclassification of HPV infection status is a possible explanation for incoherent findings in previous epidemiological studies purporting to show an etiological role for HPV in cervical cancer. Even low levels of misclassification of HPV infection can cause severe underestimation of HPV prevalence in field surveys, bias the association between HPV and sexual activity, and impair the ability to control statistically the relation between sexual activity and neoplasia by viral status [38]. Anyway, although the clinical and epidemiological studies have been criticized for a variety of technical and design shortcomings, for the most part they have independently reached the same conclusion: there is a strong association between the presence of specific types of HPV and the development of anogenital cancer. Similarly, laboratory studies clearly indicate that specific types of HPV act in concert with other cellular changes to transform a variety of cell types in vitro, including human cervical epithelial cells. These studies have stressed the need to identify important cofactors in the transformation process and determine the role of host immunity [39]. In fact, it is clear that only a minority of women with HPV 16 infection, for example, develop invasive cancer. Therefore, examination of whether sexually transmitted agents other than HPV are interacting in the genesis of cervical neoplasia is necessary. Serological methods that accurately reflect past exposure to individual agents are ideal for epidemiological studies. Sensitive and specific assays are available for HSV-1, HSV-2, Treponema pallidum, CMV, Human Immunodeficiency Virus (HIV), and Chlamydia trachomatis. Some data suggest an interaction of HSV with HPV in oncogenesis. However, at present the evidence is inadequate to prove the involvement of sexually transmitted agents other than HPV in the etiology of cervical neoplasia [40].

In conclusion, cervical cancer is an extremely common disease. Its natural history has been well described, and individual risk factors have been defined. It is clear from the epidemiologic evidence that cervical cancer has a multifactorial etiology involving infection with sexually transmitted agents such as genital HPV and cofactors such as smoking, use of hormonal contraceptives, and diet. The evidence implicating HPV as an etiologic agent of cervical cancer has come from a variety of observational laboratory studies. Genital HPV induce dysplastic lesions. Most invasive cervical cancers contain HPV DNA, as do cell lines derived from cervical cancers. Viral DNA appears to be integrated into cellular DNA, and integration involves highly conserved, transcriptionally active regions of the viral DNA [41].

HPV types 16, 18, 31, 33, 35, 39, 45, and 52 have been linked to the etiology of anogenital cancer. Experimental evidence strongly supports a role of these virus types as causative agents for cancer of the cervix, vulva, and penis. Although infection appears to be necessary for the development of malignant tumors, it is clearly not sufficient. Additional factors probably affecting host cell genes engaged in the control of HPV functions seem to be required for conversion of premalignant changes into invasive growth [42]. Numerous studies of the epidemiology of cervical cancer have shown strong associations with religious, marital, and sexual patterns. Although it is well established that women with multiple partners and early ages at first intercourse are at high risk, less is known about how these factors interact or how risk is affected by specific sexual characteristics. Recent studies indicate that number of steady partners and frequent intercourse at early ages may further enhance risk, supporting hypotheses regarding a vulnerable period of the cervix and a need for repeated exposure to an infectious agent. It is now widely accepted that HPV is the major infectious etiological agent, but whether other infectious agents play supportive or interactive roles is unclear. Of specific interest is the independent effect of HSV-2 on risk, especially given some evidence that this viral agent may interact with HPV. Other speculative risk factors for cervical cancer include cigarette smoking, OC usage, and certain nutritional deficiencies, but again it is not clear whether these factors operate independently from HPV. Although cervical cancer incidence trends correlate with the population prevalence of various venereally transmitted agents, it is not certain how disease rates are affected by other potential risk factors which have changed during recent time (e.g. exposure to HPV, cigarette smoking, high number of sexual partners, early cohabitarche, young age at first delivery, suppression and alteration of immune status, young age, and hormonal influences). In addition, a number of recent studies highlight the need for considering not only female influences on risk of cervical cancer, but also male factors, since the sexual behavior of the male consort appears to play an important role [43]. While the fact of a high number of sexual partners exclusively increases the risk of HPV infection, it is not known whether the other factors lead to either an increased risk for HPV infection and/or to HPV-associated neoplasia. Subclinical and latent genital HPV infections are highly prevalent.

The prevalence rate depends on the sensitivity of the HPV detection system used, on age and sexual activity of the population screened, and on the number of subsequent examinations performed for each subject. Sexual transmission is the main pathway for genital HPV, however vertical, peripartal, and oral transmission are also possible. Seroreactivity against genital HPV may be due to an active infection or the result of contact with HPV earlier in life. Antibodies against the HPV 16 early protein 7 (E7) indicate an increased risk for cervical cancer. Compared with humoral response, cellular immune response is probably more important for regression of genital HPV infection: impaired cellular response is characterized by depletion of T helper/inducer cells and/or Langerhans cells (LC) and impaired function of natural killer (NK) cells and/or the infected keratinocyte. In condylomata, replication and transcription of viral nucleic acids and antigen production coincide with cellular differentiation. However, the interaction between HPV and the keratinocyte on a molecular level in subclinical and latent disease is not well understood. Regression or persistence of subclinical and latent genital HPV infections as observed in longitudinal investigations show a constant come-and-go of HPV presence. Subclinical or latent cervical infections with high-risk HPV types (such as HPV 16 and 18) have an increased risk for the development of HPV-associated neoplasia [44-46].

Natural History and Pathophysiology

Despite the recent passage of coverage for Pap test screening, several aspects of the natural history of cervical cancer remain uncertain. Two central questions that affect a screening program are how long the neoplastic process takes from preinvasive disease to the development of invasive cancer, and how likely is it that a given neoplastic state observed in a woman will, in fact, progress to a more severe state [47]. As we have seen, a number of viruses, most notably HSV-2, have been suggested as etiological agents of cervical neoplasia. Studies with HPV, however, have demonstrated a remarkable association of a subgroup of these viruses with about 90% of benign, preinvasive, and invasive lesions of the cervix and anogenital tract. The oncogenic potential of HPV has been demonstrated both in laboratory animals and in cultured cells. Furthermore, susceptibility to certain HPV has been associated with a recessive genetic defect that results in SCC of the skin. HPV are difficult to study, however, because of the lack of an animal model, difficulty in developing a tissue culture system permissive for their replication, and a lack of understanding of their biology [48]. There is evidence that certain types of HPV (types 16 and 18) are associated with human genital cancer. Other virus types, such as HPV 6 or HPV 11, are more regularly found in benign genital warts. Since all viruses can be present in putative precancerous lesions of the uterine cervix (dysplasia, CIN) it has been postulated that individual HPV types have different "oncogenic potential". Expression of parts of the early region of the HPV genome in cell lines established from genital cancer supports the hypothesis that HPV are involved in inducing and/or maintaining the transformed phenotype of cancer cells [49].

Papillomaviruses are small DNA viruses that are associated with proliferative squamous intraepithelial lesions (SIL) in many higher vertebrates. In humans, over 100 distinct HPV have now been recognized, and each is associated with a specific set of clinical lesions. Approximately 15 of these viruses have been associated with benign proliferative lesions of the genital tract, and a subset of these has been regularly associated with vulvar, penile, and cervical lesions that are generally regarded as precancerous. The regular presence of this same HPV DNA in cancers of the cervix, penis, and vulva has supported the notion that these HPV may have an etiologic role in these malignancies. The biology and natural history of HPV infections have only recently been understood. In addition to the clinically apparent lesions induced, HPV-DNA can often persist latently in tissues that appear entirely normal. The cellular, hormonal, immune, and other physiologic factors involved in determining whether a HPV infection will be clinically manifest are not known. In general, there is a paucity of information concerning the host cellular and humoral immune responses to a HPV infection, though clinical observations indicate that such responses probably play a major role in the resolution of HPV-associated diseases [50]. The available evidence indicates that there are two distinct intraepithelial processes in the cervix associated with HPV. One is the classical condyloma and its counterpart in immature epithelium, atypical immature metaplasia. The other is intraepithelial neoplasia, which, like classical infection, may be mature (CIN with koilocytosis) or immature (high grade CIN or CIS). Molecular hybridization studies indicate that HPV 6 and 11 are most commonly detected in the former, whereas HPV 16 and 18 DNA are most common in the latter and in invasive cancer. From the clinical standpoint, the most important distinction is between HPV-related disease (condyloma or CIN) and reactive changes associated with other pathogens, such as Chlamydia. The former should be removed from the cervix, whereas the latter should be treated medically or followed. It is stressed that therapy should not hinge upon the histological distinction of HPV infection from neoplasia and that all lesions should be removed, by conservative means if possible. This is underscored by the fact that a high proportion of CIN lesions contain areas identical to condyloma and that lesions with deep endocervical canal involvement, including those with features suggesting condyloma, should be treated by cone biopsy to exclude the presence of invasive cancer. The management of the male partner is still unsettled. However, a large proportion of male partners of these patients has penile lesions and should be included in diagnostic and therapeutic protocols of women with genital HPV infections or neoplasms [51].

HPV are associated with a wide spectrum of epithelial lesions, ranging from benign warts to invasive carcinomas. They have been difficult to study, in part because they have not yet been propagated in tissue culture. Fortunately, advances in molecular biology have allowed characterization of HPV genomes and identification of some HPV gene functions. In addition to their clinical importance, HPV represent an important tool for exploring virus-cell interactions, gene expression, cellular differentiation, and cancer. HPV infections are not only common but also difficult to treat and prevent. Depending on the HPV type and location, the modes of HPV transmission may involve casual physical contact, sexual contact, and perinatal vertical transmission. HPV DNA genomes replicate at a low copy number in basal cells and, as most clinicians know, are difficult to eradicate. There is often a long latent period and subclinical infections, and HPV DNA can be found in normal tissue adjacent to lesions. HPV can cause widely disseminated lesions, especially in the immunocompromised host and in Epidermodysplasia verruciformis (EV). Aside from the rare carcinomas, the most serious life-threatening HPV-induced illness in children is recurrent respiratory papillomatosis. Somewhat surprisingly, in malignant lesions HPV DNA is also found as fragments incorporated into the cellular genome. Unlike retroviruses such as HIV, which integrate into the cellular genome as part of their life cycle, HPV integration is a terminal event for viral replication. Such integration may be critical, however, for viral-induced abnormal cell growth [52]. The preinvasive phase of SCC of the cervix is a continuous spectrum of abnormal epithelium, which, for convenience of classification and as a guide to management, is customarily subdivided into three grades. The histological diagnosis of CIN, as well as the distinction between the grades, depends on a combination of features embracing aspects of differentiation, nuclear changes, and mitotic activity. Grading of CIN is subjective. Generally, a minor degree of CIN would be expected to progress to a more severe form if not treated, but this progression does not seem to be inevitable. The more severe a CIN is at the time of diagnosis, the more likely it is that it will progress, both to a more severe degree of CIN and, eventually, to invasive carcinoma. Conversely, the more minor the degree of CIN is at diagnosis, the more likely it is that it will regress. True figures are not available for the rate of progression from CIN to invasive carcinoma: it is sufficient to accept that the risk of progression probably occurs in a significant proportion of cases, if not the majority. Preclinical invasive carcinoma is divided into microinvasive carcinoma and occult invasive (Stage IB) carcinoma. The definitions of these lesions have not yet been satisfactorily established: the term microinvasive carcinoma should define the maximum size of tumor that has virtually no metastatic potential and so may be treated in a conservative manner. Invasive SCC is classified histologically according to the cell type and the degree of differentiation, although it is debatable whether the cell type has any correlation with prognosis. Adenocarcinomas make up 5-10% of cervical cancers and a variety of histological types have been recognized. Adenocarcinoma in situ (AIS) is being diagnosed with increasing frequency, often in association with squamous CIN. It seems apparent that AIS is a precursor of adenocarcinoma, but little is known about its natural history [53]. When stratified into the various grades of severity, the composite data indicate the approximate likelihood of regression of CIN 1 is 60%, persistence 30%, progression to CIN 3 10%, and progression to invasion 1%. The corresponding approximations for CIN 2 are 40%, 40%, 20%, and 5%, respectively. The likelihood of CIN 3 regressing is 33% and progressing to invasion > 12%. It is obvious, from the above figures, that the probability of an atypical epithelium becoming invasive increases with the severity of the atypia, but does not occur in every case. Even the higher degrees of atypia may regress in a significant proportion of cases. As morphology by itself does not predict which lesion will progress or regress, future efforts should seek factors other than morphological to determine the prognosis in individual patients [54]. An overview of studies attempting to define the natural history of CIS of the cervix suggests that 20-30% of lesions progress to invasive carcinoma within 5-10 years. This risk of invasion and the inability to predict when invasion might occur has been reinforced by a judicial enquiry in New Zealand so that protocols that include withholding treatment are no longer justifiable. Once a diagnosis of cervical CIS is established, appropriate treatment is mandatory [55]. The vaginal smear reveals a spectrum of borderline lesions of the uterine cervix. This spectrum is the source of new clinical problems involving both the recognition and treatment of these various entities. A review of the literature of the past decades indicates that vaginal smears should be obtained regularly every year or two in all women beginning at the onset of sexual activity, but the initial smear may be falsely negative in 10% to 30% of cases. When patients have abnormal smears, the precise diagnosis can be established more accurately by cold-knife conization than by multiple punch biopsies. While hysterectomy has been considered "definitive treatment", late recurrence in the vagina occurs in 1.2% of patients so treated. Precise definition is required in treatment decisions concerning microinvasive lesions, but these may be well treated by non-radical measures [56].

Virus infection and viral gene expression emerge as necessary but obviously not sufficient factors for cancer induction. Additional modifications of host cell genes appear to be required for malignant progression of infected cells. The expression of viral oncoproteins in cells infected by "high-risk" types (e.g. HPV 16, HPV 18), in contrast to "low-risk" types (e.g. HPV 6, HPV 11), results in chromosomal instability and apparently in accumulation of mutational events. These "endogenous" modifications seem to be most important in the pathogenesis of premalignant lesions and tumor progression. Exogenous mutagens should act as additional cofactors [57]. Viral production occurs in low-grade lesions that are only slightly altered in their pattern of differentiation from normal cells. The production of viral particles, genome amplification, capsid protein synthesis, and virion assembly is dependent upon differentiation and is restricted to suprabasal cells. In carcinomas, viral DNA is usually found integrated into host chromosome, and no viral production is seen. The processes of viral transcription and replication are, therefore, intimately associated with the differentiation program of epithelial cells. In the past, studies on the life cycle of HPV have been limited due to an inability to faithfully duplicate the epithelial differentiation program in vitro. Recent advances in culture systems have overcome these problems, allowing for the propagation of HPV in vitro. In addition, insight has been gained at the molecular level regarding the mechanisms by which these viruses contribute to malignancy, centering on the action of the E6 and E7 viral oncoproteins. Evidence suggests that these oncoproteins function by inactivating the cell cycle regulators proteins 53 (p53) and retinoblastoma (pRb), thus providing the initial event in a multistep progression to malignancy [58]. Activated cellular oncogenes (i.e. myc and ras) and inactivated anti-oncogenes (p53 or pRb) participate in multistep carcinogenesis. Typification of HPV is important for clinical diagnosis. Unravelling the complexities of the immune system and understanding the biochemistry and molecular genetics of cellular oncogenes and tumor viruses have opened up new possibilities for vaccination [59].

In conclusion, HPV is a sexually transmitted virus that has been studied primarily in the context of its role as an epidemiological risk factor for cervical cancer and as a biological agent capable of modifying cellular growth and differentiation. Chronic cervical HPV infection appears to be etiologically linked to neoplastic changes of the cervix. However, it has recently become apparent that HPV is highly prevalent in the general population, including a substantial number of cytologically normal women. Although HPV detection is often transient in these individuals, it is not known whether the virus is truly eliminated or whether it remains below the threshold of detection in a latent state. Little is known about the interaction between HPV and other risk factors for cervical cancer, but variables such as pregnancy, immunosuppression, and use of OC may alter the natural history of HPV infection [60]. During the past 40 years, > 100 genotypes of HPV have been identified. Most of them are found in benign proliferations. However, several have been discovered in malignant tumors. Specifically, cancer of the cervix, other anogenital cancers, but also some cancers of the skin, the oral and nasal cavity, and the rare periungual carcinomas have been linked to specific HPV infections. The pathogenesis of cancer of the cervix has been particularly well studied. Specific viral genes (E6 and E7) of high-risk HPV (types 16, 18, and others) act as oncogenes. Their expression emerges as necessary but not sufficient factors for malignant conversion. Besides stimulating cell proliferation, they are responsible for the genetic instability of the infected cells. Their transcriptional and functional activity is regulated by host cell genes. Mutational modifications of the latter appear to be required for malignant progression [61-66].

Molecular Biology and Genetics

Viruses are becoming increasingly recognized as a major etiological agent in the development of numerous forms of human cancer. HPV have been associated with a number of neoplastic lesions, most notably cervical cancer, which is one of the major forms of cancer worldwide. Of the over 100 types of identified HPV, types 16, 18, 31, and 33 are the most commonly associated with malignant carcinomas. These viruses contain double stranded DNA that code for about eight gene products, some of which are oncogenic when introduced into cultured rodent or human cells. In particular, both the E6 and E7 gene products have different oncogenic capabilities and these genes are selectively retained within the genome of cervical carcinoma derived cells. The E7 gene product has immortalizing capabilities in primary cells and is able to co-operate with an activated ras oncogene to fully transform primary rodent cells. The E7 gene product from HPV type 16 is also capable of complexing in vitro to the anti-oncogene product, pRb. Similar complexes occur with Adenovirus E1 (E1A) and Simian Virus (SV) 40 large T proteins, which may suggest a shared mechanism of transformation used by HPV type 16, E1A, and SV40. Transformation studies using primary human cells and nontumorigenic HeLa/fibroblast hybrid cells have also suggested that chromosome 11 may be important in suppressing the HPV transformed phenotype. The transformed phenotype may therefore also involve an impaired intracellular control of persisting HPV oncogenic sequences. Although there exists no solid evidence that a cytotoxic T-lymphocyte (CTL) reaction is mounted against HPV transformed cells, there is evidence that both NK cells and activated macrophages can preferentially kill HPV transformed cells in vitro [67]. The HPV 16 E7 protein has recently been shown to be a multi-functional protein possessing both transcriptional modulatory and cellular transforming properties similar to those described for E1A proteins. E7 is able to transactivate the Adenovirus E2 (E2A) promoter and can cooperate with an activated ras oncogene to transform primary baby rat kidney cells. The N-terminal 37 amino acids of all of the E7 proteins of the genital associated HPV contain regions which are highly conserved and which are quite similar to portions of conserved domains 1 and 2 of E1A. These domains in E1A are critical for cellular transformation properties and contain the amino acid sequences involved in binding the product of the pRb. Results from a collaborative study have shown that the E7 oncoprotein of HPV 16 can associate with the pRb in vitro. The ability of the E7 proteins encoded by various HPV to bind pRb has been examined using an in vitro complexing assay. E7 is not sufficient for transformation of human keratinocytes. The co-operation of the HPV 16 E6 and E7 genes has been shown to be important for transformation of these cells [68]. Increasing evidence points to the existence of a host-mediated intracellular control which down-regulates these HPV genes in replicating normal cells. This control appears to be interrupted in HPV-positive carcinoma-cells, probably due to structural modifications of the respective host cell genes acquired during the period of viral DNA persistence. Factors affecting genes seem to be responsible for geographic differences in anogenital cancer incidence, since HPV infections appear to occur worldwide at similar frequency [69, 70].

Cytometric methods allow a division of tumors into a near diploid and an aneuploid group. In most carcinomas, aneuploidy has been associated with poor prognosis, but as regards SCC of the uterine cervix, the results are conflicting. The introduction of flow cytometry, a reliable and rapid method for determination of ploidy level and S-phase rate, has resulted in a renewed interest in cytometric studies of cervical carcinomas. In summary, aneuploidy is more common in stages III and IV and correlates to aggressive histopathology, but because of a higher degree of radioresponsiveness, the biological differences between aneuploid and near-diploid tumors are not consistently reflected in prognosis. High S-phase rates are correlated both to aggressive histopathology and to impaired short-term prognosis [71]. Chromosomal localization of HPV 16 and 18 on human cervical carcinomas and epithelial cell lines obtained after HPV transfection has uncovered a nonrandom association of viral integration and specific genome sites. Fragile sites appear to be preferential targets for viral integration because of their structural and functional characteristics through which chromosomal anomalies, alterations in proto-oncogene activity, and gene amplification can occur. Individually or in association, such changes lead to the acquisition of an unlimited cell growth potential but not tumorigenicity. Genetic instability and uncontrolled cell division resulting from HPV integration increase the cell's susceptibility to other exogenous carcinogenic factors that may complete the process of neoplastic development [72]. Recognizing cervical cancer as a natural stochastic phenomenon, that is in the first stage of its self-organization into a new biological dissipative structure (initiation) and sustaining its development in the second stage (promotion), is a basic requirement in conquering cancer and preventing neoplastic disease, i.e. the third stage of neogenesis (progression). A dissipathogenic state inside an organism is the only common primary cause of neoplasia. Thus, medical thermodynamics clarifies why so many non-specific factors enable the origin of cervical cancer, that is can cause cervical dissipathogenic states. This thermodynamical theory abolishes opposition and unites the heretofore-cellular neoplastic theories by bringing them to an atomic level. Diagnosis and treatment of dissipathogenic processes implies true causal prophylaxis of cancer, therapy of which always has to encompass its environment [73].

In conclusion, in the past years new data have been published on the molecular biology of HPV infections and their relationship to cervical neoplasia. As molecular techniques have become more sophisticated and as the molecular knowledge of HPV infections has been pursued in greater depth, it is increasingly apparent that this human tumor DNA virus is similar to a number of other oncogenic DNA viruses that have been described and well studied. These viruses appear to act through a common pathway of producing oncogenic proteins that interfere with key signaling elements that normally control the process of cell division [74]. Transformation involves a multi-step process and requires additional factors besides high-risk HPV infection. High-risk HPV are capable of immortalizing primary human keratinocytes in tissue culture, but such cells become transformed only after certain chromosomal changes take place, possibly having to do with oncogene activation. The DNA of high-risk HPV is frequently (if not always) integrated into the genome of cancer cells, while it is normally episomal in premalignant lesions. Integration disrupts the E2 and E5 genes and viral gene regulation. Cells containing integrated viral DNA show excessively high levels of E6 and E7.

While there is some conflicting evidence, it appears that the p53 and pRb tumor-suppressor genes are more frequently mutated in HPV-negative tumors than they are in HPV-positive tumors, suggesting that for tumor formation to proceed the p53 and pRb must be inactivated either by interaction with the viral proteins or by mutation. The presence of an activated oncogene in a cell lacking functional p53 or pRb may then be sufficient to cause tumor progression [75]. Progression of an HPV-infected cell clone to invasive growth involves consecutive modifications of a set of host cell genes. Some of these modifications suppress viral oncogene functions post-transcriptionally, and others suppress transcription via a signaling pathway stimulated by activated macrophages and possibly by additional cells. A scheme tries to unify available data by postulating the existence of two intracellular signaling pathways in the control of latent HPV infections [76]. Significant advances have been made toward the understanding of the initiation and progression of cervical dysplasia and neoplasia at the molecular level. To date, this has not translated into improvements in diagnosis or treatment although it is a realistic expectation that this will occur. Significant variation in the proportion of tissue specimens that exhibit genetic alterations is striking. This may be attributed to different methods of analysis, different methods of tissue fixation, which influence antigen preservation, and the analysis of small numbers of samples per report, which introduces the possibility of sampling error. In spite of the variation among published reports, it is clear that several genetic alterations occur in preneoplastic and early-stage invasive cervical neoplasms. It remains to be determined which alterations of genetic structure or expression contribute to tumor initiation. The prognostic applicability of oncogene mutations is a particularly interesting area of investigation that is the closest to clinical application, although additional research involving larger numbers of patients is critical.

The development of convenient methods of tissue fixation that preserve the myc oncoprotein, the synthesis of specific antibodies that provide consistent results, and the application of computer-assisted image analysis to quantitate results will be particularly important in this regard [77]. With a better mechanistic knowledge, it should be possible to design new therapeutic approaches to treating HPV-associated disease that are directed toward specific cellular events such as turning off the production of E6 and E7 proteins or restoring the activity of pRb or p53. Increased attention has also been turned to immunologic aspects of HPV infections, making real the possibility of using simple office-based procedures to detect specific proteins encoded for by the HPV open reading frames in an attempt to determine who has been infected, is actively infected, and has proteins being produced that are indicative of neoplasia. From the clinical point of view, the use of outpatient excisional techniques such as the LEEP is rapidly supplanting ablative techniques because of their superior ability to identify early invasive carcinomas and AIS that have not been detected by colposcopy [74, 78, 79].

Cytohistopathology

Use of the Pap smear for screening patients for cervical cancer has reduced the mortality of invasive cervical SCC. The continuum of cellular abnormalities leading to invasive carcinoma has been carefully studied through cytologic evaluation. Through this process, terminology has changed, and the concept of CIN has developed. Improved reporting of the cytologic abnormalities will not only lead to institution of appropriate therapy, but also to a reduction in the number of false-negative results of cytologic studies. Improved communication between the cytopathologist and the attending clinician, as recommended by the Bethesda system (Table 1), attempts to refine the process of appropriate patient care in the detection and treatment of cervical carcinoma and its precursor states [80]. Currently used histological and cytological classification systems for cervical lesions suffer from poor inter- and intra-observer reproducibility, and do not allow accurate identification of which mild lesions will progress towards cancer. It is postulated that low-grade and high-grade SIL (L-SIL and H-SIL) might represent distinct entities with different potential for progression rather than necessary stages of a continuum leading to cervical cancer. Improved understanding of the etiological role of HPV types in cervical cancer and of the natural history of L-SIL and H-SIL might result in more suitable clinical treatment of low-grade lesions [81].

The Bethesda Pap smear system and its 1991 and 2001 revisions aim to simplify Pap smear reporting and make it more reproducible. It redefines the Pap smear request as a medical consultation. The pathologist consultant is required not only to provide the smear reading but also its clinical recommendation. The Bethesda system insists on a detailed Pap smear report assessing specimen adequacy and types of epithelial changes. Squamous cell abnormalities are grouped according to their biologic potential. Both CIN 1 (mild dysplasia) and HPV lesions are grouped together as L-SIL, while moderate and severe dysplasia (CIN 2 and 3) belong to the H-SIL category.

Table 1. The Bethesda system

SPECIMEN TYPE:
- Conventional smear (Pap smear)
- Liquid-based preparation
- Other

SPECIMEN ADEQUACY:
- Satisfactory for evaluation (describe presence or absence of endocervical/transformation zone component and any other quality indicators, e.g. partially obscuring blood, inflammation, etc.)
- Unsatisfactory for evaluation... (specify reason)
- Specimen rejected/not processed (specify reason)
- Specimen processed and examined, but unsatisfactory for evaluation of epithelial abnormality because of (specify reason)

GENERAL CATEGORIZATION (optional):
- Negative for intraepithelial lesion or malignancy conventional smear (Pap smear)
- Other: see interpretation/result (e.g. endometrial cells in a woman ≥ 40 years of age)
- Epithelial cell abnormality: see interpretation/result (specify "squamous" or "glandular" as appropriate)

INTERPRETATION/RESULT:
- NEGATIVE FOR INTRAEPITHELIAL LESION OR MALIGNANCY: when there is no cellular evidence of neoplasia, state this in the general categorization above and/or in the interpretation/result section of the report, whether or not there are organisms or other non-neoplastic findings
- ORGANISMS:
    * Trichomonas vaginalis
    * Fungal organisms morphologically consistent with Candida spp.
    * Shift in flora suggestive of bacterial vaginosis
    * Bacteria morphologically consistent with Actinomyces spp.
    * Cellular changes consistent with HSV
- OTHER NON NEOPLASTIC FINDINGS (optional to report; list not inclusive):
    * Reactive cellular changes associated with:
        - Inflammation (includes typical repair)
        - Radiation
        - Intrauterine contraceptive device (IUD)
    * Glandular cells status post hysterectomy
    * Atrophy

Table 1. (Continued)

OTHER:
- Endometrial cells (in a woman ≥ 40 years of age): specify if "negative for squamous intraepithelial lesion (SIL)"
- EPITHELIAL CELL ABNORMALITIES:
    - SQUAMOUS CELL:
        * Atypical squamous cells:
    - Of undetermined significance (ASC-US)
    - Cannot exclude H-SIL (ASC-H)
        * Low grade SIL (L-SIL) (encompassing: HPV/mild dysplasia/cervical intraepithelial neoplasia [CIN] 1)
        * High grade SIL (H-SIL) (encompassing: moderate and severe dysplasia, carcinoma in situ [CIS]/CIN 2 and CIN 3):
    - With features suspicious for invasion (if invasion is suspected)
        * Squamous cell carcinoma (SCC)
    - GLANDULAR CELL:
        * Atypical:
    - Endocervical cells (not otherwise specified [NOS] or specify in comments)
    - Endometrial cells (NOS or specify in comments)
    - Glandular cells (NOS or specify in comments)
        * Atypical
    - Endocervical cells, favor neoplastic
    - Glandular cells, favor neoplastic
        * Endocervical adenocarcinoma in situ (AIS)
        * Adenocarcinoma:
            - Endocervical
            - Endometrial
            - Extrauterine
            - NOS
- OTHER MALIGNANT NEOPLASMS (specify)

ANCILLARY TESTING: provide a brief description of the test methods and report the result so that it is easily understood by the clinician

AUTOMATED REVIEW: if case examined by automated device, specify device and result

EDUCATIONAL NOTES AND SUGGESTIONS (optional): suggestions should be concise and consistent with clinical follow-up guidelines published by professional organizations (references to relevant publications may be included)

Adapted from: International Agency for Research on Cancer (IARC), 2013.

Atypical squamous cells of undetermined significance (ASC-US) and atypical glandular cells (AGC) need further qualification as to whether they favor either a reactive or a neoplastic process [82]. ASC-US and AGC are two acronyms introduced in 1988 by the

Bethesda system for reporting borderline cytological changes in cervical cytology. ASC-US and AGC categories should be subclassified. Five ASC-US subgroups were proposed:

1) ASC-US due to processing defects;
2) with "mature" cytoplasm;
3) in post-menopausal women:
   a) in the setting of atrophy; and
   b) with estrogen stimulation;
4) atypical metaplasia; and
5) ASC-US with keratinized cytoplasm.

AGC subgroups may be subcategorized in endometrial or endocervical based on origin. Endocervical AGC should be further qualified, but the analysis of AGC may be difficult and the conclusive diagnosis is frequently "AGC not otherwise specified (NOS)". The subclassification of ASC-US and AGC is useful for an appropriate clinical management, but pertinent patient information (such as age, date of last menstrual period, mechanical therapies, tamoxifen therapy, and others) is needed to avoid an overdiagnosis and consequently an overtreatment. In fact, various subgroups require different clinical management. Therefore, an effective communication between cytopathologists and referring physicians is essential in the analysis of squamous and glandular atypias [83].

The human uterine cervix offers a unique opportunity to study the early lesions of SCC, i.e. CIS and dysplasia (combined as CIN). In vivo, the patients with CIN have the epidemiological common denominators or "markers" of early onset of coitus, multiple sexual partners, first delivery before age 20, and antibodies to HSV-2 more frequently than do controls. The lesions themselves have specific epithelial and vascular changes observable with the colposcope in addition to the usual histological markers from biopsy specimens. The chromosomes and DNA content of cells in these lesions are abnormal. In vitro, the cells from CIN have characteristics somewhat between normal and invasive carcinoma. They lack contact inhibition and may be transferred for several generations, in contrast to normal cervical epithelial cells. The fibroblasts from areas adjacent to CIN are different from normal fibroblasts. The mitotic mechanism in cells cultured from CIN has a significantly prolonged prophase and telophase when compared to similar normal cells. The surface of CIN cells, unlike normal cells, has numerous microvilli when examined by scanning electron microscopy and has characteristic differences from normal cells with numerous elongated, irregular microvilli. With the transmission electron microscope, an increase in microvilli and a decrease in desmosomes and tonofibrils are seen in CIN cells. Some of these markers are being used clinically to manage patients with CIN [84]. It is clear that the relation between HPV infection and cervical neoplasia is more complex than initially realized. Preliminary molecular virologic data suggest preferential distributions of low- and high-risk HPV types in CIN that tend to correlate with the morphologic appearance. Thus, mild and moderate dysplasias (CIN 1 and 2) contain a diverse distribution of HPV types, including a minority that has a high risk of malignant potential. HPV, therefore, appears to play a major role as a promoter. Neoplastic transformation is probably determined by specific HPV types but, in addition, requires initiation by some other carcinogenic stimulus, e.g. HSV-2 and cigarette smoking. Despite numerous studies performed during the past 50 years, the long-term behavior of dysplasia remains uncertain. The natural history of HPV-associated lesions is unknown. Until this information is available, it is recommended that the conventional dysplasia, CIS, or CIN nomenclature be used. The presence of associated viral changes can be considered and added to the diagnosis, e.g. "moderate dysplasia (CIN 2) with evidence of HPV infection". Treatment should be the same for all intraepithelial lesions, regardless of the presence of morphologic evidence of HPV. In the future, it may be necessary to modify the classification of precancerous lesions of the cervix if it is shown that a specific HPV type induces a characteristic morphologic alteration or that the HPV type, in and of itself, has greater prognostic significance. Until then, confusion will be minimized and management optimized if the conventional dysplasia, CIS, or CIN nomenclature is employed [85]. Microinvasive carcinoma is the transition stage from intraepithelial growth to clinical invasive cancer. The early invasive growth must be accepted as an indication that the lesion is significant: it may be self-healing but its objective evidence of progression and invasion remains the most significant indication of malignancy. The subjective changes of CIS, nuclear enlargement, pleomorphism of nuclei, altered nuclear-cytoplasmic ratio, etc. are transcended and the recognition and diagnosis of microinvasive carcinoma should be facilitated for the pathologist. Treatment that tends to be conservative is more widely accepted, but the disease can be lethal and the most serious complication appears to be, like CIS, vaginal recurrence [86].

The identification of a specific marker cell, the koilocyte, has led to initial studies of frequency and biologic significance of neoplastic lesions of the uterine cervix associated with HPV [87]. HPV induces pathognomonic abnormality of squamous cells, known as koilocytosis, which may precede or accompany various manifestations of cancerogenesis including invasive cancer. Still, recent studies suggest that HPV infection is quite common in normal people and may prove to be ubiquitous. Hence, the activation of the virus and its ability to interact with cervical epithelium is likely to be due to "patient factors" rather than the presence of the virus per se [88]. It is suggested that cervical lesions be diagnosed as flat condyloma if they contain HPV types 6 or 11 and as CIN if they are confined to the epithelium and contain HPV types 16 or 18 or other types associated with neoplasia. Patients with a Pap smear or clinical evidence of HPV infection in the genital tract should be examined colposcopically, invasive cancer should be excluded, and the HPV-induced lesions should be identified and eradicated [89]. Pathologic and epidemiologic studies performed over the past five decades have provided evidence that the development of SCC of the cervix is a multistep process involving a precursor preinvasive stage. Infection by a variety of HPV types may result in active viral intranuclear replication without integration into the cellular genome. This episomal form of infection is manifested morphologically by the development of mild dysplasia (CIN 1 with koilocytosis and acanthosis). Approximately 20 different HPV types have been associated with CIN 1 lesions, whereas high-grade dysplasia and CIS (CIN 2 and 3) are associated with only a few viral types (mainly HPV 16, 31, 33, and 35). Low-grade lesions are differentiated and have a low risk of progression to cancer, whereas high-grade lesions are characterized by nearly complete or complete loss of squamous maturation and a higher risk of progression to invasive cancer. Based on the biologic dichotomy of an infectious and a neoplastic process and the segregation of HPV types into two groups, a modification of the CIN classification into L-SIL and H-SIL in accordance with the Bethesda system has been proposed. HPV plays a significant role in the development of cervical neoplasia, and the value of identifying HPV DNA by such molecular techniques as Southern blot analysis, ISH, and the polymerase chain reaction (PCR) in the early detection of preinvasive lesions has now been determined and their routine use is at present recommended [90].

Although the incidence of SCC of the cervix has declined in recent years, it remains the most common type of cervical cancer in our society. Early invasive, International Federation of Gynecology and Obstetrics (FIGO) stage IA carcinoma has been a source of controversy in diagnosis and therapy for many years. Specific requirements must be met in order to make this diagnosis.

Most importantly, the cervical conization specimen must be handled properly, so that the features of tumor dimensions, vascular involvement, and completeness of excision can be correctly evaluated. The risk of lymph node metastasis in lesions with depths of invasion up to 3 mm is < 1%. This risk increases significantly with deeper levels of invasion. In the area of frankly invasive SCC of the cervix, certain pathologic features have been shown to be clinically relevant. These include the extent of local disease, cell type, and the presence of vascular or lymphatic invasion. Regarding cell type, it is critical to distinguish between poorly differentiated small cell squamous carcinoma and small cell undifferentiated carcinoma, as the prognosis for these tumors may differ. Finally, as several rare but pathologically distinct variants of SCC of the cervix often have different natural histories than typical SCC, correct diagnosis of these lesions is vital [91]. It is possible to distinguish the various epithelial types in the normal cervix based on their keratin expression patterns. Reserve cells display a bidirectional keratin pattern, comprising keratins typical of both squamous and simple types of differentiation, reflecting the bipotential nature of these cells. CIN can be divided into two subpopulations, one characterized by the reserve cell keratin phenotype and the other by a keratin phenotype typical of nonkeratinizing squamous epithelia. The first population also contains the simple keratins, the relative percentage of which increases with increasing degree of dysplasia. It is therefore suggested that these lesions are progressive in nature. Carcinomas show a differentiation-related keratin expression pattern in addition to the basic reserve cell keratin phenotype. Adenocarcinomas also have been shown to express most of the reserve cell keratins. The latter observation indicates a common progenitor for both carcinoma types [92].

Adenocarcinomas and related tumors now account for approximately 15% of carcinomas of the uterine cervix. There is new information about the microscopic features, differential diagnosis, and subtypes of these neoplasms such as adenoma malignum, and villoglandular, mesonephric, adenoid basal, and adenoid cystic carcinomas. These tumors may cause considerable diagnostic difficulty, sometimes being difficult to distinguish from non-neoplastic glandular proliferations. Their correct identification has major prognostic implications [93].

The past four decades have seen an increase in the incidence of endocervical carcinoma. Numerous studies have increased understanding of these tumors: hormonal therapy, HPV, and other cofactors have been implicated in the etiology of endocervical carcinoma. Early diagnosis is difficult: precursor lesions to AIS are still poorly defined and understood, and there may be a rapid transit time from in situ to invasive carcinoma. The definition of microinvasive adenocarcinoma is not uniformly agreed upon, and at this time the recommendation is not to use the term. Histologic typing and grading of adenocarcinoma may be useful in the prediction of prognosis for patients. Therapy is based upon stage of disease, the most beneficial results being obtained from either radical surgery or combination surgery and radiation therapy [94-96].

Immunology

Numerous studies have demonstrated an altered antigenicity in the carcinomatous cervix. Whether the neoplasia-associated antigens are of viral origin, are actually normal antigens expressed in elevated levels, or are true tumor-associated antigens has not been precisely determined, since evidence has been presented for all of these possibilities. These antigens associated with cervical SCC have been demonstrated not only biochemically and by raising antisera to the tumors in animals, but also by studies of the humoral and cell-mediated immune responses of cervical cancer patients. Immunodiagnosis of cervical cancer with the use of these antigens has, to date, not been feasible, although several of the assays appear potentially useful [97]. Polyclonal and monoclonal antibodies to cytokeratin polypeptides were used to study the expression of these intermediate filament proteins in normal, squamous metaplastic, and neoplastic epithelium of the uterine cervix, in order to investigate the morphogenesis of early epithelial changes preceding cervical SCC. A polyclonal keratin antiserum showed a positive reaction in all different epithelial cell types of the uterine cervix. A positive reaction was also found in subcolumnar reserve cell hyperplasia, in squamous metaplastic and dysplastic cells, and in squamous CIS. A monoclonal antibody specific for columnar epithelium (RGE 53) gave a positive reaction in endocervical columnar cells and in some immature metaplastic cells but was negative in subcolumnar reserve cells, squamous metaplastic cells, dysplastic cells, and most cases of CIS. Another monoclonal cytokeratin antibody (RKSE 60) pointed to early keratinization in light microscopically nonkeratinizing squamous metaplastic and dysplastic epithelium. A possible overlap in staining patterns of RGE 53 and RKSE 60 was seen in some cases of immature metaplasia. Morphologic changes occurring in the transformation zone upon dedifferentiation are accompanied by alterations in cytokeratin expression. Similarities in cytokeratin expression were found between dysplasia and CIS on one hand and subcolumnar reserve cell hyperplasia and squamous metaplasia on the other. This study favors an epithelial origin and a squamoid nature of subcolumnar reserve cells [98].

Epithelial antigen immunostaining in the uterine cervix has been claimed to be helpful in the identification and classification of rare lesions, evaluation of basement membrane integrity, study of atypical condylomas, immunodetection of proliferating processes, and early diagnosis of malignant transformation [99]. Although cervical cancer is the most common malignancy of the gynecologic system, very few tumor markers have been specially prepared for this disease. TA-4, a tumor antigen of cervical SCC, has currently been widely used in clinical practice [100]. Studies of cervical secretions as well as cells composing the endocervix have provided evidence for a functional and potentially important immunological system in the mucosa of that organ. The availability of the tools of cell biology as well as three agents that may be used as probes to infect cervical mucosa experimentally has made possible a detailed approach to define the structural and functional characteristics of local cervical immunity. A long-term goal of these studies is to determine how the cervical immune response may be regulated to reduce local viral replication and virus-associated diseases. With LC for antigen presentation, cervical immune responses generally remain detectable for > 30 days, are predominantly of the immunoglobulin A (IgA) isotype, can be influenced by estrogen or progesterone, and are best elicited by local rather than systemic exposure to antigen. Cervical immune responses to HPV are of particular importance in this regard, because this virus is associated with cervical neoplasia. While responses in serum to HPV 16 late proteins 1 (L1), E4, and E7 has been found in up to 78% of persons with HPV-associated cervical neoplasms, data showing that a local response of comparable frequency consistently occurs have yet to be confirmed. The current status of local HPV 16-specific Ig as a potentially useful indicator of HPV 16-related infection or pre-cancer is controversial, and is confounded by several potentially important factors, including patient age, estrogen /progesterone level, smoking status, and sample admixture with serum Ig [101].

Cell surface carbohydrates serve as differentiation and developmental markers characteristic of different cell and tissue types. Expression of these carbohydrate antigens is often significantly altered in tumors, particularly in those arising from epithelial tissues. In normal cervical uterine epithelium, the result shows that the glycosylation of metaplastic squamous cells is different from that of original squamous cells, indicating that the regulation and differentiation of the epithelium in the transformation zone is different from that of the original squamous epithelium. This variation in expression of carbohydrates seen in the metaplastic epithelium may be of importance for the development of carcinomas in this area [102]. Infection appears to begin in the basal cells. Early gene expression is associated with acanthosis, and late gene expression is associated with appearance of structural antigens and virions in nuclei of cells of the granular layer, usually koilocytotic cells. Malignant transformation of warts and papillomas appears to be related to a variety of factors:

1) infection by certain HPV types (HPV 5, HPV 8, HPV 16, HPV 18, HPV 31);
2) decreased cellular immunity to HPV-associated antigens; and
3) interaction with cofactors such as other micro-organisms or sunlight.

Spontaneous regression or successful treatment of the benign lesions appears to depend on either naturally acquired or iatrogenically related stimulation of HPV type-specific immunity. The humoral antibody response to HPV particles may be important in preventing infection. In contrast, the local events surrounding regression of warts and condylomata are primarily associated with specific cell-mediated immunity. Local cell-mediated immune responses, particularly cell-associated soluble mediators and stationary macrophage-like cells, may be especially important in the host's immune response to mucosal infections [103].

The presence of HPV DNA in the genital tract and the genotype of the infecting HPV are now widely employed as biochemical markers in epidemiological studies of cervical cancer. Additional HPV markers could be utilized in future investigations. The amount of HPV DNA is likely to be higher in case specimens than in control specimens, viral genome would be integrated frequently in cases but almost never in controls, and early region transcripts may be relatively more abundant in cases than in controls. When valid serological markers for past HPV infection become available (very likely, antibodies to HPV capsid proteins), they will be useful to estimate lifetime exposure to HPV. Serological markers for HPV-associated neoplasia (very likely, antibodies to early proteins) may prove useful for surveillance and have prognostic value. A serological marker capable of detecting past HSV-2 infection permits an analysis of the role of this virus in cervical cancer, either as an independent risk factor or in interaction with HPV. Other possible biomarkers include activation of oncogenes and inactivation of tumor-suppressor genes, assays for serum micronutrients, and analysis of leukocytes for human leucocyte antigens (HLA). These should provide insights into the sequence of events that lead to cervical cancer and help to explain the geographic distribution of the disease [104]. NK lymphocytes, an important defence against viral diseases, are present in most HPV-associated lesions and CIN. HPV-positive cervical cancer cells and HPV-immortalized human cervical epithelial cells which possess properties similar to cervical dysplasia, however, are resistant to NK but are sensitive to lymphokine-activated killer (LAK) lymphocyte lysis. Sensitivity can be enhanced by treatment of cervical cells with leukoregulin, a cytokine secreted by lymphocytes. Combination treatment with leukoregulin and a chemotherapeutic drug, e.g. cisplatin, further enhances sensitivity of HPV-infected cells to LAK lymphocyte lysis. In contrast, gamma-interferon (IFN) treatment of cervical cells can result in decreased sensitivity to LAK lysis, illustrating the potential balance cytokines can exert in the immunologic control of cervical cancer [105-107].

Cell-mediated immunity likely plays an important role in prevention of HPV-associated disease, and HPV-associated SCC has been shown to occur with increased frequency among iatrogenically immunosuppressed individuals. Similarly, individuals with HIV-associated immunodeficiency have been shown to have a high prevalence of anogenital HPV infection as well as a high prevalence of HPV-associated lesions that are thought to be cancer precursors. Thus, HIV-positive women have a high prevalence of CIN, and HIV-positive men have a high prevalence of anal intraepithelial neoplasia (AIN). The risk of disease in these populations appears to increase as the degree of immunosuppression increases, and these individuals are likely at risk for development of invasive SCC. Because these diseases are preventable, women should be screened on a regular basis with cervical Pap smears, followed by colposcopy if the Pap smear is abnormal. Although preliminary studies indicate that anal Pap smears may also be useful for screening, further trials need to be performed and, at this time, HIV-positive men should be assessed on a regular basis with anoscopy. Lesions that are detected should be biopsied for histopathologic assessment. Thorough assessment of the entire anogenital region should be performed because of the multicentric nature of HPV-associated diseases. Following treatment, rigorous follow-up should be maintained because of the high recurrence rate of HPV-associated disease in these populations [108]. As individuals with advanced immunosuppression live longer due to improvements in the medical therapy for HIV infection, it is expected that the incidence of HPV-associated neoplasia, as well as that of other tumors, will continue to increase [109].

An increasing body of information permits certain conclusions to be drawn about the nature and magnitude of the interactions between HPV and HIV infections and their influence on the genesis of intraepithelial neoplasia and, to a lesser extent, cancer. Importantly, findings tend to be consistent across a number of independent studies. While HPV infection probably does not significantly alter the course of HIV infection, HIV-induced immunosuppression does increase the severity and duration of anogenital warts, increase their infectiousness and reduce treatment efficacy. However, in developed countries the countervailing effects of enhanced HPV infectiousness and declining rates of unsafe sexual behavior have resulted in stable or declining incidence rates of anogenital warts. Advanced immunosuppression due to HIV infections results in highly significant increases in rates of HPV-associated CIN and AIN. In developed countries, population-based secular trend analyses point to increasing incidence rates of anal cancer in single men in areas of high HIV prevalence, but not yet of cervical cancer in women [110]. Available data on the association between acquired immunodeficiency syndrome (AIDS) and cervical neoplasia have practical implications for gynecological care. All controlled studies reported a significant association between HIV infection and cervical neoplasia. The summary odd ratio (OR) indicated that the odds of HIV-infected women having cervical neoplasia are 4.9 (95% confidence interval [CI], 3.0-8.2) times that of HIV-negative women. Research is needed to clarify etiological relationships and the role of HPV in the causal pathway of the observed association. Meanwhile, available data are sufficient to encourage regular Pap smear screening of HIV-infected women, and HIV testing and counseling of women with cervical neoplasia considered at risk for HIV infection [111].

This association is not completely due to immunosuppression. It is likely that HPV pathogenesis is altered in HIV-infected women. Preinvasive cervical neoplasia likely occurs more frequently in HIV-infected women because of several factors, including immunosuppression, viral interactions, and alterations in viral pathogenesis. As new treatments prolong the life of HIV-infected individuals, we must continue to be aware of and reactive to an increasing number of opportunistic complications of HIV infection, such as HPV infection and associated diseases [112]. With heterosexual transmission of HIV becoming the primary mode of transmission to women in the USA and a high rate of HPV and cervical neoplasia in HIV-infected women, obstetrician-gynecologists have become primary care providers for HIV-infected women. Reports of a high rate of recurrence and progression of cervical neoplasia in this population suggest that gynecologists must strive to identify those women with cervical neoplasia who are HIV-infected. Alterations in local immune response of the genital tract caused by HIV infection may be responsible for higher prevalence, recurrence rates, and progression rates of cervical neoplasms in these women [113]. Cervical and anal neoplasia are likely to become more common manifestations of HIV disease as patients with profound immunodeficiency, who would have succumbed to opportunistic infections earlier in the epidemic, are now surviving for extended periods of time because of increasingly effective antiretroviral, prophylactic, and antimicrobial therapies. Cervical cancer in the setting of HIV infection appears to be a more aggressive disease, less likely to be successfully treated by standard therapies, and consequently associated with a poorer prognosis than in comparable non-HIV-infected women. Anecdotal observations suggest that anal cancer in HIV-infected persons may share these features. Strategies need to be developed for earlier detection and treatment of neoplasia and anogenital cancer in the setting of HIV-induced immunodeficiency [114]. Recent technical advances localizing virus DNA and gene products in situ will provide new avenues for investigation, allowing us to go beyond correlations and to clarify the mechanisms of interaction between the two viruses in individual patients. As we have said, with improved antiretroviral therapy and prophylaxis for HIV-associated opportunistic infection and prolonged survival of women with HIV, HPV infection and its most serious consequence, cervical cancer, are likely to assume greater significance in the clinical management of HIV-infected women throughout the world. A better understanding of the role of HIV in promoting the clinical manifestation of HPV infection will be essential to the control of this disease [115]. Taking into account these data, the Centers for Disease Control (CDC) since 1993 have included invasive cervical carcinoma among the AIDS-defining conditions. A primary means by which HIV infection may influence the pathogenesis of HPV-associated cervical pathology is by molecular interaction between HIV and HPV genes. Although these have not been well defined, an upregulation of HPV E6 and E7 genes expression by HIV proteins (such as tat) has been postulated by some authors. Cervical cytology appears to be adequate as a screening tool for CIN in HIV-positive women, but the high recurrence rate and multifocality of this disease reinforces the need for careful evaluation and follow-up of the entire anogenital tract in these women. Probably, in the next few years cervical tumors will represent one of the most frequent complications of HIV infection, a part of progression through AIDS. This points to a need for greater interdisciplinary co-operation for a best disease definition and for the development of effective prevention measures [116-118].

Pregnancy

Cancer in pregnancy requires the careful consideration of multiple complex issues to achieve the most favorable outcome for mother and fetus [119]. Carcinoma of the cervix is the most common gynecologic cancer found during pregnancy. Management and treatment of this condition depend on cancer stage, estimated gestational age, and ethical, religious, and personal desires [120]. Because of the uncommon synchronous occurrence of pregnancy and invasive cervical carcinoma, this disease entity remains poorly understood. In addition, inconsistent reporting has precluded meaningful meta-analysis. About 1 in 2000 pregnancies is associated with cervical cancer and pregnancy is a complication in approximately 3% of patients with cervical cancer. There is little evidence to suggest that pregnancy has an influence on prognosis. Although not firmly established, vaginal delivery may have an adverse effect on outcome. Timing of delivery must be individualized inasmuch as there is a role for delaying treatment in order to achieve fetal lung maturity. Surgery and radiotherapy should be utilized in the same stage-dependent manner as in nonpregnant patients, but management should be individualized and undertaken by a multidisciplinary team [121].

Pregnancy represents an ideal time for cervical cancer screening, and all pregnant women presenting for prenatal care should be carefully examined. The management of the abnormal smear in pregnancy remains a challenge to the modern colposcopist. Colposcopy in pregnancy is difficult. Anatomic variants can mimic disease. Significant cytologic overall detection of L-SIL demands an increased understanding of physiologic variants in pregnancy. Possible recent increases in cervical cancer incidence in younger women require comprehensive knowledge of warning signs of early invasion. Modern management approaches must temper the need for accurate exclusion of cancer with the risk of overly aggressive interference in patients without disease or with minor atypia [122]. Most patients with pregnancy-associated cervical cancer present with early-stage disease. The prognosis for pregnant patients after stratification for stage is similar to that for nonpregnant patients. Patients with early-stage squamous cancers diagnosed in the late second and early third trimester may have cancer treatment delayed to increase the likelihood of fetal maturity without compromising maternal prognosis. Cesarean section (CS) in patients with pregnancy-associated cervical cancer should be the delivery method of choice. Early-stage cervical cancer should initially be treated surgically. In patients with advanced disease, primary radiation therapy is a safe and effective modality. In the first and second trimester, radiation therapy should be performed without hysterotomy [123]. Incorporating effective screening into preventive health care for women would theoretically eliminate the diagnosis of cervical cancer in pregnancy. Until this goal is reached, our management decisions are limited by the relatively small and retrospective studies that form the basis for our pertinent knowledge and the ethical issues that would complicate randomized controlled trials (RCT) of treatment in pregnancy. Limited data suggest that radical hysterectomy with pelvic lymphadenectomy might carry a more favorable therapeutic index than radiation therapy in early-stage disease. In general, improvements in neonatal management may allow earlier intervention, shortening the time between diagnosis and treatment in hope of improving maternal outcome. The actual survival impact of this information remains to be demonstrated. At many institutions, the rate of "atypical" or other nonspecified cytologic abnormalities exceeds 10%, and low-grade dysplastic changes are common and less threatening. These conditions place the responsibility for cervical cancer detection firmly upon the clinician and his index of suspicion that a significant abnormality exists. Those directing prenatal care must remain compulsive in the proper use of cytologic screening and careful clinical examination. A diagnosis should be rapidly and vigorously pursued when a cancer is suspected, with timely referral when needed. These practices may have an immediate impact upon both maternal and fetal outcome when facing cervical cancer in pregnancy [124]. As we have said, radical hysterectomy and pelvic lymphadenectomy are indicated for the treatment of cervical carcinoma that is localized clinically to the cervix and upper vagina. Intraoperative complications have been reported in 1.1-7.4% of patients. Long-term complications include bladder dysfunction (2% at 3 years), urinary fistula (vesical, 0.8%; ureteral, 1.2%), stress urinary incontinence (29%), ureteral stricture (1%), rectal dysfunction (80%), severe constipation (5.3%), lymphocysts (20% by ultrasonography, 2% clinically), and lymphedema (10%). The operative mortality is 0.7%. The 5-year survival rate for patients with stage IB disease is 85.7% and for stage IIA is 69.6%. The recurrence rate is 27.2%. Recurrences are distributed equally between the pelvis and extrapelvic sites. Radical hysterectomy affords termination or delivery of the pregnancy at the same time that the treatment is provided. For patients with stage I disease treated with radical hysterectomy, the survival rate is 92.1% [125].

In conclusion, cervical cancer is one of the two most frequently encountered malignancies during pregnancy with breast cancer. Cervical cancer is generally diagnosed in its early stages, therefore the physician must have a high index of suspicion and must aggressively pursue the diagnosis in pregnant women to try to detect the disease as early as possible. Premalignant lesions of the cervix must be evaluated thoroughly. Therapy for this cancer is similar to the treatment of nonpregnant women, with some modifications made due to fetal considerations and informed maternal desires. Pregnancy does not affect the progression or prognosis of the disease significantly. Pregnancy following the treatment for cervical cancer is unlikely, if not impossible, because current standard therapies will render these women infertile. There have been, however, some recent reports describing trachelectomy followed by laparoscopic lymph node dissection for the treatment of early-stage cervical cancer in an attempt to preserve future fertility [126]. Triage of the abnormal Pap smear in pregnancy requires colposcopic evaluation and directed biopsy. If histologic CIN is confirmed, the patient can be managed with observations and can be re-evaluated in the postpartum period. If evidence of microinvasion is present, conization must be performed. For patients with invasive disease, a delay in therapy until fetal maturity is achieved does not compromise survival [127]. The management of abnormal cytology during pregnancy has changed dramatically during the last three decades. The goal has been and remains timely diagnosis of and treatment planning for invasive carcinoma of the cervix. Because therapy for preinvasive disease can safely be postponed until the postpartum period, the ability to distinguish CIN from invasive cancer without cone biopsy has been a major step forward in the management of cervical disease in pregnancy. The data demonstrate the safety and accuracy of the more conservative approach of colposcopy and biopsy. The use of cone biopsy during pregnancy, associated with substantial morbidity, has been significantly reduced by the diligent application of colposcopy. As is true in the nonpregnant state, cone biopsy is necessary when colposcopic examination is nonsatisfactory. Cone biopsies cannot be considered therapeutic during pregnancy, owing to the high incidence of positive margins and residual disease on postpartum evaluation. For this reason, the importance of postpartum re-evaluation cannot be overemphasized [128-130].

Clinics

The early stages of cervical cancer are generally asymptomatic and the most common symptoms often can be linked to other diseases of non-tumor type. Among the warning signs that may raise suspicion of cervical cancer there are, for example, abnormal bleeding (after a sexual intercourse, between two menstrual cycles, or in menopause) and vaginal discharge without blood or pain during sexual intercourse. Then, we can find dysmenorrhea, hematuria, strangury, incontinence, while because of the development of metastases we can have dyspnea and hepatomegaly. In later stages, the symptoms vary depending on which organs are involved: we can also observe rectal urgency or proctorrhage. In the course of the disease, renal failure with uremia can occur. Among the other complications are copious bleeding and respiratory failure for metastatic involvement of the lungs.

Screening

Cancer of the uterine cervix is one of the most common female cancers and a major source of premature female mortality. UK deaths exceed 2000 women-year (WY). To reduce these rates, national screening programs have been introduced using the Pap method. By far, the most difficult and underestimated component of the complex detection system leading to the discovery and treatment of precancerous lesions and early cancer of the uterine cervix is the screening and interpretation of cervical (Pap) smears. Cytological examination of cervical smears employs the Pap staining technique and cell morphology to detect abnormal cells from the susceptible transformation zone of the cervix. The Pap smear has been used to screen women for cervical cancer since 1940. The annual Pap test became a recommended standard for American women without ever having been subjected to RCT to estimate its efficacy and effectiveness. After > 70 years of routine use, the Pap test fails to meet most of the generally accepted criteria for a mass screening program. The policy persists, however, because the nation's ideology supports the maximum utilization of new technologies, and special interest groups have promoted the test as the major weapon against cancer [131]. Therefore, Pap smear screening for cervical cancer has become an established practice in most developed countries. This is because the cervix is relatively accessible to investigation and treatment, and early stages in the morphogenesis of cervical cancer are both recognizable and easily treated. The Pap smear is a valid test. It is simple, relatively inexpensive, reliable, and free of risk. Although the test has far from perfect sensitivity, it has high specificity, and false-positive results are rare. In most reported series, the majority of false-negative results have been found to be attributable to collection errors rather than laboratory errors. Despite the importance of Pap smear screening, controlled prospective trials have not been undertaken to determine its efficiency in reducing cervical cancer incidence and mortality. However, countries with well-organized programs, wide population coverage, and correct follow-up appear to have had some impact on mortality from cervical cancer. Nevertheless, coverage of high-risk groups, particularly women over 40 years of age, remains the greatest problem. Recommendations on the frequency of testing vary considerably. Statistical models indicate triennial testing may deliver almost all of the effectiveness of annual testing at a substantially reduced cost, but the numerous reports of false-negative results argue strongly in favor of annual screening. These problems may be solved by increasing the sensitivity of the test and/or by the use of additional tests [132]. Anyway, the Pap smear is a safe, easy, and inexpensive method for the screening of large numbers of sexually active women for the presence of neoplasia of the cervix. When the Pap smear is reported as being abnormal, it is highly accurate. Unfortunately, some cytology laboratories report lesions as "class II" or "atypical". These reports are not helpful to the clinician and require further evaluation. Most sexually active women are at "high risk" for the development of cervical neoplasia because of early sexual activity for multiple sexual partners. All women at high risk should have annual Pap smears. If a woman has a Pap smear that suggests the presence of CIN (dysplasia or CIS), colposcopy should be performed. This office procedure allows for the detection of the areas causing the abnormal cytology. Colposcopy can often allow outpatient therapy of CIN lesions. Conization should be performed only when the colposcopic examination is unsatisfactory or patient or lesion factors are not favorable for office therapy. Hysterectomy is not recommended for treatment of cervical dysplasia or CIS [133].

A clinical trial to evaluate Pap smears was never undertaken. However, evidence gradually accumulated from time trend analyses and from cohort and case-control studies showed the incidence and mortality of cervical cancer to be reduced by organized screening programs. The risk of cervical cancer following different screening histories was estimated in a study of the International Agency for Research on Cancer (IARC). Screening with 1-year and 3-year intervals was estimated to reduce the incidence of SCC by 94% and 91%, respectively. Cervical cancer is rare in young women, and little was estimated to be gained from including women below the age of 25 years in organized screening programs. The age distribution of cervical cancer has changed: a substantial proportion of cases now occur in the older generations of women, who have never been offered organized screening. Computerized pathology registration systems may serve as a tool for integration of the total smear-taking activity and, thus, ensure that a high percentage of women are screened regularly at minimized costs. The planning of a screening program should include both the smear-taking activity and the treatment [134]. Cytologic case finding may fail because of inadequate samples, insufficient time devoted to screening, or human fatigue. Other weak points of the system are an inadequate clinical component, inadequate patient compliance, poor reproducibility of diagnoses, and ineffective aftercare. For example, obtaining a second smear to confirm or refute a diagnosis of cellular atypia is often a misleading practice. Although this cancer detection system has been shown to be effective in reducing the rate of morbidity and mortality from invasive cervical cancer in appropriately screened populations, there is no evidence that the Pap test has succeeded anywhere in complete eradication of this theoretically preventable disease. It is important to inform the public about the potential failures of the system and the reasons for them [135].

The essential controversy about cervical cancer screening is not whether or not it should be done, but who should be screened, how often they should be screened, and how to obtain the best sample for the screen [136]. Population screening with annual cervical (Pap) smears after beginning sexual activity until age 35 and at 5-year intervals after that can reduce both incidence and mortality rate from invasive cervical cancer. Benign, premalignant, and malignant conditions may be identified in smears. The term CIN reflects better the continuum of change in precursor lesions and is preferred over the older dual terminology of dysplasia/CIS for precursors of cervical cancer. Colposcopy is essential for evaluation of all patients with abnormal cervical smears. Colposcopy is used to identify the site, severity, and extent of abnormality as well as to aid directed biopsy, plan treatment, and allow use of conservative methods to treat the precursor lesions. Colposcopy, however, has no role as a primary screening procedure for cervical cancer, but instead cervical smears are used for screening [137]. Indirect evidence indicates that cervical cancer screening should reduce the incidence and mortality of invasive cervical cancer by about 90%. In the absence of screening, a 20-year-old average-risk woman has about 250 in 10,000 chances of developing invasive cervical cancer during the rest of her life, and about 118 in 10,000 chances of dying from it. Screening at least every 3 years from 20 to 75 years of age will decrease these probabilities by about 215 in 10,000 and 107 in 10,000, respectively, and will increase a 20-year-old woman's life expectancy by about 96 days. The particular age at which screening is begun (for example, 17 or 20 years), the requirement of several initial annual examinations before reducing the frequency, and screening every 1 or 2 years compared with every 3 years improves the effectiveness by < 5%. Screening is recommended at least every 3 years from about age 20 to about age 65 years [138].

The earlier optimistic predictions that invasive carcinoma of the uterine cervix could be totally eradicated by means of Pap screening have failed. Experiences from different countries give evidence, however, that a considerable reduction of incidence and mortality can be gained with this type of secondary prevention. Improved knowledge of the epidemiology of carcinoma of the uterine cervix and of its natural history could be anticipated to give a better basis for the planning of preventive measures. Maintenance of a high laboratory standard, a good technique for taking of smears, improved communications between laboratories and the doctor or nurse taking the smear and the doctor or clinic performing the treatment, and an adequate reaction to the report from the laboratory with adequate treatment of the precancerous stages are supposed to improve the effect of the screening programs [139]. All physicians performing Pap smears need to be aware of the risk factors for the development of cervical cancer. There is a continuing controversy concerning the significance of certain Pap smear findings, the timing of colposcopic intervention, and the management of abnormal findings on these tests. Clinical decisions should be based on the newer concepts of degrees of dysplasia, cytological and descriptive findings, and the potential for rapid progression of lesions [140]. The Department of Health and Human Services (HHS) and the American Cancer Society (ACS) invited a working group to review the 1985 recommendations on cervical screening. Minor modifications have been made to the earlier recommendations in the light of more information about the effectiveness of different screening policies, and in the expectation that comprehensive cytology registers to ensure recall and follow up of abnormalities will be in place shortly. All women from the age of 20 up to 70 years should be offered cervical screening every three years. Any woman who has never had sexual intercourse or who has had a hysterectomy with complete removal of the cervical epithelium for a benign condition need not be screened. Women should have a second smear within one year if they have never had a smear before or if > 5 years have passed since their last smear. However, recall through the register should not be more frequently than three yearly for women with a history of normal smears [141].

The main obstacles to the success of cervical screening are organizational, i.e. the inaccuracy of address registers. Some ways of encouraging uptake include appropriately worded invitations and educational material, personalized approaches from members of the primary health care team, and flexible surgery hours [142]. Cytology screening programs have suffered from an inability to cover whole populations, particularly less affluent and/or socially disadvantaged groups, which are most at risk. Despite this difficulty, the magnitude of the problem makes it necessary to continue its study. In particular, efforts are needed in developing countries to study incidence, to better define high-risk groups, and to devise economical ways of detecting more cases in the earlier stages [143]. With passage of the Breast and Cervical Cancer Mortality Prevention Act of 1990, significant activity has emerged in the development, implementation, and evaluation of cervical cancer screening programs targeting underserved populations. This activity has prompted health educators and program planners to identify barriers to cervical cancer screening specific to low-income and minority women, those traditionally underserved by cancer control programs, and to develop strategies that address these barriers [144].

The Pap smear, unquestionably, is a successful screening test for cervical cancer. However, recent advances in technology have raised questions regarding whether the conventional Pap smear is still the standard of care. Perhaps nowhere in medicine is clinical decision making being more strongly influenced by market and other external forces than in cervical cytopathology [145]. Refinements are continually being made in the terminology used to define the gradations of disease, in the classifications used to describe test results, and in the appropriate technique for performing the test [146]. In screening for cancer, the examination of specimens is an intensive and expensive task. Its high cost has led to a number of attempts to automate the process, either fully or partially. Over the last 50 years, various experimental prescreening systems have been developed for the diagnosis of cytological samples, including the use of image processing techniques [147]. In an effort to reduce the false-negative rate of cervical cytologic findings, several new technologies have recently evolved. Automated cytologic testing (PapNet, AutoPap 300 QC) proposes to rescreen negative conventional cytologic findings to identify smears likely to be false negative. Fluid-based monolayers (ThinPrep, CytoRich) propose to reduce the false-negative rates by optimizing the collection and preparation of cells. HPV DNA testing by Hybrid Capture has been proposed for a variety of screening and triage roles. Visual screening after application of acetic acid is done by cervicography by use of a photographic technique, whereas in speculoscopy the screening is done by direct visualization of the cervix by the primary care provider. Polarprobe uses biophysical parameters and a computer algorithm to give an instantaneous prediction of the likelihood of cervical disease [148]. Cervicography is not a surrogate for colposcopy. Its easy availability and economy maximize the predictive potential of the existing screening test, the Pap smear. It can also be used as a triage tool for women "at risk" for cervical HPV infections, such as women with a history of vulvar condylomata. It is not colpophotography, as the magnification and focus are stable, and the operator cannot manipulate the position of the cervix and change focus and light settings. Cervicography cannot replace Pap smears in detection programs, but can augment the predictive value of screening when used in tandem, and can push cervical cancer detection rates closer to 100%. What cervicography does provide are a screening tool with great potential and a way to attack the troubling death rates from cervical cancer still facing us in the 21st century [149].

At the beginning of its use, there was the doubt that HPV testing should not replace cervical cytology as the first-line approach in screening for cervical cancer, as HPV testing was not considered sufficiently reliable. Even though there are many unanswered questions about the validity of HPV tests, it is timely to consider that HPV testing might improve the management of the substantial number of women whose smears are neither clearly normal nor abnormal, but are described as atypical, suspicious, or mildly dyskaryotic. The efficacy and costs of incorporating HPV testing into a cervical cancer-screening program has been evaluated in RCT with very good results [150]. With the development of the PCR, it has become possible to detect small numbers of HPV genomes in clinical samples. The sensitivity and specificity of this technique, together with the possibility of performing the test on crude cervical scrapes, makes PCR the method of choice for screening. The question arises whether screening for diagnostic purposes must include all the HPV types associated with infections of the genital tract or only those which are strongly associated with cervical cancer (HPV 16 and HPV 18) [151]. Now, the latter is the standard procedure.

In conclusion, screening with Pap smears should begin at age 18 or at the age of first sexual intercourse and should be repeated every one to three years, depending on individual risk factors, until age 65. Screening may be discontinued in women over age 65 that have had normal findings on two consecutive Pap smears. Use of a spatula and Cytobrush for cervical sampling will improve the chances of collecting an adequate sample containing endocervical cells. In women with cervical or genital HPV infection and persistent inflammatory cervical changes unresponsive to appropriate therapy, colposcopy is necessary to screen for underlying dysplasia [152]. Population screening for cervical cancer resulted in significant reduction in the morbidity and mortality from cervical cancer. An increased understanding of the relationship of HPV infection with cervical cancer and the natural history of cervical cancer precursor lesions further solidifies and expands the biological basis for cervical cancer screening. Pap tests in asymptomatic women remain the cornerstone of cervical cancer screening. Clinicians should be cognizant of the significant false-negative rate of Pap smears. Meticulous attention to proper Pap smear technique is necessary to maximize the sensitivity of the test [153]. Recently, a number of new technologies have been developed to improve the detection of cervical cancer and its precursors. The current literature reflects three routes toward improving cervical cancer screening. The first is to improve the test qualities of cytology-based screening. The use of liquid-based cytology and computerized analysis of Pap tests are examples of attempts at this approach. Secondly, through various combinations of parallel or sequential tests, either the sensitivity or the specificity of a given test could be improved depending on the tests chosen and the order in which they were performed (e.g. Pap test followed by HPV test or vice versa). Several excellent studies have been published on the use of HPV DNA testing as a primary screening modality and as an adjunct to the triage of mildly abnormal cytologic findings. The recent literature also reflects increasing interest in visual inspection of the cervix and self-collected samples for HPV testing as an equally effective and viable alternative to cytology in low-resource settings. A third possibility is to make use of advances in digital and spectroscopic techniques. In these cost-conscious times, a significant number of articles address the cost-effectiveness of these technologies and the real value of cervical cancer screening [154]. However, there is substantial controversy about whether the new tests offer meaningful advantages over the conventional Pap smear. Ideally, these new tests will increase the early detection of meaningful Pap smear abnormalities, reduce the number of unsatisfactory smears and provide fewer ambiguous results. It is also hoped that these new screening methods will not increase the number of false-positive results, but will improve the productivity of cytology laboratories without substantially increasing costs. The new tests include liquid-based/thin-layer preparations to improve the quality and adequacy of the Pap smear, computer-assisted screening methods to improve Pap smear interpretation, and new-generation HPV testing methods that may be useful in triaging patients with ASC-US or L-SIL [155-157].

Diagnosis

There has been remarkable improvement in the early diagnosis of cervical carcinoma in recent years. There is, however, disagreement regarding the definition and treatment of microinvasive carcinoma of the uterine cervix [158]. The use of cytology in evaluating the state of the uterine cervix is well recognized and accepted [159]. Diagnostic problems arise because of overlap of cytologic criteria of some squamous and glandular lesions of the female genital tract, lack of experience, or an overzealous attempt to interpret some features. Sampling techniques greatly influence the pathologist's ability to interpret the material [160]. From surveys conducted, it is concluded that the best and most acceptable quality control methods in cytology are those from within the laboratory. Most of these have results that can be reported centrally. Where the overall control and codes of practice are high, there the results are the most reliable, as sources of error from whatever cause are quickly brought to light [161]. The visual inspection of cellular specimens and histological sections through a light microscope plays an important role in clinical medicine and biomedical research. The human visual system is very good at the recognition of various patterns but less efficient at quantitative assessment of these patterns. Some samples are prepared in great numbers, most notably the screening for cervical cancer, which results in hundreds of millions of samples each year, creating a tedious mass inspection task. Numerous attempts have been made over the last 60 years to create systems that solve these two tasks, the quantitative supplement to the human visual system and the automation of mass screening. The most difficult task, the total automation, has received the greatest attention with many large-scale projects over the decades. The main reason for this difficulty is the great pattern recognition capabilities needed to distinguish between cancer cells and all other kinds of objects found in the specimens: cellular clusters, debris, degenerate cells, etc. Improved algorithms, the ever-increasing processing power of computers, and progress in biochemical specimen preparation techniques made useful automated prescreening systems become available. Meanwhile, much less effort has been put into the development of interactive cell image analysis systems. Still, some such systems have been developed and put into use at thousands of laboratories worldwide. In these, the human pattern recognition capability is used to select the fields and objects that are to be analyzed while the computational power of the computer is used for the quantitative analysis of cellular DNA content or other relevant markers. Numerous studies have shown that the quantitative information about the distribution of cellular DNA content is of prognostic significance in many types of cancer. Several laboratories are therefore putting these techniques into routine clinical use. The more advanced systems can also study many other markers and cellular features, some known to be of clinical interest, others useful in research. The advances in computer technology are making these systems more generally available through decreasing cost, increasing computational power, and improved user interfaces [162].

The increasing frequency of cervical neoplasia among younger women and the increased invasiveness of these tumors have led to a considerable growth in research into this disease. Conventional methods (epidemiology, cytology, and immunology), while being extremely useful, also have significant limitations. Recent advances in techniques for the manipulation of DNA now make it possible to analyze tissues for the presence of viral genomes [163]. HPV types 16 and 18 viral DNA were molecularly cloned and used as probes to screen a large number of genital tumors by Southern blot analysis. HPV 16 or HPV 18 sequences were found in a high percentage of cervical carcinomas, but only in a small number of condylomata acuminata or flat condylomas. The majority of the latter lesions, however, contained HPV 6 or HPV 11 sequences, respectively, which, in contrast, were detected only rarely in CIS or invasive carcinomas. A similar distribution of the different HPV was observed when cell scrapings taken from the cervix were tested by ISH [164,165]. A number of validation experiments have compared the most commonly used HPV hybridization methods with the accepted gold standard, Southern blot hybridization. The methods are filter ISH (FISH), dot blot hybridization (ViraPap/ViraType), and PCR. FISH now appears to be too inaccurate to be recommended for future epidemiological studies. ViraPap/ViraType compares well to Southern blot, but is limited to the detection of seven genital HPV types. PCR-based methods may be more sensitive than Southern blot and are likewise capable of detecting the most known genital HPV types. Currently, there is no perfect method for HPV testing, because Southern blot itself is prone to some errors in performance and interpretation. Given that the scientific and clinical usefulness of HPV tests depends on the repeatability and accuracy of the assays, more intra- and inter-assay comparisons should be done to establish reference standards applicable to this area of molecular diagnostics [166]. PCR-based hybridization methods have been used to show that some women with normal cytology are carriers of HPV DNA of the types strongly related to cervical cancer. Reports which have estimated type-specific HPV prevalence in relation to the presence or absence of morphological signs of HPV infection indicate that among women who were identified as carriers of HPV DNA (by PCR-based methods) and who also had a normal cytological smear, the HPV type detected in the majority of instances was a high-risk viral type for cervical cancer (HPV types 16/18 = 44.7%, HPV types 31/33/35 = 8.1%, other and unknown types = 37.9%). This suggests that screening programs which include PCR-based HPV detection could reduce the false-negative rates currently reported by screening programs based on cytology alone [167].

In summary, the issue of determining which HPV is present in a clinical specimen (typing specimens for HPV) has received attention because HPV cause condylomata acuminata and are associated with the continuum of disease which ranges from dysplasia to invasive genital cancer. Morphological inspection of precancerous lesions is not sufficient to determine which lesions will progress and which will not. A number of research tools based primarily on DNA hybridization have been developed. These permit identification and typing of HPV in genital tract scrapings or biopsies. Some HPV types (e.g. HPV 16 and HPV 18) have been identified in high-grade dysplasias and carcinomas more commonly than other types (e.g. HPV 6 and HPV 11) and have been designated "high-risk" types for cervical cancer. Thus, the question arises whether HPV typing would improve patient management by providing increased sensitivity for detection of patients at risk or by providing a prognostic indicator. Analysis of the typing data indicates that, while HPV types can be designated high risk and low risk, these designations are not absolute and thus the low-risk group should not be ignored. In addition, interpretation of the data is complicated by finding high-risk types in individuals with no indication of disease [168]. The technology of detecting viral nucleic acids in genital fluids brought with it initial hopes that it would serve to identify women at risk for having or developing precancers or cancers of the cervix. Subsequent studies, however, have demonstrated limitations of the technology for predicting future disease. Recently, molecular immunology has complemented these prior efforts, with the intent to identify serological indices of exposure to HPV and perhaps delineate individuals at risk [169]. A variety of serological assays to detect antibodies to genital-type HPV has been developed. Bacterially expressed fusion proteins, synthetic peptides and HPV 11 virus propagated in a xenograft system have been the most commonly used antigen targets in either Western blot assays or enzyme-linked immunoabsorbent assays (ELISA). HPV antibodies have been readily detected and most studies suggest that they are type-specific. Primarily, antibodies appear to be directed against the capsid antigens. The presence or titer of antibodies to the HPV 16 E7 protein is strongly associated with cervical cancer in approximately 25% of cases. The significance of antibodies to other HPV antigens or of antibodies that recognize conformational epitopes is less clear. Attempts to validate the sensitivity and specificity of serological assays are still ongoing [170]. However, only DNA analysis accurately detects and determines the type of infection. The variety of molecular methods for detection of HPV DNA primarily reveals whether or not a lesion is in fact associated with HPV infection. For minor grade cervical squamous lesions or equivocal Pap smear results, HPV detection and typing can help identify patients at increased risk for cervical carcinoma. Cervical colposcopy and biopsy are indicated for definitive diagnosis [171].

The colposcope was developed in 1925 and is well established in clinical gynecologic practice for defining and delineating cytologically detected lesions mainly of the cervix but also the vagina and vulva, enhancing the cytologic detection and histologic verification of precancerous and cancerous lesions. The cost-effectiveness of colposcopy and its applicability, particularly in countries with a limited health budget, is a major issue. Automated cytology can interface with colposcopic examination in a number of significant ways. Automated cytologic analysis of conventional cervical smears can potentially direct colposcopic examination by predicting the nature of a lesion, assist in determining which patients should receive colposcopy, and thereby reduce, in some settings, the number of colposcopies. Potentially, various combinations of automated cytology and colposcopy may be used to generate screening protocols that might result in more effective and inexpensive screening. The role of cervicography, or high-resolution cervical photography, as a screening device remains to be defined. Sensitivity for high-grade lesions is generally no greater than that in cytology, and specificity appears lower. The interpretation of cervical photographs in triage of mildly abnormal cytology may prove to be useful in countries with established cytology programs. In areas of the world where cytology-screening programs are not in place, the interpretation of cervical photographs may have its most dramatic effect. Cost-effectiveness analyses are needed. There are, at present, insufficient data for the evaluation of speculoscopy, a procedure using chemiluminescent illumination of the cervix for visualization of acetowhite areas. Basic training in colposcopy should be integrated into the residency programs of obstetrics and gynecology. Criteria for the adequate training of colposcopists should be developed. Continuing education programs in colposcopy should be developed when they are not already in existence. The cost-effectiveness of integrating colposcopy as a primary screening technique should be evaluated. Following an H-SIL cytology result, colposcopically directed punch biopsy should be taken with or without endocervical curettage.

This generally should precede the LEEP. However, in certain circumstances direct LEEP may be indicated. LEEP under colposcopic vision is an efficient way to treat an H-SIL lesion of the cervix, because the histologic extent and margins can be determined, unlike with laser surgery or cryosurgery. It is also more cost-effective than cold knife conization, because general anesthesia and an operating room are unnecessary. Following LEEP, the endocervical canal should be examined colposcopically for any evidence of involvement. Lesions in the endocervix can then be removed with a different-shaped loop. Further research into Raman spectroscopy as a diagnostic aid in cervical pathology is needed, as is the use of micrococolpohysteroscopy for in vivo cytologic analyses, especially of the endocervical canal and transformation zone. Hysteroscopy is the most direct method for the diagnosis and treatment of intrauterine diseases. Hysteroscopic endometrial biopsy is more accurate than conventional biopsy methods. Cervical invasion of endometrial cancer can be detected by hysteroscopy. The depth of invasion, however, is more accurately determined by magnetic resonance imaging (MRI) or CT [172].

Clinicians have long looked for an imaging modality that can provide accurate and useful information on cervical carcinoma. In the past 30 years, MRI has come to play an important role in evaluating patients with this disease before treatment and in monitoring them afterward. Before treatment, MRI can accurately depict tumor size (volume) and extension [173]. MRI is also useful for demonstrating enlarged retroperitoneal lymph nodes. MRI evaluation of the parametria appears promising, but further studies are necessary to elucidate the optimal imaging parameters and to better define the overall accuracy of MRI compared to the clinical evaluation of the parametria [174]. MRI thus has the potential to supplant the traditional clinical FIGO staging system for this disease, which is based on clinical findings and is inherently subjective. Promising areas of research include endorectal, endovaginal, and phased-array coils [173].

In conclusion, the exact histologic diagnosis of CIN lesions is essential for a differentiated therapy. These data indicate that mild and moderate CIN lesions are detected more frequently by Pap smear and colposcopically directed punch biopsy than by cervical smears alone. Histological diagnosis and HPV-typing offer the possibility to establish a differentiated therapy, e.g. by way of close follow-up, local destruction, or cone biopsy. Main attention should be directed at early detection of dysplasia, at timely institution of follow-up programs, and a possibly conservative therapeutic management [175]. Since infection of the genital mucosa by HPV includes a wide variety of viral types, it is essential to recognize the specific HPV type eventually present in a genital lesion to ensure an appropriate follow-up of the patient. A PCR-based assay differentiates in a single amplification reaction the "malignant" HPV genital types from the "benign" ones. It is possible to design and use a PCR-based assay for the simultaneous detection of various genital agents from a single genital swab. This assay can be a model for the development of additional multidetection systems of microorganisms potentially involved in similar pathologies [176].

Minor cytologic abnormalities of the cervix, such as ASC-US, are vastly more common than H-SIL or invasive cancer. Current guidelines for the management of ASC-US include repeating the Pap smear at specific intervals, referring all patients for colposcopy, or using an adjunctive test such as Hybrid Capture HPV testing or cervicography. The usefulness of the Pap smear is limited by its considerable false-negative rate and its dependence on clinician and laboratory performance. Colposcopy is a highly sensitive procedure, but many patients with ASC-US have normal colposcopic findings. The Hybrid Capture test not only measures quantitative HPV load, but also detects both oncogenic and nononcogenic HPV types, thereby increasing the probability that serious cervical disease is not missed. Hybrid Capture sampling is simple to perform and positive results are strongly associated with cervical dysplasia. HPV testing in women with ASC-US can be used as an adjunctive test to identify those with HPV-associated disease. It can also serve as a quality assurance measure. Together, repeat Pap smears and HPV testing should identify most patients with underlying cervical dysplasia. Combined testing may also minimize the number of unnecessary colposcopic examinations in women who have no disease [177]. New technologies are trying to make significant changes in the way we perform the Pap smear test, a test that has undergone no significant modification since its inception. Efforts have focused on improving sampling with liquid-based methods, improving detection of abnormal cells with automated screening, and improving the detection of HPV with assays practical for use in routine clinical material. Taken together, these technologies can have a positive impact on cervical disease detection and intervention [178-180].

Staging

In cancer of the uterus, the morphologic factors influencing the choice of therapy and patient prognosis are tumor size, depth of invasion, presence of lymph node metastasis, and stage (Table 2). Clinical staging is often inaccurate with resultant suboptimal therapy, thereby invalidating comparison between treatment options. The available cross-sectional imaging modalities of ultrasound (US), CT, and MRI, have significantly improved the staging of malignant disease. In the pelvis, MRI offers several advantages over the other imaging modalities.

In particular, MRI has excellent soft tissue contrast resolution, allowing direct multiplanar imaging with evaluation of tumor extension in all three directions, and has variable imaging parameters (TR/TE), characteristics of the echo patterns, to facilitate optimal tumor detection. It is a non-invasive technique with an ability to visualize blood vessels without the need for contrast injection and is independent of body habitus. However, MRI is not tissue-specific and a histological diagnosis is required in all cases. In the post-radiotherapy patient, MRI has the ability to demonstrate radiation tissue change and the potential to differentiate radiation fibrosis from recurrent/residual tumor. Its non-invasive nature and lack of ionizing radiation make it suitable for assessing treatment response and as an adjunct for patient monitoring [181].

Table 2. FIGO cervical cancer staging

- Stage 0 (Tis, N0, M0):
The cancer cells are only on the surface of the cervix, without invading deeper tissues of the cervix. This stage is also called carcinoma in situ (CIS) which is part of cervical intraepithelial neoplasia grade 3 (CIN 3). Stage 0 is not included in the FIGO system.

- Stage I (T1, N0, M0):
In this stage, the cancer has invaded the cervix, but it is not growing outside the uterus. The cancer has not spread to nearby lymph nodes (N0) or distant sites (M0).
    o Stage IA (T1a, N0, M0):
    This is the earliest form of stage I. There is a very small amount of cancer, and it can be seen only under a microscope. The cancer has not spread to nearby lymph nodes (N0) or distant sites (M0).
    o Stage IA1 (T1a1, N0, M0):
    The cancer is < 3 mm deep and < 7 mm wide. The cancer has not spread to nearby lymph nodes (N0) or distant sites (M0).
    o Stage IA2 (T1a2, N0, M0):
    The cancer is between 3 mm and 5 mm deep and < 7 mm wide. The cancer has not spread to nearby lymph nodes (N0) or distant sites (M0).
    o Stage IB (T1b, N0, M0):
    This stage includes stage I cancers that can be seen without a microscope as well as cancers that can only be seen with a microscope if they have spread deeper than 5 mm into connective tissue of the cervix or are wider than 7 mm. These cancers have not spread to nearby lymph nodes (N0) or distant sites (M0).
    o Stage IB1 (T1b1, N0, M0):
    The cancer can be seen but it is not larger than 4 cm. It has not spread to nearby lymph nodes (N0) or distant sites (M0).
    o Stage IB2 (T1b2, N0, M0):
    The cancer can be seen and is larger than 4 cm. It has not spread to nearby lymph nodes (N0) or distant sites (M0).

- Stage II (T2, N0, M0):
In this stage, the cancer has grown beyond the cervix and uterus, but has not spread to the walls of the pelvis or the lower part of the vagina.
    o Stage IIA (T2a, N0, M0):
    The cancer has not spread into the parametria. The cancer may have grown into the upper part of the vagina. It has not spread to nearby lymph nodes (N0) or distant sites (M0).
    o Stage IIA1 (T2a1, N0, M0):
    The cancer can be seen but it is not larger than 4 cm. It has not spread to nearby lymph nodes (N0) or distant sites (M0).
    o Stage IIA2 (T2a2, N0, M0):
    The cancer can be seen and is larger than 4 cm. It has not spread to nearby lymph nodes (N0) or distant sites (M0).
    o Stage IIB (T2b, N0, M0):
    The cancer has spread into the parametria. It has not spread to nearby lymph nodes (N0) or distant sites (M0).

- Stage III (T3, N0, M0):
  The cancer has spread to the lower part of the vagina or the walls of the pelvis. The cancer may be blocking the ureters. It has not spread to nearby lymph nodes (N0) or distant sites (M0).
  o Stage IIIA (T3a, N0, M0):
     The cancer has spread to the lower third of the vagina but not to the walls of the pelvis. It has not spread to nearby lymph nodes (N0) or distant sites (M0).
  o Stage IIIB (T3b, N0, M0; or T1-3, N1, M0): either:
     The cancer has grown into the walls of the pelvis and/or has determined hydronephrosis, but has not spread to lymph nodes or distant sites. Or:
     The cancer has spread to lymph nodes in the pelvis (N1) but not to distant sites (M0). The tumor can be any size and may have spread to the lower part of the vagina or walls of the pelvis (T1-T3).

- Stage IV:
  This is the most advanced stage of cervical cancer. The cancer has spread to nearby organs or other parts of the body.
  o Stage IVA (T4, N0, M0):
     The cancer has spread to the bladder or rectum (T4). It has not spread to nearby lymph nodes (N0) or distant sites (M0).
  o Stage IVB (any T, any N, M1):
     The cancer has spread to distant organs beyond the pelvic area, such as the lungs or liver.

Adapted from: American Cancer Society (ACS), 2013.

Clinical staging has serious limitations and is inaccurate in about 50% of patients with cervical cancer. Operative staging, although invasive, has significant advantages in identifying patients with metastatic disease: identification of this group will allow the extension of normal pelvic treatment methods and the more appropriate targeting of studies to assess therapy protocols for this difficult management group [182]. Clinical experience of the value of surgical-pathological staging in planning adequate treatment and in prognosis of uterine cancer, some new concepts concerning early stage definition, aggressiveness of tumors factors, and adequate surgical strategy or integrated therapy draw the conclusion that surgical-pathological staging in every uterine cancer is mandatory [183]. Most patients will be upstaged based on surgical exploration, usually because of occult nodal metastases. Data from surgical staging indicate that the incidence of positive para-aortic nodes is about 7% for patients with Stage I disease, about 17% for Stage II, and 28% for Stage III. Extended field radiation, to the level of T12, can salvage about 25% of patients with positive para-aortic nodes. About 40% of patients having extended field radiation develop distant metastases, and about 25% develop a pelvic recurrence. These data suggest the need for prospective clinical trials to evaluate the role of chemoradiation for improved local control, prophylactic extended field radiation for improved regional control, and prophylactic chemotherapy for improved systemic control [184]. According to other authors, clinical staging does not define the true extent of disease in approximately one-third of the patients with early cervical cancer. Unless clear nodular tumor extension into the parametria is palpable, a patient should be considered for surgical therapy. This involves a thorough staging laparotomy, including the exploration of the pelvic retroperitoneal spaces and para-aortic node dissection. If the disease appears to be confined to the cervix, a radical hysterectomy and pelvic lymphadenectomy is performed.

If gross tumor invasion into the parametria, the bladder, or rectum muscularis is documented, the patient is treated with pelvic radiation. If microscopic distant metastases to the para-aortic nodes are found, extended field radiation and possible chemotherapy is the treatment of choice. Survival is determined mostly by the extent of disease at the time of treatment. Therapy has to encompass the whole region affected by disease in order to provide the patient with a chance of cure. For disease beyond the cervix, regional radiation makes more sense if microscopic disease beyond the cervix is found after a radical hysterectomy. However, additional radiation adds morbidity, length of therapy, and cost. Unless there is clear proof that adequate primary radiation is inferior to surgery and postoperative radiation, it is recommended radiation for cancer of the cervix with proven Stages IIB and above [185].

Noninvasive radiologic methods to detect para-aortic lymph node metastases are reliable when combined with fine needle aspiration (FNA) of enlarged lymph nodes. However, the sensitivity is low, and undetected microscopic metastases leads to treatment failure. These patients with para-aortic lymph node metastasis are not treated with extended-field radiation, and they all die within 3 years. The CT scanning is probably the best diagnostic method to evaluate cervical cancer, because it can assess the primary tumor, the urinary tract, gastrointestinal tract, liver parenchyma, and retroperitoneum. It also permits the guidance of FNA and the arrangement of radiation ports. Surgical staging provides the direct assessment of the peritoneal cavity and the retroperitoneal spaces. Metastatic tumor, including enlarged lymph nodes, can be resected, but this is of dubious benefit. The operative morbidity is acceptable, with fewer intestinal complications when the extraperitoneal approach is used, and long-term morbidity is minimal when appropriate para-aortic radiation doses are employed (< 5,000 cGy). Surgical staging has provided data on the frequency of para-aortic lymph node metastasis by stage of cervical cancer, and thus, treatment strategies can be better developed. Extended-field radiation results in 5-year survival rates of 20-25% in patients with microscopic para-aortic lymph node metastasis, patients who would not survive without the treatment. However, surgical staging has produced only a modest boost in survival rates, because of the high rate of pelvic and systemic failure. When extended-field radiation is used prophylactically or in patients with probable lymph node metastasis seen on radiographic studies, survival rates are similar to patients irradiated after surgical staging finds para-aortic lymph node disease. As our ability to predict, and detect nonsurgically, positive para-aortic node disease improves, extended radiation (or other adjuvant therapy) could be used more frequently without operation in patients who are at high risk for metastatic disease. In a study, prophylactic para-aortic radiation was given to patients at high risk for para-aortic metastasis. In patients with a high probability of local disease control, para-aortic radiation significantly reduced the incidence of para-aortic and distant metastases. Patients with known para-aortic lymph node metastases frequently have occult systemic metastases. In these same patients, pelvic failure is also common. Thus, until effective systemic therapies emerge, a marked improvement in survival is unlikely in patients who have para-aortic lymph node metastasis [186]. CT scans and MRI techniques are unlikely to replace surgical staging in the near future due to their lack of sensitivity and specificity, yet these techniques combined with FNA of suspicious abdominal or pelvic lymph nodes can assist the oncologist in determining the necessity for extended field radiotherapy. In the absence of positive findings by FNA, young healthy patients with large volume tumors should be offered extraperitoneal surgical staging to aid in treatment planning. Radical surgery for early Stage (IB, IIA) tumors is as likely to result in cure as surgery combined with radiotherapy or chemotherapy, although the availability in the future of more sensitive chemotherapeutic agents may allow such systemic adjuvant therapy to play a larger role. Exenterative surgery still has a place as salvage therapy in this disease but as radiotherapy becomes more effective, its role diminishes [187]. Thus, CT scanning has been found to be no more accurate than examination for staging of early cervical cancer. Several studies have evaluated risk factors for recurrent disease in patients treated for early-stage cervical cancer, including a prospective surgical pathologic study by the Gynecologic Oncology Group (GOG). The risk of ovarian metastases in patients with early-stage cervical cancer is very low for both SCC and adenocarcinoma. Lateral transposition of the ovaries at the time of radical hysterectomy for cervical cancer has significant potential benefits but also risks [188,189].

Therapy

In the past decades, neoadjuvant and concomitant multimodality therapies have been studied in patients with cervical cancer. The past years has witnessed more pilot studies confirming the feasibility of multimodality therapy. It is now time to evaluate prospective RCT to determine the effects on disease-free intervals, to examine survival rates, and to define the ideal chemotherapeutic regimen and relationship to radiation therapy or surgery [190].

The surgical therapy of cancer of the cervix has historically been a mainstay of treatment for this malignancy. Surgery maintains an important role in the diagnosis and treatment of premalignant as well as early invasive and recurrent cervical cancer. Although the indications for and benefits of surgical staging remain to be determined, specific procedures frequently are necessary to manage treatment-related complications [191]. During the last 50 years, there have been major changes in the methods used to diagnose and manage cervical cancer precursors. Early detection of precursors through mass cytologic screening programs and the eradication of these precursors when detected are currently the cornerstone of policies aimed at reducing cervical cancer. These policies have been successful, resulting in a marked reduction in both the number of cases and deaths from cervical cancer in North America and Western Europe. Recently, however, significant controversy has arisen over several aspects of the diagnosis and management of CIN. Two of the most important of these controversies are whether all patients with low-grade CIN lesions require therapy and what the appropriate role is for the newly introduced LEEP in managing patients with CIN [192]. Over the past decades, the management of intraepithelial lesions of the visible portion of the female genital tract has substantially changed with the introduction of cryosurgery and the carbon dioxide (CO_2) laser. Although cryosurgery and the CO_2 laser are very effective in eradicating preinvasive disease, the selection of patients by colposcopy and appropriate biopsies is more important than the treatment techniques. Failure to properly evaluate women with genital tract neoplasia can result in disasterous consequences for the patient. The CO_2 laser shows considerable promise in managing dysplasia and CIS of the vagina and vulva. The laser combines the accuracy of the operating microscope and the precision and control of the photon beam. Post-treatment sequelae are minimal, and scarring is absent [193]. The laser has provided a relatively easy and safe method for treating all types of CIN. The advantages of lasers include great conservatism due to tissue sparing, great precision because of microsurgical method, combination of excisions and vaporization possible, suitable for therapy of multifocal disease, uncluttered field, and good hemostasis. Although other modalities have also been used successfully in the therapy of this disease, it appears that none is as versatile as CO_2 laser or possesses its ability to accurately treat the multifocal disease that may involve large surface areas of the lower reproductive tract. It seems unlikely that any of the cervical ablation methods (chemical destruction, hot cautery, diathermy electrode, cryoprobe, laser, and diathermy loop) will completely disappear from use in the near future. Ablation is an attractive alternative to cold-knife excision in properly triaged patients, since it is usually an outpatient procedure done without anesthesia or with only local anesthesia. Most importantly, a large number of patients have completely visible lesions of a severity less than that of CIS: they really do not need excisional conization by any technique and benefit by quick ablation of the transformation zone. A conization, to be diagnostic and therapeutic, must remove the entire transformation zone to the proper depth. This procedure is usually attended by a higher morbidity rate than is simple ablation. Laser excisional conization and the large loop excision of the transformation zone procedure are similar in a number of respects, because the operator must have certain capabilities and a through understanding of the disease to be treated to perform the operation correctly [194]. The conservative management of CIN is available and applicable to many patients. Regardless of the definitive therapy used in CIN, it is mandatory that proper pretreatment evaluation be performed. This includes cytology, colposcopy, colposcopy-directed biopsies, and clinical examination to rule out invasive cancer. If this can be done according to the stated criteria, one may proceed with outpatient treatment. If performed accurately, such treatment can be very effective, saving the patient a major surgical procedure. This is of tremendous benefit to the patient in time and money saved, as well as to the saving of hospital bed space and operating room time. For the young patient who has not yet completed her family or the patient who is pregnant, outpatient evaluation is probably the optimal method. If the techniques are unavailable or the physician managing the patient does not have the expertise to perform them, standard management by means of conization, which historically has been used in this disease, should continue to be used. The consequence of inadequate outpatient management of CIN can be catastrophic. If the procedures are properly followed, then the patient with CIN can be managed safely and effectively [195].

Stage I and Stage IIA disease are adequately treated with a radical hysterectomy. Morbidity and mortality in the last five decades has been reduced to a minimum. The extent of the radical surgical procedure called radical hysterectomy has been tailored to the extent of the disease by the use of modern knowledge of spread patterns [196]. Wertheim's radical operation aimed, by removing the parametrial tissue far from the tumor, to achieve margins free of disease. The paratissues contain the lymphatic channels draining the cervix. They run to the pelvic wall and are interspersed by lymph nodes scattered throughout the parametrium. If lymphadenectomy is to be curative, then the entire parametrium must be removed. To this end, the resection of the cardinal ligament was pushed to its limit by dissection directly at the pelvic wall. The surgical technique is guided by the anatomy of the pelvic fascia. The gaine hypogastrique lies just beneath the peritoneum and facilitates the opening of the paravesical space. The order in which the surgical steps are carried out is important. The paraspaces are opened first. The ureter is identified and lymphadenectomy is performed. The rectum is dissected off the vagina and the uterosacral ligaments are identified and removed. Only then is the vesico-uterine fold opened. The bladder is dissected off the vagina and the anterior parametrium is clamped and divided. Now the cardinal ligament is completely exposed. The bladder, rectum, and ureter have been mobilized so that the parametrium can be divided sharply directly at the pelvic wall, clipping the vessels step-by-step. The paracolpium is clamped and divided according to the proposed vaginal cuff. Thus, the entire lymphatic drainage can be removed. The value of this extension of radical abdominal hysterectomy lies especially in the treatment of large, voluminous tumors [197]. If there is no vascular involvement, survival from microscopic SCC is maximized by conservative treatment if tumor invasion is < 3 mm, while treatment by radical surgery results in maximal survival rates if the tumor invasion is over 3 mm. Radical surgery also maximizes survival for smaller lesions where lymph channel involvement is present, especially if a surgical mortality at the lower end of the reported range is assumed. These conclusions are still valid regardless of the patient's relative preference for death from surgery or death from cancer. However, the wish to preserve fertility sharply reduces the overall net benefit of surgery. Conservative treatment becomes the preferred option for all microinvasive lesions even for patients who are prepared to trade-off a small (e.g. 2%) risk of death in order to retain their fertility [198]. The main value of decision analysis is that it makes the trade-offs involved in a decision explicit. When depth of invasion is < 3 mm with no vascular or lymphatic involvement, the risk of spread is so low that radical surgery is not warranted. When the lesion involves lymphatics but does not penetrate the basement membrane > 1 mm, conservative therapy is still recommended if the operative mortality rate of radical treatment is at least 3.5 per 1000. However, in units with a low operative mortality rate, radical treatment offers the greatest survival advantage if fertility is not an issue. These statements refer only to optimizing survival chances and the decision is one of probabilistic dominance where correct treatment is determined entirely by probabilities rather than utility. For a young potential mother who accepts some risk to preserve fertility, the situation is different. Conservative therapy may be preferable despite lymphatic or vascular involvement if there is no > 1 mm depth of invasion. Where invasion exceeds 5 mm, or where it exceeds 3 mm with vascular involvement, the risk of spread increases exponentially and there must be very few patients for whom conservative therapy is appropriate [199].

Over the past decades, the role of surgery in the management of patients with advanced disease has been studied with a view toward a more precise extent of disease evaluation prior to definitive therapy. The role of pelvic exenteration in the treatment of recurrent cervical cancer has been established for > 50 years [200]. A survey of the literature over a 50-year period suggests that exenteration operations have not been widely accepted or perhaps not commonly reported except in the USA. Even in the USA, the series reported are usually of very small numbers. The reasons for this are difficult to explain except to say that carcinoma of the cervix has been decreasing in incidence as far as the more advanced stages are concerned. It is being detected at an earlier stage with a greater chance for cure without recurrence. It must be stated that in cases where pelvic exenteration is indicated, and these are highly selective ones, there is no other equally curative form of therapy that exists for the distressing problem of recurrent pelvic cancer. With the new stapling techniques and the use of clips along the pelvic wall to control bleeding from the blood vessels in this area, it is possible to perform a pelvic exenteration with much less blood loss and in considerably less time than previously. The improved methods of monitoring these patients with a Swan-Ganz catheter and a better understanding of the metabolic and physiologic process has reduced the mortality rate to less the 5%. Having given these patients a quantity of life, it is important to give them a quality of life. These patients should be rehabilitated and, if needed, a vagina should be reconstructed and the patient encouraged leading a normal life. Perhaps these patients cannot be described as happy, but at least given a second chance for life they can become well adjusted and make significant contributions to their family and the community [201].

Carcinoma of the cervix is most commonly treated with radiotherapy when the disease is locally advanced. Tumor bulk often limits the efficacy of this therapy, as does the tolerance of adjacent healthy tissue. The conventional treatment for carcinoma of the uterine cervix is a combination of external teletherapy and low dose-rate (LDR) intracavitary brachytherapy. Recently, however, there has been an increasing trend toward the use of high dose-rate (HDR) brachytherapy, in combination with external irradiation. The question is addressed of designing HDR treatments that will produce equivalent results to the more conventional protocols. It is argued that for the unique case of radiotherapeutic treatment of carcinoma of the cervix, the criterion for producing an equivalent treatment should be based on the matching of early, not late, effects. In essence, this is because the dose to the tissues at risk for late effects is usually significantly smaller than the prescribed dose. When this effect is factored in with the different shape of dose-response curves for early and late effects, it is concluded that, in the majority of cases, late effects will be no worse in a HDR regimen than a LDR regimen, if the corresponding doses have been matched to produce equal early effects [202]. HDR remote afterloading intracavitary brachytherapy has been widely used in the treatment of carcinoma of the cervix in Europe and Asia since the 1960s. Recently, there has been an increase of interest in the use of this technique in North America. Most of the non-randomized studies suggest similar survival, local control, and complication rates using fractionated HDR remote afterloading intracavitary brachytherapy combined with external beam irradiation compared to historical or concurrent LDR controls. However, the techniques as well as the dose fractionation schedules used in different institutions are variable [203]. HDR brachytherapy demonstrates certain advantages over historical LDR treatments. HDR intracavitary treatment improves radiation safety, lessens treatment times, allows for outpatient treatment regimens, and has improved packing and retraction techniques, which can decrease rectal and bladder doses. Although retrospective studies of HDR treatment show survival rates comparable with those of historical LDR intracavitary treatment, there have been few randomized, prospective studies to support the use of HDR techniques. LDR and HDR comparisons are further complicated by the lack of standardized fractionation schemes and dose prescriptions for HDR treatment. Recent data showing decreased local control in advanced cervical cancer with the prolonged overall treatment time of LDR treatment suggest the practical advantage of outpatient HDR intracavitary brachytherapy, which uses fractionated regimens and shortens overall treatment times. Although HDR treatment has not been shown to improve survival compared with LDR treatment, its practical advantages account for its increasing use [204].

Chemotherapy of cervical cancer is a difficult problem. The cancer is chemosensitive but the ability to express that chemosensitivity may be modified by previous radiotherapy and inadequate renal function. Regimens are available which will produce remissions with increase in survival in patients with advanced disease. Now, chemotherapy is used more frequently in the initial management of the patient prior to potentially curative surgery or radiotherapy in the hope of improving overall survival [205]. Cisplatin has emerged as the most active agent in the treatment of patients with advanced cervical cancer. Cisplatin's documented radiopotentiating effects have led to many studies of cisplatin-based regimens before or concurrent with definitive radiation therapy to the pelvis for advanced, previously untreated disease. Encouraging results have led to trials of this combined-modality approach that have irrevocably changed the management of patients with previously untreated, advanced cervical cancer [206]. However, cervical cancer is a relatively drug-resistant disease and prolonged cisplatin treatment appears to induce multiple mechanisms of tumor resistance. The majority of objective responses to cisplatin are partial and relatively short-lived and, therefore, have little impact on survival duration. Complete responses to cisplatin are seen predominantly in patients with extrapelvic metastases rather than pelvic recurrences [207].

The role of carboplatin in cervical cancers has been assessed through clinical trials. Results indicate some activity against these gynecologic tumors. Carboplatin has also been integrated into combination regimens with other active drugs. In the treatment of cervical cancer, it is used as part of combined-modality regimens prior to radiotherapy. Patients have shown better subjective tolerance to carboplatin than to cisplatin. This finding has facilitated the widespread implementation of carboplatin-based combinations [208]. As we have seen, cytotoxic chemotherapeutic agents have been used with concomitant radiotherapy. Extensive data are available on dose and schedule tolerance for cisplatin, 5-fluorouracil, and a number of combination regimens. Hydroxyurea, an S-phase-specific inhibitor of ribonucleotide reductase, lacks single-agent activity against metastatic, cervical SCC [209]. There is clearly a need for effective chemotherapy for early-stage, high-risk patients with carcinoma of the uterine cervix, and for those with advanced disease. Results to date have been disappointing. Cisplatin is active but overrated. Ifosfamide and dibromodulcitol are of interest, but unproven in this disease. Vinblastine and etoposide deserve further evaluation. New drug combinations require careful study, with the initial focus on women with little or no prior chemotherapy, and with adequate sample size. Patient selection needs to be precise with respect to prognostic factors for response and survival, so that results will be more reproducible. Trials of neoadjuvant chemotherapy in locally advanced disease should be randomized, non-randomized trials should be discouraged [210]. In fact, although radiation therapy and surgery form the basis for treatment of disease limited to the pelvis, those who have advanced disease or recurrences after locoregional therapy depend on systemic treatment for any hope of disease control. Currently, no combinations have been shown to be better than single agents are. No chemotherapy for advanced or recurrent carcinoma of the cervix is more effective than single-agent cisplatin. The major thrust of current and future investigation seeks to identify additional active agents and to develop combinations that offer greater patient benefit [211]. Based on the ability of numerous cytotoxic agents to induce regressions in advanced and recurrent cervical cancer, there is now a trend toward early use of these drugs. The efficacy of cisplatin-containing regimens, in particular, suggests that new strategies combining chemotherapy and surgery may result in improved survival rates in patients with high-risk cervical cancer. The administration of neoadjuvant chemotherapy to patients with local and locally advanced cervical cancer allows radical surgery to be performed in many patients who otherwise would be considered inoperable. In these patients, there also appears to be a decrease in the incidence of pelvic and distant recurrences and possibly an improvement in survival rates. Adjuvant chemotherapy after radical surgery for patients at high risk for recurrence appears to provide a survival advantage in some high-risk patients [212]. Drug therapy for cervical cancer is slowly undergoing evaluation in early disease stages, in which it is more likely to make an impact. Cisplatin has been the principal drug used in systemic therapy for all stages, with the possible exception of the radiosensitizer hydroxyurea. Nevertheless, current studies use cisplatin in this role as well. To a limited extent, substitution of carboplatin for cisplatin also has been explored. Conflicting interpretations of carboplatin trials nonetheless support continued study of this drug: its activity is reproducible and it can be combined with radiation therapy in practical dose schedules [213].

The recent surge of interest in the mechanisms of action of biomodulators, also known as biological response modifiers, offers a new avenue of approach in the treatment of cancer. The in vitro antitumor activities of these agents, such as IFN, when combined with chemo- or radiotherapy, have generated enthusiasm among clinicians for developing clinical trials. In recent years, many antineoplastic agents have been investigated as neoadjuvant or adjuvant therapy for patients with cervical cancer in an attempt to improve local control and to decrease incidence of metastasis. Normal tissue tolerance limits the potential combinations of standard cytotoxic chemotherapeutic agents with radiation [214].

The incidence of non-squamous carcinoma of the cervix, relative to SCC, seems to have been increasing over the past 40 years, and adenocarcinomas currently constitute 10% to 18% of cervical cancers. Uncertainties regarding the clinical behavior and management of women with non-SCC persist. Certain cell types and grade of adenocarcinomas play a role in prognosis and treatment selections. Treatment via irradiation or radical surgery for Stage I, small, garden-variety cervical adenocarcinomas will result in excellent survival. Conversely, survival may be poor in early stage non-squamous lesions if they are of high grade or of certain cell types, such as adenosquamous carcinoma. Patients with advanced cancers of other organ systems can now achieve an increase in progression-free interval with neoadjuvant chemotherapy or concomitant irradiation/chemotherapy. Such treatments might also benefit patients with non-SCC [215]. Although mortality from cervical cancer has decreased substantially the incidence of recurrent disease, at 35-50%, remains unaltered. Many more young patients are seen with recurrent cervical cancer today. Newer, more objective prognostic indicators based on molecular understanding of cancer cells are hopeful means through which patient selection and treatment could be improved in the future. In the developing world where persistent or recurrent disease is more common, the situation is unlikely to improve soon [216].

In conclusion, since the early 1940s, the incidence of cervical cancer has dramatically decreased due in large part to the work of Papanicolaou and Traut. Successful treatment can now be done using simple or radical surgical intervention for early invasive lesions and radiation therapy for more advanced lesions. However, despite current advances in screening and early treatment, local recurrences still happen and are difficult to treat. The natural history of cervical cancers is that of a slowly growing, locally invasive tumor. As such, it lends itself to radical surgical resection in selected patients prior to distant metastasis. Current advances in intraoperative and postoperative monitoring, as well as improved surgical techniques and devices, have decreased the morbidity and mortality of radical surgical procedures to acceptable levels [217]. Neither radiation nor surgery is clearly superior. The benefits of surgery include:

1) emotional satisfaction that the tumor has been removed;
2) accuracy of surgical staging;
3) preservation of the ovaries;

4) no secondary uterine cancer (a very uncommon problem); and

5) complications that are more readily correctable.

Radiation offers the major advantages of being useful in most patients regardless of age or medical condition and is the choice for large cancers. Stage IB cervical cancer is a very diverse pathological entity with a number of potential prognostic factors (including cell type, depth of invasion, tumor volume, lymphatic space involvement, and occult lymph node metastases), and because patients present with a number of other conditions (including excess weight, advanced age, prior pelvic surgery or infection, and severe medical illness). In general, the following have proven the most expedient treatments:

1) simple hysterectomy (class I), for microinvasive cancer of 3 mm invasion or less without lymphatic space involvement;

2) modified, extended hysterectomy (class II) and pelvic lymphadenectomy for lesions of 3 mm and lymph vascular space involvement or when the lesion seems to just exceed 3 mm and for very early adenocarcinoma;

3) radical hysterectomy (class III) and pelvic lymphadenectomy for larger IA2, IB, and IIA lesions that are < 4 cm, particularly for the pregnant or younger patient, and when ovarian conservation is desired;

4) radiation therapy is used for lesions over 4 cm and for women with severe medical illness making extended hysterectomy too hazardous; and

5) combination therapy and chemotherapy are now reserved for study in poor prognosis patients with very large lesions (> 6 cm), occult metastases, and unfavorable histologic criteria [218].

The advantages and risks of radical surgery, radiation therapy, and combined treatments bring to no clear conclusion being found. Advanced or recurrent cervical cancers may be treated with radiation, chemotherapy, or ultraradical surgery depending on the clinical setting. Early studies of combination therapies are given for these difficult situations [219]. It would appear that, stage-for-stage, the cure rate has not improved in the treatment of carcinoma of the cervix in the last six decades. However, the overall survival rate has improved, and this has been due to the number of cases that have been diagnosed at an earlier stage. It is obvious that new methods must be explored for the treatment of carcinoma of the cervix [220-222].

Follow-up

In inflammatory cytology without suspicion of cervical neoplasia, a pelvic examination is done in order to exclude a macroscopic visible tumor. After treatment of an inflammation, a repeat cytology and a colposcopy is performed preferably 8 to 12 weeks later. If the cytology or the colposcopy is abnormal, if the colposcopy is inconclusive, or if the inflammation is of viral origin, the patient is referred to colposcopy-directed biopsies and endocervical curettage like the patients with an initial cytology suspicious of cervical neoplasia. A histologically verified CIN 1 is treated as soon as it proves itself stable, that is if biopsies or endocervical curettage 3 to 6 months after the initial ones again show CIN 1. In very young women, treatment may be postponed another 3 to 6 months. Histologically verified CIN 2 and 3 are treated without postponement. In CIN 1 and 2, treatment by means of destruction is recommended if the neoplasia is located on the exocervix and the preoperative endocervical curettage is normal and if colposcopy can exclude microinvasion. A CIN 3 fulfilling the same criteria may be destructed too, preferably by the CO_2 laser, partly because of the well-defined and precise destruction especially with regard to the depth into the stroma and partly because the laser contrary to the cryoapparatus is very suitable of treating CIN involving large areas of the exocervix, including neoplasias extending into the vagina. In this connection, the combined excision and destruction by the laser should be mentioned, a treatment modality made accessible by the appearance of the laser [223]. The accuracy of cervicovaginal cytology following radiotherapy for cervical cancer is compromised by the anatomical and tissue changes resulting from irradiation. Collection of representative samples may be more difficult, and benign radiation changes, post-irradiation dysplasia, and the frequent occurrence of repair cells and active stromal cells in post-irradiation smears may cause diagnostic problems. Nevertheless, cytology is a valuable tool for the detection of locally recurrent cervical cancer. It is simple and economical to perform at the time of clinical follow-up examination, and may detect occult tumor recurrence. Awareness of the cellular changes resulting from irradiation, and the varied composition of post-irradiation smears may lead to a more accurate interpretation of the cytological findings [224-226].

Prognosis

Cancer of the uterine cervix accounts for 80-85% of all female genital tract malignancies in the developing countries and remains a major problem for oncologists in other parts of the world. A major concern regarding the disease is the lack of specific tumor markers for early detection, for accurate prediction of biological behavior, and for accurate assessment of prognosis. A new and exciting answer to this issue may now be available with the description of specific oncogenes and oncoproteins associated with this malignancy. On a clinical level, these genes and their products may allow us to improve our understanding of disease etiology, and provide a more precise diagnostic, prognostic, and therapeutic characterization of individual tumors. The possibilities of using altered expression of oncogenes and their products in neoplastic tissue as markers for the diagnosis and prognosis of cervical cancer support the view that detailed analysis of such gene expression has the potential to predict tumor behavior [227]. While advances in radiation therapy and surgical techniques have made the treatment of cervical carcinoma impressive, limitations to successful management remain. In fact, the 5-year survival rate, stage for stage, has not improved in the USA or world wide in the past 60 years. With an estimated half a million women developing this disease annually, this lack of improved survival poses an international unresolved health problem. Immune response has been shown to be a major factor involved in the course of the disease for this cancer. Immunologic monitoring was also shown to be of effective value in assessing the prognosis for cervical carcinoma [228]. It is believed that HPV are important etiological factors and their detection in precancerous lesions is a risk factor for malignant transformation. If these viruses seem to have a role in the initiation of cervical cancer, other factors may be necessary to the malignant transformation. Among those, certain proto-oncogenes (c-myc and c-Ha-ras) seem to be involved in the development and progression of cancer. Detection of gene alterations (mutation, deletion, and amplification) and gene overexpression in early invasive cancers could be useful to establish a more reliable prognosis. A better surveillance of these high-risk patients and a more appropriate treatment could then be selected [229].

Stage I cervical cancer encompasses a wide range of clinical disease from microscopic microinvasive tumors to bulky lesions measuring as much as 10 cm in diameter. Tumor volume and lymph node status are the most important predictors of recurrence and survival. Assessment of tumor volume using the parameters of clinical substage, depth of stromal invasion, and cervical diameter are currently used to determine primary therapy. Patients with positive lymph nodes are at high risk for recurrence and should be treated aggressively. Features that may be predictive of treatment failure in node-negative patients include nonsquamous histology, poor histologic differentiation, lymphatic space invasion, and altered host immune responses. Further investigation of stage I patients should focus on the determination of an optimal management approach for high-risk patients with lymph node involvement of bulky tumors, and identification of secondary prognostic features that can target low-risk patients who might benefit from adjuvant therapy [230]. Microinvasive cervix cancer (Stage IA) is the earliest stage of squamous carcinoma, and has a 98% 5-year survival. The important prognostic factors for treatment planning are depth of invasion, lateral extent of invasive tumor, and lymphvascular space invasion. Conservative management is appropriate in selected cases with the goal of preserving fertility [231]. The following factors can be clearly identified as independent risk factors for an increased incidence of recurrence and decreased survival in patients with early (Stages IB and IIA) cervical cancer:

1) nodal metastases:
   a) multiple nodes or node groups; and
   b) bilateral nodes or node groups;
2) size of tumor $\geq$ 4 cm; and
3) depth of invasion into the cervix $\geq$ 10 mm or invasion into the outer one-third of the cervix.

Risk factors which may be important but which are not clearly established as being independent of other factors are:

1) histological cell type;
2) histological grade;
3) lymphvascular invasion;
4) extension to the corpus uteri;
5) age of the patient at diagnosis; and
6) stage IIA.

It is thus clear that patients with nodal metastases, patients who have large primary tumors, and patients with deep invasion into the cervix should be identified for adjunctive therapy [232]. It seems useful to define subgroups of patients according to tumor characteristics, determined after surgical treatment and accurate histologic examination of the surgical specimen. Patients with one or more of these tumor features need additional treatment to improve survival. Data in the literature suggest that particularly patients with para-aortic or multiple pelvic lymph node metastasis (> 3) have already developed distant metastases at the time of primary treatment and therefore need adjuvant systemic therapy. Patients with tumors > 4 cm in diameter, differentiation grade III, lymph-blood vessel invasion, or cervical invasion (> 70%) seem to have high recurrence rates at both pelvic and distant sites, indicating that there is also a need for better pelvic control [233].

Some studies have suggested that the presence in tumors of nucleic acids from HPV constitutes a prognostic marker of disease severity in cervical cancer. There are two conflicting lines of evidence in this regard. First, the presence of HPV 18 is equated to rapid progression through early disease stages, possibly resulting in a more aggressive clinical course. Although fragmentary, in terms of the clinical and epidemiological basis, this line of evidence has some experimental support. Second, the absence of HPV from the tumor would confer a worse prognosis than if any viral types were present. Unlike the former, the latter line of evidence is not bolstered by experimental data but emerged from persuasive clinical studies, which had adequate sample sizes, used survival end points, and controlled for confounders. The absence of HPV in some tumors could indicate that they originated through different oncogenic mechanisms, perhaps resulting in different cell proliferation rates and, consequently, distinct clinical behavior. On the other hand, HPV detectability could simply be a correlate of other genuine prognostic characteristics, which would explain its association with survival. Both the nature and the mechanism of the prognostic role for HPV in cervical cancer remain to be elucidated. The paucity of studies can be attributed to the labor-intensive nature of assays for HPV. The advent of the PCR method has facilitated the conduct of retrospective studies of archival histopathology specimens and survival information [234-236].

Prevention

Since SCC of the cervix is preceded by a spectrum of easily detectable and treatable premalignant changes, it is very preventable [237]. As our understanding of genital precancers has evolved, it has become clear that HPV are intimately related to the spectrum of precancerous change. Traditional approaches to removing these lesions have centered on destruction of the neoplastic epithelium and careful cytological follow-up. This approach has met with success in preventing cancer, but has not addressed patients who present with invasive cancer whose precancer went undiscovered. With the realization that HPV is closely associated with precancers and invasive cancers of the female genital tract, efforts have centered on developing methodologies which would identify specific HPV types in high-risk women or in the general population that might reduce the number of missed carcinomas. This approach, although attractive, has met with problems due to the high prevalence rate of HPV infections in general in the population and the knowledge that certain cofactors, either environmental or host related, play a part in selecting a subset of women who will eventually develop cancer. The impact of HPV screening on detecting and preventing the rarer forms of aggressive cancer, such as adenosquamous carcinoma and small cell carcinomas, is yet unclear. The possibility that genital cancer may be prevented by a vaccine to HPV is supported by the identification of a host response to specific HPV products. Efforts have been made to characterize the early and late gene products associated with HPV infection, identify the specific epitopes commonly recognized by the host, and initiate studies to determine the spectrum of the population displaying an immune response to these infections [238].

Population screening by cervical cytology, if properly carried out, can substantially reduce mortality and morbidity due to cancer of the cervix. The technique of smear taking requires careful attention as well as maintenance of high standards in cytology screening laboratories. Patients with abnormal cytology are at high risk for cervical cancer and should be managed appropriately and followed-up indefinitely [239]. Currently, SIL is diagnosed by cytology, evaluated by colposcopy, and treated preferentially with cone biopsy. Prophylactic removal of the cervix does not eliminate the risk of cancer: it may shift the risk to the vaginal epithelium. The cervix has a role in sexual arousal and orgasm, probably due to stimulation of the Frankenhauser uterovaginal plexus. Bladder and bowel dysfunction following total hysterectomy may be related to loss of nerve ganglia closely associated with the cervix. Increased operative and postoperative morbidity, vaginal shortening, vault prolapse, abnormal cuff granulations, and oviductal prolapse are other disadvantages of total hysterectomy. The cervix is not a useless organ and should not be removed during hysterectomy without a proper indication [240]. Yet, supracervical hysterectomy, commonly performed in the earlier decades of this century, is rarely performed in contemporary practice. The desire to prevent future cervical cancer initially underlay the advocacy of total hysterectomy. Cervical cytologic screening and effective outpatient treatment of preinvasive cervical disease are commonly available. Cancer of the cervical stump is an uncommon and largely preventable occurrence. Removal of the normal cervix reportedly may have adverse effects on bladder, bowel, and sexual function. Reduced operating time and a shorter recovery period may be associated with a supracervical procedure. The risk of subsequent cervical cancer may not outweigh the benefits of supracervical hysterectomy, which should be offered as an option to selected patients. Supracervical hysterectomy by minilaparotomy is within the capability of practicing gynecologists and may be adaptable to outpatient short-stay surgery, offering a cost-effective alternative for a variety of gynecologic conditions [241-243].

Viruses are responsible for approximately 15% of human cancer worldwide. HPV and HBV/HCV are the recognized agents of cervical and liver cancer, respectively, which together constitute 80% of all virally induced cancers. If measures could be found to bring viral infection under control, a great proportion of human cancer would be greatly reduced. Vaccines have been developed against HPV. In principle, two different types of vaccine could be envisaged: prophylactic vaccines, that would elicit virus-neutralizing antibodies and would prevent infection, and therapeutic vaccines, that would induce regression of established lesions before progression to malignancy took place. The research on vaccines against HPV was hampered by the difficulties encountered in growing the virus in tissue culture and by the unacceptable nature of experimentation in humans. Effective vaccines, both natural and genetically engineered, have been developed against BPV and cottontail Rabbit Papillomavirus (RPV). The success obtained with the animal models supported the optimistic prediction that in the relatively near future vaccines would be available against the most problematic or potentially dangerous forms of papillomatosis in humans [244]. Vaccines that protect against HPV infection or induce tumor regression are beneficial in the treatment of recalcitrant warts and in preventing malignant progression. Successful prophylaxis and rejection of epidermal and alimentary canal tumors have been achieved in cattle with both conventional and genetically engineered vaccines. Successful vaccination in animals has important implications for the management of HPV-associated tumors in humans, particularly laryngeal papillomas and cervical carcinomas [245]. A prophylactic vaccine has been developed to induce neutralizing antibodies to HPV 16 and HPV 18 virions in genital secretions, and a therapeutic vaccine could be developed to elicit cytotoxic T-cell responses against early proteins in established lesions (CIN and cervical cancers) [246]. Although significant advances have been achieved, problems remain before the latter vaccines can be used routinely [247]. As we have seen, the technical problems of developing cheap, effective vaccines against HPV associated tumors have been formidable, but they were by no means insuperable. Experiments in cows with BPV-2 showed that both therapeutic and prophylactic vaccines worked to some extent and the immunogens used were by no means the best that could be envisaged. There are still both practical and ethical problems, as with any STD, but the main problem is one of support [248]. Development of a subunit vaccine against high-risk genital HPV was a desirable and, it appeared, an increasingly feasible long-term goal. The viral E6 and E7 oncoproteins were selectively maintained and expressed in progressed HPV tumors and have been targets for therapeutic vaccines. The L1 major virion structural proteins have recently been shown to self-assemble into virus-like particles (VLP) when expressed in insect cells [249]. The ability of the L1 major capsid protein of HPV to self-assemble into VLP that could, when inoculated systemically, induce high levels of neutralizing antibodies and protect animals against experimental viral challenge made L1 VLP an excellent candidate subunit vaccine. VLP have the limitation of inducing type-specific immunity [250]. In addition, the strongly immunogenic characteristics of VLP rose the possibility that they could also serve as vehicles for inducing therapeutic responses against HPV-induced neoplasia and other diseases [251]. However, these particles served as the basis for a prophylactic vaccine to prevent genital HPV infection. The design of such vaccines has evolved from an understanding of the nature of HPV infections and their consequences, together with evaluation of the efficacy of different approaches to vaccination in animal models. These studies have culminated in the production of several different vaccine preparations. The justification for the widespread implementation of prophylactic HPV vaccines depended on the outcome of larger scale studies of vaccine efficacy that took into account the epidemiology of HPV infections and associated disease. The usefulness of therapeutic HPV vaccines requires evidence that they can substantially augment or substitute for the effectiveness of currently available treatments [252]. Although the effectiveness of these vaccines cannot be evaluated in small studies, they constitute an important step toward the development of therapeutic uterine cervix cancer vaccines. A polytope DNA vaccination approach combined with immunomodulatory cytokines may offer an excellent strategy to reduce the risk of relapse and metastasis following conventional therapies [253].

In conclusion, because of several recent advances in molecular biology, the association between HPV infection and cervical cancer has been firmly established, and the oncogenic potential of certain HPV types has been clearly demonstrated. Several lines of evidence suggest the importance of the host's immune response, especially cellular immune response, in the pathogenesis of HPV-associated cervical lesions. These observations formed a compelling rationale for the development of vaccine therapy to combat HPV infection. Efforts to develop prophylactic vaccines against viruses that cause cancer have been a major research engagement. Vaccinology, the science of vaccines, engaged the sciences of immunology and of microbiology, both relying heavily on molecular biology. Successful development of vaccines relied on extensive knowledge of immunology and vaccinology.

Although HPV infections are not very immunogenic, there is evidence that the immune system controls the spread of virus and the development of diseases associated with such infections. Efforts to develop vaccines against cervical cancer caused by HPV have been focused on use of the structural antigens L1 and L2 of the virus and on the oncoproteins E6 and E7. Since the viral oncoproteins E6 and E7 are constitutively expressed within the tumor cells, they were considered as suitable targets for attack by T-lymphocytes. Several approaches to specifically trigger a cell-mediated immune response have been successful in experimental animals, leading to suppression of HPV-induced tumors. First clinical trials rose hopes that a similar effect could also be achieved by therapeutic vaccination of humans. Work on HPV vaccines has been brilliantly conceived and executed and some of vaccines are now in clinical utilization [254, 255]. Both prophylactic and therapeutic HPV vaccine strategies have been developed. Prophylactic strategies focus on the induction of effective humoral immune responses against subsequent HPV infection. In this respect, impressive immunoprophylactic effects have been demonstrated in animals using VLP. VLP are antigenic and protective, but are devoid of any viral DNA that may be carcinogenic to the host. For treatment of existing HPV infection, techniques to improve cellular immunity by enhancing viral antigen recognition have been studied. For this purpose, the oncogenic proteins E6 and E7 of HPV 16 and 18 are the focus of current clinical trials for cervical cancer patients. The development of successful HPV-specific vaccines offers an attractive alternative to existing screening and treatment programs for cervical cancer [256-258].

Health Policy Issues

Screening programs for cervical cancer have been credited with reducing the incidence of and mortality from cervical cancer. The main components of these screening programs are:

1) their level of organization;
2) the age at which women begin screening;
3) the age at which women discontinue screening;
4) the interval between repeat screens;
5) the frequency at which the programs provide screening; and
6) the response to an abnormal screening test.

However, not all screening programs are equally efficient and differences in program components can result in big differences in their cost-effectiveness. Studies that employ cost-effectiveness analysis to examine the efficiency of different program components can inform the development of cost-effective programs. Cost-effectiveness studies of cervical cancer screening consistently find that certain types of programs are more cost-effective than others. Programs that are centrally organized and implemented by the public sector are reported to be more cost-effective than those that use public funds for screening at other medical visits (convenience screening), or those that provide guidelines for healthcare professionals and the public to promote spontaneous discretionary screening. There is also substantial agreement about the cost-effectiveness of other program components. When multiple screenings are possible, studies report that they should generally begin at age 25 to 35 years and end at age 65 to 70 years, although it is important that older women have three normal Pap smears before the discontinuation of screening. The interval for repeat screens that is reported to provide the best balance between cost and life-years saved is between 3 and 5 years. However, when a choice must be made between screening more women fewer times, or screening fewer women more times, most studies indicate that it is more cost-effective to prioritize resources to obtain at least one screening for each woman. The screening of previously unscreened and high-risk populations has been shown to be especially cost-effective. Despite this agreement, many studies report that models of the cost-effectiveness of screening for cervical cancer are sensitive to a number of parameters. Changes in the attendance rate of the program, the quality of the Pap smear, and the cost of the Pap smear can markedly change the cost-effectiveness of a screening program [259].

There is essentially no debate about the benefits of cervical cancer screening. The current debate centers around periodicity, the appropriate interval for repeated testing, and the age at which screening should be discontinued. As the frequency of screening is increased within a defined population, there is a gain in survival (life-years) depending upon the risk status of the population segment screened. However, each increment in survival comes at an increasingly high cost. Significant gains have been made in improving screening and detection services through widespread availability of the Pap test. However, there has been concern raised that the cost-effectiveness of cervical cancer screening has not been clearly demonstrated. A relatively small group of studies was located which directly addressed the cost-effectiveness question. All of the studies attempted in some manner to describe the relationship between benefits of cervical cancer screening and costs. Two studies reported a program design with net positive monetary benefits, while one estimated that the direct cost of medical care avoided through screening was approximately equal to the cost of the screening program. In general, however, screening for cervical cancer is viewed as an investment in extending life (a net cost per year of life gained). Most analysts ascribe a net monetary cost to cervical cancer screening programs. Then, the question becomes one of cost-effectiveness, designing a program so as to optimize the result obtained. With respect to optimizing screening, the literature leaves no doubt of the value of cervical cancer screening in general. From a cost-effectiveness perspective, screening no more frequently than every 3-5 years appears reasonable. It is important to think in terms of a total program and how effectively the population at risk is being reached. The literature spans a period of more than 40 years and reflects studies across the globe. While the quality is uneven, from this body of work a consensus emerges: screening is effective, but the frequency of screening in the USA is probably too high. In addition, those who are most intensively screened are probably at the lowest risk. Outreach and targeting of at-risk population groups needs to be addressed in order to improve cost-effectiveness of cervical cancer screening. The effectiveness of the screening technology (Pap test) is taken for granted, but this may be a mistake [260]. The mathematic models used to assess the benefits and cost-effectiveness of cervical screening reveal little consistency in the definition of disease status, the basic assumptions made, or the data used in the model. Conclusions derived from the models often are model and data dependent. Several authors have used simplified models and unrealistic assumptions, such as the failure to differentiate between different grades of dysplasia or 100% sensitivity for the screening test. The Markov process assumes that the rate of transfer between states is independent of the duration of time spent in one state, and this assumption may be unsound. The difficulty with all models is in interpreting the appropriateness of the parameter values. Some are well documented, for example, stage-specific survival rates for treated patients or attendance for screening. Many, however, cannot be given a fixed value. The large number of factors that appear implicated in the incidence of and mortality from cervical cancer can lead to many feasible sets of parameter values that generate output that approaches the observed data [261].

Consideration of cost-effectiveness has guided public and insurers' decisions about preventive services for almost 20 years. Legislative decisions on coverage of specific cancer screening tests under Medicare and Medicaid have traditionally followed studies of their cost-effectiveness. Cost-effectiveness analysis is a stylized form of investment analysis, where the returns on the investment are measured in improvements in health rather than in dollars and consider society as a whole as the relevant investor. Cost-effectiveness studies of screening for two common cancers, cervical and colorectal, illustrate the strengths and weaknesses of cost-effectiveness analysis. Dependence on models of the disease process, which may be sketchy, and uncertainty about costs and benefits of screening are inherent in the methodology. Although economic evaluations of both cervical and colorectal cancer screening have found them to be relatively cost-effective compared with doing nothing, such studies have not resolved the uncertainty about the best screening strategy for either disease. With cervical cancer, evidence about the relationship between HPV and high-grade neoplasia suggests the need for new models of the disease process that can support additional cost-effectiveness analyses. Despite uncertainty and contradictions in existing studies of screening, investment models force clinicians and decision-makers to consider all important consequences for health care costs and outcomes [262]. To determine the potential effects on costs and outcomes of changes in sensitivity and specificity with new screening methods for cervical cancer, using a Markov model of the natural history of cervical cancer, estimates of conventional Pap test sensitivity of 51% and specificity of 97% were obtained from a meta-analysis. The effect of reducing false negative rates has been estimated from 40-90% and increasing false positive rates by up to 20%, independently and jointly. When specificity was held constant, increasing sensitivity of the Pap test increased life expectancy and costs. When sensitivity was held constant, decreasing specificity of the Pap test increased costs, an effect that was more dramatic at intervals that are more frequent. Decreased specificity had a substantial effect on cost-effectiveness estimates of improved Pap test sensitivity. Most of those effects are related to the cost of evaluation and treatment of low-grade lesions. Policies or technologies that increased sensitivity of cervical cytologic screening increased overall costs, even if the cost of the technology was identical to that of conventional Pap smears. These effects appear to be caused by relatively high prevalence of low-grade lesions and are magnified at frequent screening intervals. Efficient cervical cancer screening requires methods with greater ability to detect lesions that are most likely to become cancerous [263].

In conclusion, cost-effectiveness analyses are an important source of information for the design and evaluation of policies to reduce cervical cancer. The recommendations of a panel on cost-effectiveness studies convened as part of the International Consensus Conference on the Fight Against Cervical Cancer (FACC) include:

1) the use of reference case methods to support comparisons across studies;
2) the use of a consistent standard of evidence on the clinical effectiveness of different screening strategies;
3) further research into the cost-effectiveness of different screening and treatment strategies for cervical cancer;

4)　further research into screening and treatment strategies in a wide range of countries;
5)　easily accessible and detailed descriptions of the methods and supplementary analyses underlying published studies;
6)　greater use of newly developed models of cervical cancer; and
7)　greater revelation of potential conflict of interest by researchers [264-266].

Psychological Issues

Current research evidence convincingly links the presence of HPV to the development of cervical cancer, suggesting that bringing together knowledge from the Pap smear screening and HPV infection research may help formulate a new approach that bridges primary and secondary prevention strategies. Bringing together, these two areas of research involve an understanding of the psychosocial factors that underlie both [267]. It is argued that the etiological model employed for cervical cancer takes little account of psychological and psychophysiological factors. Both of these factors are now thought to play important roles in disease processes. A new etiological model for cervical cancer incorporates existing epidemiological and medical formulations into a new multifactor framework. It is suggested that psychological interventions could play a much greater role than they had in the past [268]. However, significant progress has been made in understanding the psychologic and behavioral aspects of cervical cancer. Descriptive data indicate acute trauma and disruption with the diagnosis and treatment, yet the majority of women return to precancer life. The notable exception to this is sexual functioning, which remains an area of significant morbidity. Future research will need to test variables that predict which women will be vulnerable to sexual dysfunction. Sexual self-concept (sexual self-schema), which is the extent to which a woman has a positive view of her own sexuality, appears to provide valuable information. The identification of such variables is an important step toward designing interventions for enhancing quality of life for patients with cervical cancer [269].

The long, tedious search for the causes of and cure for cancer has not resulted in one astounding breakthrough discovery. Instead, researchers have slowly and painstakingly made small inroads into the understanding of the way cell growth goes awry and becomes malignant, destroying tissues and, if unchecked, spreading to other organs of the body and eventually causing death. One of those inroads is the discovery that a cancer of the uterine cervix is almost certainly caused by a virus transmitted through sexual contact. A slowly progressive preinvasive lesion, dysplasia, which can be detected by a screening test, the Pap smear, and effectively treated with organ-preserving local therapy, usually precedes cancer of the cervix. Because dysplasia and early invasive cancer usually develop in young women, the need for conservative management is of utmost importance to preserve a woman's ability to have children. The social and psychological impacts of a cancer occurring in young women are enormous and are further magnified by the fact that this cancer may be caused by a sexually transmitted virus. Sexual practice patterns, number of sexual partners, smoking, and other behavioral aspects contribute to the complexity of this disease. However, early detection of preinvasive and invasive cancer is possible with fairly simple and inexpensive means, and curative therapy is available. The disastrous impact of cervical cancer theoretically could be contained if patients at risk regularly participate in early detection programs. In addition, the disease could largely be prevented altogether through healthful behavior and sexual practices.

The social challenge is to provide this information to the public in a nonthreatening, nonmoralistic fashion. We especially need to help young people to accept that sex within a caring, responsible relationship is a healthy human response and, at the same time, understand that there are dangers associated with transmittable diseases that can have profound effects on their ability to have children and on their lives [270]. The UK cervical screening program has been successful in securing participation of a high proportion of targeted women, and has seen a fall in mortality rates of those suffering from cervical cancer. There remains, however, a significant proportion of unscreened women and, of women in whom an abnormality is detected, many will not attend for colposcopy. Reasons for non-participation in the screening program include administrative failures, unavailability of a female screener, inconvenient clinic times, lack of awareness of the test's indications and benefits, considering oneself not to be at risk of developing cervical cancer, and fear of embarrassment, pain, or the detection of cancer. The receipt of an abnormal result and referral for colposcopy cause high levels of distress owing to limited understanding of the meaning of the smear test: many women believe the test aims to detect existing cervical cancer. The quality of the cervical screening service can be enhanced by the provision of additional information, by improved quality of communication, and by consideration of women's health beliefs. This may result in increased participation in and satisfaction with the service [271]. Combining the data from the studies suggests default rates of 3%, 11%, and 12% for assessment/treatment visits, first review, and second review, respectively. The intervention studies suggested a need to tailor the intervention to the population and the type of information to suit the individual. Varying definitions make comparison of default rates difficult, and the use of a crude non-attendance rate may result in an overestimate of default rates. The vast majority of women invited to colposcopy eventually attend. It is questionable if there is a need for interventions to increase compliance. Where necessary, greater cooperation across the primary/secondary care interface and use of the extended primary care team may be a more cost-effective means of increasing compliance [272]. Psychosocial associations have been observed with level of cervical dysplasia or "pre-cancer" and invasive cervical cancer (related to HPV infection). Psychoneuroimmunological relationships have been observed in HIV-1 infection, which is being described in an increasing number of women. Relationships of psychosocial factors and level of cervical dysplasia were similarly observed with reference to immunological and health status in asymptomatic and early symptomatic HIV-1 infected homosexual men, suggesting that a potentiating effect may occur in HIV-1 and HPV co-infected women. Consistency of relationships across studies appeared to be enhanced by the use of a biopsychosocial model integrating the effects of life stressors, social support, and coping style as well as psychiatric disorders. Research is indicated on the relationships between psychosocial factors, immunological status, and clinical health status in this group of women. Because of the high prevalence of psychosocial risk factors for chronic psychological distress in these women and the known immunological and health status decrements occurring with progression of these two infections, a clinical screening program based on the biopsychosocial model is recommended as a means of secondary prevention. If effective in generating treatment referrals, such a program would likely improve quality of life and could aid in the determination of relationships with immunological and health status as well [273-275].

Counseling

The success of screening programs for cervical cancer partly depends on women's acceptance and take-up of the service. Uptake of preventive health care programs appears to be related to people's underlying motivations and attitudes, not only towards the disease in question, but towards health and illness generally. The perceived costs to the individual of embarking on particular courses of action also have to be taken into consideration. These attitudes and motivations vary between social groups. Unless the reasons for non-participation in preventive health care and screening programs is understood, programs will be misdirected and inappropriately designed. However, the failure of any one theory to account for most of the variance in health behavior between social groups emphasizes the importance of health education and provision of information about health and prevention on a personal basis. General practitioners and practice-based nurses are in a good position to be able to elicit the fears, prejudices, and priorities of patients in this area, and thus provide more effective health education and information about preventive and screening services [276-278].

Medico-Legal Issues

Public expectation for the eradication of death from carcinoma of the cervix has not been realized. It is imperative to educate the public as to the value and limitations of screening for cervical cancer by the Pap smear and to develop reasonable practitioner standards for the performance of the test. The current climate of increasing litigation over alleged false negative Pap smears has the potential to reduce the use and availability of this test which is still considered the most effective cancer screening test devised [279]. The cervical cancer-screening program has an emerging litigation problem. Some recent initiatives taken to address the problem include the establishment of registries of women being screened, education to promote an appreciation of the limitations of screening, and the introduction of outcome standards for laboratories reporting cervical cytology. An international evidence-based definition of the standard of care is the most pressing need in the immediate future [280]. Malpractice claims against pathologists for misdiagnosis have been sharply rising, especially in the areas of breast FNA and cervical (Pap) smears. Communication is one of the best medical malpractice prevention tools. In the areas of brest FNA and cervical smears, dissemination of diagnostic error rates in the cytology report is recommended. This would help safeguard against malpractice liability being imposed without showing a deviation by the cytopathologist from reasonable practice standards [281]. Cytologists need to critically evaluate their practices and practice settings to ensure that what they do and how they document what they do will withstand both regulatory and legal scrutiny. Any individual involved in cytology as a laboratory owner, operator, director, supervisor, technical or staff employee, independent agent, or customer representative is a potential target of cytology malpractice litigation. All of these individuals must participate in the risk management process. For the laboratory as a corporate entity, business and technical practices, including quality control and quality assurance procedures, must be contemporary, legitimate, and justifiable. Sound scientific evidence and well-subscribed standards of practice supporting an individual's or laboratory's conduct are the best defenses to malpractice claims. For the near future, litigation will continue to focus on false negative Pap smears on a case-by-case basis. Laboratories and individuals can reduce the risk of malpractice liability by directing their attention to proactive quality control and quality assurance methods. Nevertheless, in the final analysis, consumer education about the benefits and limitations of the Pap test is key to limiting malpractice claims [282]. The Clinical Laboratory Improvement Amendments (CLIA) of 1988 requires a 5-year retrospective review of negative or normal smears in patients with diagnoses of H-SIL or cancer, and amended reports are required when discrepancies that would affect current patient care are found. Notwithstanding the requirements of the CLIA, one laboratory has been required by a State HHS to issue amended reports even when the discrepancy did not affect current patient care. The implications of notifying the patient and her physician of any discrepancy in a Pap smear may lead to media attention and litigation. Amended reports and/or correspondence to patients and physicians can be utilized to generate media attention and litigation [283]. General definitions of quality assurance and quality control (QA/C) have existed in many forms for decades, and a new discipline guides their application to diverse industrial and recently medical processes without much fanfare. However, in the field of cervical cytology screening, the range of QA/C options has recently broadened and become controversial. With the advent of new systems of terminology, larger-scale laboratories and new technologies, plus strong governmental and legal pressures in some nations, the range of extremely difficult and sometimes expensive QA/C choices our community faces is greater than ever. The basic definitions of QA/C posed little difficulty. Presentation of the range of methods in use today and of those based on new technologies where use is proposed or has just begun also was achieved with little or no dispute. However, there was lack of consensus on exactly how QA/C methods are to be assessed. Indeed, there was little consistency in the use of different outcome measures with which we can judge success or failure of specific QA/C options. In addition, the tension between pressure to adopt sometimes uncertain or expensive method enhancements and pressure to maintain affordability and the widest possible access for populations that most need cervical cytology screening is greater than ever. More data are required that would enable assessment of QA/C options with the clearest possible understanding of cost/benefits and current or new assumptions of risk. Other task forces, such as medico-legal, cost/benefit, and those devoted to new technologies, are our essential partners in meeting the challenges described above [284].

In conclusion, increasing litigation over alleged false negative cervical cytologic smears threatens the viability of this test for cervical cancer detection. The problem appears to be largely American but is beginning to appear in some other countries. In the vast majority of cases, there is either a settlement or a jury verdict for the plaintiff based largely on the testimony of expert witnesses. Cases are judged on an individual basis without significant consideration of the general performance of the cervical cytologic smear in laboratories operating in compliance with a wide array of laboratory regulations and with documented and comprehensive quality control practices in place. It is acknowledged that there are problem laboratories and cytology practitioners. There is an emerging issue of automated preparation and screening devices and issues of informed patient consent. Cytology professionals have done an extraordinary and commendable job of educating the public about the benefits of the cervical cytologic smear. We have been less successful and conscientious about explaining and defining the limitations of the cervical cytologic test. There is a need for public and professional education as to the benefits and limitations of the cervical cytologic smear for cervical cancer detection. The process suggested is to work with women's groups, public health agencies, government agencies, and state and national legislatures and to coordinate professional committees working on liability issues. Contextual information could be included with the cervical cytologic smear report to indicate that a negative report confers a low probability of developing cervical cancer. It is suggested that appropriate language and a menu of statements be developed. Increased efforts should be directed to physician education with respect to informed consent concerning the benefits and limitations of cervical cytologic smear testing and the application of new technology to improve smear accuracy. The process should include development of appropriate statements on the use of alternative technology. The profession should develop "process guidelines" for review of cervical cytologic smears in the context of possible litigation, including standardized methods for blind slide review of smears that reduce or eliminate context and outcome bias. It is suggested that review panels be anonymous, that the process be standardized and that there be limitations on liability for participating organizations. Professional cytopathology and pathology societies should formulate acceptable guidelines for expert witnesses. The standards should be applicable to both defendant and plaintiff experts. All materials to the practical extent, including consultant opinions, should be available for peer review. Professional cytopathology and pathology societies should monitor expert testimony for objectivity and scientific accuracy. For the near future, litigation will continue to focus on false negative cervical cytologic smears on a case-by-case basis. Laboratories and individuals can reduce the risk of malpractice liability by directing their attention to proactive quality control and quality assurance methods. In the final analysis, consumer education about the benefits and limitations of the test is key to limiting malpractice claims. To stem the tide of continued medico-legal challenges to the integrity of cytology practice, the cytology community has now focused its efforts on developing and utilizing standards that convey to patients, attorneys, and cytologists the contemporary status of and reasonable expectations for the practice of cytology. Guidelines such as those for uniform reporting terminology and clinical management of cervical abnormalities form the basis of cytology practice standards on which legal standards of practice can be based [285-287].

Conclusion

The identification of the close association of certain types of HPV with the development of cervical cancer should lead to an extensive revision of appropriate health policies. Having taken into account the drawbacks inherent in the existing data (stemming from the use of varying nomenclature, diagnostic methods and reliability, registration, and screening practices) it is possible to conclude that the incidence of HPV infections, all premalignant and malignant stages of cervical cancer are, or will soon be, increasing in several countries. This rate of increase is fastest for the younger age groups and is despite the introduction of various forms of screening. These trends therefore indicate an urgent need to adopt policies to avert an unnecessary increase in fatalities due to cervical cancer. It is therefore recommended to:

1) establish a routine diagnostic method which can identify either the type of HPV present or the lesions which are progressing;

2) determine the incidence of HPV infections in the general population;
3) disseminate to medical personnel, teachers, and other members of society existing knowledge concerning the dangers associated with this virus and relevant to preventing its further spread;
4) introduce an effective population screening campaign for all sexually active women, preferably involving a yearly examination at a colposcopy clinic; and
5) intensify basic and applied HPV research, especially that which leads to a deeper understanding of viral transmission and infection, identification of cofactors which promote cervical lesion progression, or to the production of vaccines [288].

During the last decades, much has been learned about the biology of HPV and many progresses have been made in the development of rational and effective patient management strategies. With stronger evidence supporting a causal role for HPV in the development of genital tract and anal cancers, and without the availability of effective therapies, it is recommended widespread screening for detection of HPV DNA or ribonucleic acid (RNA) with the molecular hybridization tests available commercially. Pap smear screening for detection of early precancerous changes of the cervix and referral for colposcopy and biopsy of areas of epithelium that are suspicious for intraepithelial neoplasia of the cervix, vagina, vulva, penis, or anus remain the cornerstones of genital tract and anal cancer prevention. The patient care implications of subclinical persistent HPV infection of the genital tract are not well understood. For this reason, and because none of the available therapies are curative, treatment of large areas of normal-appearing genital tract epithelium cannot be recommended at this time. It is hoped that, with the growing research focus on therapies that have the potential for virologic cure, someday effective treatment for subclinical infection will be available. Until that time, patients with recalcitrant or recurring genital warts may benefit most by the sequential application of different treatment modalities [289]. Screening for cervical cancer and its precursors has traditionally been performed by Pap smear. As cost considerations have become more important and as developing countries have begun to initiate screening programs, other approaches to screening have been considered. Cervical cancer screening using unaided or aided visual approaches, HPV DNA testing and typing, cervical photography, and automated Pap smear screening instruments are all potentially valuable when used alone or in combination, depending on the country. New techniques will make it possible to screen high-risk and low-income populations for cervical cancer and its precursors and to do so more cost-effectively than is possible using conventional Western approaches. In addition, the latest technology can enhance the screening methods traditionally used in industrialized countries and can increase the positive and negative predictive value of the screening method [290]. Adjunctive diagnostic procedures for the detection of HPV infection could increase the sensitivity of primary and secondary screening of cervical cancer. HPV testing could also improve the specificity of screening programs resulting in avoidance of overtreatment and saving of costs for confirmatory procedures. Progression of HPV infection is associated with the persistence of HPV infection, involvement of high-risk HPV types, high HPV viral load in specimens, integration of viral DNA, and possibly the presence of cofactors. The design of HPV diagnostic tests will need to take into account these parameters of disease progression. HPV DNA detection techniques based on signal-amplification are standardized, commercially available, and detect several high-risk HPV types. They increase the sensitivity of screening for high-grade and low-grade lesions.

Although they may yield false negative results in the presence of significant HPV-related disease, new test formats could resolve this weakness. Amplification techniques are ideal instruments for epidemiologic purposes, since they minimize misclassification of HPV infection status and allow for the detection of low-viral burden infections [291].

Based on rigorous interpretation of current evidence, systemic therapy has two roles in the management of carcinoma of the uterine cervix. In patients with advanced or recurrent disease, single-agent chemotherapy constitutes the treatment of choice. The most extensively studied agents are the platinum compounds. Either cisplatin or carboplatin represent a reasonable choice for first-line treatment. There appears to be no significant influence of either dose or schedule on patient benefit. Other agents with clear-cut activity include ifosfamide, dibromodulcitol, and doxorubicin. In patients with locoregionally advanced disease (stages IIIB or IVA), radiation plus either hydroxyurea or a combination of cisplatin plus 5-fluorouracil offers an advantage over radiation alone in terms of progression-free interval and survival. In patients with more limited disease, there is no defined role for systemic therapy now. Three goals constitute the focus for current investigational efforts:

1) continued efforts to identify additional highly active drugs are needed;
2) the development of effective combination chemotherapy depends on the use of logically designed combinations of active drugs in well-designed trials with single-agent therapy as the control; and
3) trials seeking more effective combinations of systemic therapy with surgery and/or radiotherapy should continue for not only locoregionally advanced disease but also for more limited carcinoma of the cervix [292-295].

References

[1]   Brenner, DE. Carcinoma of the cervix – A review. *Am. J. Med. Sci.* 1982; 284: 31-48.
[2]   Marcial, VA. Carcinoma of the cervix: present status and future. *Cancer* 1977: 39: 945-958.
[3]   Singh, P. Cervical cancer: aetiology, earlier diagnosis and treatment. *Ann. Acad. Med. Singapore* 1990; 19: 255-263.
[4]   Richart, RM; Wright, TC Jr. Pathology of the cervix. *Curr. Opin. Obstet. Gynecol.* 1991; 3: 561-567.
[5]   Boronow, RC. Advances in diagnosis, staging, and management of cervical and endometrial cancer, stages I and II. *Cancer* 1990;65: 648-659.
[6]   Lizano, M; Berumen, J; García-Carrancá, A. HPV-related carcinogenesis: basic concepts, viral types and variants. *Arch. Med. Res.* 2009: 40: 428-434.
[7]   zur Hausen, H. Papillomaviruses causing cancer: evasion from host-cell control in early events in carcinogenesis. *J. Natl. Cancer Inst.* 2000;92: 690-698.
[8]   zur Hausen, H. Papillomaviruses and cancer: from basic studies to clinical application. *Nat. Rev. Cancer* 2002; 2: 342-350.
[9]   Erickson, BK; Alvarez, RD; Huh, WK. Human papillomavirus: what every provider should know. *Am. J. Obstet. Gynecol.* 2013; 208: 169-175.

[10] Piver, MS. Invasive cervical cancer in the 1990s. Semin Surg Oncol 1990; 6: 359-363.

[11] Himmelstein, LR. Evaluation of inflammatory atypia. A literature review. *J. Reprod. Med.* 1989; 34: 634-637.

[12] Adelusi, B. Carcinoma of the cervix: can a viral etiology be confirmed? *IARC Sci. Publ.* 1984; 63: 433-450.

[13] Syrjänen, KJ; Syrjänen, SM. Human papilloma virus (HPV) infections related to cervical intraepithelial neoplasia (CIN) and squamous cell carcinoma of the uterine cervix. *Ann. Clin. Res.* 1985; 17: 45-56.

[14] Syrjänen, KJ. Human papilloma virus (HPV) infections of the female genital tract and their association with intraepithelial neoplasia and squamous cell carcinoma. *Pathol. Annu.* 1986; 21 Pt 1: 53-89.

[15] Moscicki, AB. Human papillomavirus infections. *Adv. Pediatr.,* 1992; 39: 257-281.

[16] Williams, C. Ovarian and cervical cancer. *BMJ* 1992; 304: 1501-1504.

[17] zur Hausen, H. Papillomaviruses – To vaccination and beyond. *Biochemistry* (Mosc) 2008; 73: 498-503.

[18] Oaknin, A; Díaz de Corcuera, I; Rodríguez-Freixinós, V; Rivera, F; del Campo, JM; SEOM (Spanish Society of Clinical Oncology). SEOM guidelines for cervical cancer. *Clin. Transl. Oncol.* 2012; 14: 516-519.

[19] Beral, V; Hermon, C; Muñoz, N; Devesa, SS. Cervical cancer. *Cancer Surv.* 1994; 19-20: 265-285.

[20] Brinton, LA; Fraumeni, JF Jr. Epidemiology of uterine cervical cancer. *J. Chronic Dis.* 1986; 39: 1051-1065.

[21] Hulka, BS. Risk factors for cervical cancer. *J. Chronic Dis.* 1982; 35: 3-11.

[22] Reid, BL. The causation of cervical cancer. Part I: A general review. *Clin. Obstet. Gynaecol.* 1985; 12: 1-18.

[23] Chou, P. Review on risk factors of cervical cancer. *Zhonghua Yi Xue Za Zhi* (Taipei) 1991; 48: 81-88.

[24] zur Hausen, H. Viruses in human cancers. *Science* 1991; 254: 1167-1173.

[25] Josey, WE; Nahmias, AJ; Naib, ZM. Viruses and cancer of the lower genital tract. *Cancer* 1976; 38: 526-533.

[26] Maitland, NJ. The aetiological relationship between herpes simplex virus type 2 and carcinoma of the cervix: an unanswered or unanswerable question? *Cancer Surv.* 1988; 7: 457-467.

[27] Stevenson, K; Macnab, JC. Cervical carcinoma and human cytomegalovirus. *Biomed. Pharmacother.* 1989; 43: 173-176.

[28] Reid, R. Genital warts and cervical cancer. II. Is human papillomavirus infection the trigger to cervical carcinogenesis? *Gynecol. Oncol.* 1983; 15: 239-252.

[29] Okagaki, T. Female genital tumors associated with human papillomavirus infection, and the concept of genital neoplasm-papilloma syndrome (GENPS). *Pathol. Annu.* 1984; 19 Pt 2: 31-62.

[30] Syrjänen, KJ. Human papillomavirus (HPV) infections and their associations with squamous cell neoplasia. *Arch. Geschwulstforsch.* 1987; 57: 417-444.

[31] Syrjänen, KJ. Biology of human papillomavirus (HPV) infections and their role in squamous cell carcinogenesis. *Med. Biol.* 1987; 65: 21-39.

[32] Muñoz, N; Bosch, X; Kaldor, JM. Does human papillomavirus cause cervical cancer? The state of the epidemiological evidence. *Br. J. Cancer* 1988; 57: 1-5.

[33] Koutsky, LA; Galloway, DA; Holmes, KK. Epidemiology of genital human papillomavirus infection. *Epidemiol. Rev.* 1988; 10: 122-163.

[34] McCance, DJ. Human papillomavirus (HPV) infections in the aetiology of cervical cancer. *Cancer Surv.* 1988: 7: 499-506.

[35] Muñoz, N; Bosch, FX. HPV and cervical neoplasia: review of case-control and cohort studies. *IARC Sci. Publ.* 1992; 119: 251-261.

[36] Vousden, KH. Human papillomaviruses and cervical carcinoma. *Cancer Cells* 1989; 1: 43-50.

[37] Franco, EL. Viral etiology of cervical cancer: a critique of the evidence. *Rev. Infect. Dis.* 1991; 13: 1195-1206.

[38] Franco, EL. Measurement errors in epidemiological studies of human papillomavirus and cervical cancer. *IARC Sci. Publ.* 1992; 119: 181-197.

[39] Wright, TC Jr; Richart, RM. Role of human papillomavirus in the pathogenesis of genital tract warts and cancer. *Gynecol. Oncol.* 1990; 37: 151-164.

[40] Lacey, CJ. Assessment of exposure to sexually transmitted agents other than human papillomavirus. *IARC Sci. Publ.* 1992; 119: 93-105.

[41] Reeves, WC; Rawls, WE; Brinton, LA. Epidemiology of genital papillomaviruses and cervical cancer. *Rev. Infect. Dis.* 1989; 11: 426-439.

[42] zur Hausen, H. The role of papillomaviruses in anogenital cancer. *Scand. J. Infect. Dis. Suppl.* 1990; 69: 107-111.

[43] Brinton, LA. Epidemiology of cervical cancer – Overview. *IARC Sci. Publ.* 1992; 119: 3-23.

[44] Schneider, A. Pathogenesis of genital HPV infection. *Genitourin. Med.* 1993; 69: 165-173.

[45] Castellsagué, X; Díaz, M; de Sanjosé, S; Muñoz, N; Herrero, R; Franceschi, S; Peeling, RW; Ashley, R; Smith, JS; Snijders, PJ; Meijer, CJ; Bosch, FX; International Agency for Research on Cancer Multicenter Cervical Cancer Study Group. Worldwide human papillomavirus etiology of cervical adenocarcinoma and its cofactors: implications for screening and prevention. *J. Natl. Cancer Inst.* 2006; 98: 303-315.

[46] Ciesielska, U; Nowińska, K; Podhorska-Okołów, M; Dziegiel, P. The role of human papillomavirus in the malignant transformation of cervix epithelial cells and the importance of vaccination against this virus. *Adv. Clin. Exp. Med.* 2012; 21: 235-244.

[47] Mandelblatt, J; Schechter, C; Fahs, M; Muller, C. Clinical implications of screening for cervical cancer under Medicare. The natural history of cervical cancer in the elderly: what do we know? What do we need to know? *Am. J. Obstet. Gynecol.* 1991; 164: 644-651.

[48] Lancaster, WD; Jenson, AB. Natural history of human papillomavirus infection of the anogenital tract. *Cancer Metastasis Rev.* 1987; 6: 653-664.

[49] Gissmann, L; Schwarz, E. Persistence and expression of human papillomavirus DNA in genital cancer. *Ciba Found Symp.* 1986; 120: 190-207.

[50] Howley, PM; Schlegel, R. The human papillomaviruses. An overview. *Am. J. Med.* 1988; 85: 155-158.

[51] Crum, CP; Levine, RU. Human papillomavirus infection and cervical neoplasia: new perspectives. *Int. J. Gynecol. Pathol.* 1984; 3: 376-388.

[52] Cripe, TP. Human papillomaviruses: pediatric perspectives on a family of multifaceted tumorigenic pathogens. *Pediatr. Infect. Dis. J.* 1990; 9: 836-844.

[53] Anderson, MC. The pathology of cervical cancer. *Clin. Obstet. Gynaecol.* 1985; 12: 87-119.

[54] Ostör, AG. Natural history of cervical intraepithelial neoplasia: a critical review. *Int. J. Gynecol. Pathol.* 1993; 12: 186-192.

[55] Chang, AR. Carcinoma in situ of the cervix and its malignant potential. A lesson from New Zealand. *Cytopathology* 1990; 1: 321-328.

[56] Jones, WE. Carcinoma in situ of the uterine cervix. A review of some present clinical problems. *Calif. Med.* 1968; 109: 353-362.

[57] zur Hausen, H. Human papillomaviruses in the pathogenesis of anogenital cancer. *Virology* 1991; 184: 9-13.

[58] Laimins, LA. The biology of human papillomaviruses: from warts to cancer. *Infect. Agents Dis.* 1993; 2: 74-86.

[59] Rangel, LM; Ramírez, M; Torroella, M; Pedroza, A; Ibarra, V; Gariglio P. Multistep carcinogenesis and genital papillomavirus infection. Implications for diagnosis and vaccines. *Arch. Med. Res.* 1994; 25: 265-272.

[60] Morrison, EA. Natural history of cervical infection with human papillomaviruses. *Clin. Infect. Dis.* 1994; 18: 172-180.

[61] zur Hausen, H; de Villiers, EM. Human papillomaviruses. *Annu. Rev. Microbiol.* 1994; 48: 427-447.

[62] zur Hausen, H. Papillomaviruses in anogenital cancer as a model to understand the role of viruses in human cancers. *Cancer Res.* 1989; 49: 4677-4681.

[63] zur Hausen, H. The role of papillomaviruses in anogenital cancer. *Scand. J. Infect. Dis. Suppl.* 1990; 69: 107-111.

[64] zur Hausen, H. Human papillomaviruses in the pathogenesis of anogenital cancer. *Virology* 1991; 184: 9-13.

[65] zur Hausen, H. Papillomaviruses in human cancers. *Proc. Assoc. Am. Physicians* 1999; 111: 581-587.

[66] Syrjänen, K. Mechanisms and predictors of high-risk human papillomavirus (HPV) clearance in the uterine cervix. *Eur. J. Gynaecol. Oncol.* 2007; 28: 337-351.

[67] Matlashewski, G. The cell biology of human papillomavirus transformed cells. *Anticancer Res.* 1989; 9: 1447-1456.

[68] Howley, PM; Münger, K; Werness, BA; Phelps, WC; Schlegel, R. Molecular mechanisms of transformation by the human papillomaviruses. *Princess Takamatsu Symp.* 1989; 20: 199-206.

[69] zur Hausen, H. Host cell regulation of HPV transforming gene expression. *Princess Takamatsu Symp.* 1989; 20: 207-219.

[70] Reid, R; Campion, MJ. The biology and significance of human papillomavirus infections in the genital tract. *Yale J. Biol. Med.,* 1988; 61: 307-325.

[71] Strang, P. Cytogenetic and cytometric analyses in squamous cell carcinoma of the uterine cervix. *Int. J. Gynecol. Pathol.* 1989; 8: 54-63.

[72] Popescu, NC; DiPaolo, JA. Preferential sites for viral integration on mammalian genome. *Cancer Genet. Cytogenet.* 1989; 42: 157-171.

[73] Klimek, R. Cervical cancer as a natural phenomenon. *Eur. J. Obstet. Gynecol. Reprod. Biol.* 1990; 36: 229-238.

[74] Richart, RM; Wright, TC Jr. Human papillomavirus. *Curr. Opin. Obstet. Gynecol.* 1992; 4: 662-669.

[75] Swan, DC; Vernon, SD; Icenogle, JP. Cellular proteins involved in papillomavirus-induced transformation. *Arch. Virol.* 1994; 138: 105-115.

[76] zur Hausen, H. Disrupted dichotomous intracellular control of human papillomavirus infection in cancer of the cervix. *Lancet* 1994; 343: 955-957.

[77] Baker, VV. Oncogene expression in cervical cancer. *Cancer Treat. Res.* 1994; 70: 43-51.

[78] Crum, CP. Contemporary theories of cervical carcinogenesis: the virus, the host, and the stem cell. *Mod. Pathol.* 2000; 13: 243-251.

[79] Johansson, C; Schwartz, S. Regulation of human papillomavirus gene expression by splicing and polyadenylation. *Nat. Rev. Microbiol.* 2013; 11: 239-251.

[80] Oren, A; Fernandes, J. The Bethesda system for the reporting of cervical/vaginal cytology. *J. Am. Osteopath. Assoc.* 1991; 91: 476-479.

[81] Kiviat, NB; Critchlow, CW; Kurman, RJ. Reassessment of the morphological continuum of cervical intraepithelial lesions: does it reflect different stages in the progression to cervical carcinoma? *IARC Sci. Publ.* 1992; 119: 59-66.

[82] Nguyen, HN; Nordqvist, SR. The Bethesda system and evaluation of abnormal pap smears. *Semin. Surg. Oncol.* 1999; 16: 217-221.

[83] Cenci, M; Vecchione, A. Atypical squamous and glandular cells of undetermined significance (ASCUS and AGUS) of the uterine cervix. *Anticancer Res.* 2000; 20: 3701-3707.

[84] Wilbanks, GD. In vivo and in vitro "markers" of human cervical intraepithelial neoplasia. *Cancer Res.* 1976; 36: 2485-2494.

[85] Brescia, RJ; Jenson, AB; Lancaster, WD; Kurman, RJ. The role of human papillomaviruses in the pathogenesis and histologic classification of precancerous lesions of the cervix. *Hum. Pathol.* 1986; 17: 552-559.

[86] Fennell, RH Jr. Microinvasive carcinoma of the uterine cervix. *Obstet. Gynecol. Surv.* 1978; 33: 406-411.

[87] Koss, LG. Cytologic and histologic manifestations of human papillomavirus infection of the female genital tract and their clinical significance. *Cancer* 1987; 60: 1942-1950.

[88] Koss, LG. Cytologic and histologic manifestations of human papillomavirus infection of the uterine cervix. *Cancer Detect. Prev.* 1990; 14: 461-464.

[89] Richart, RM. Causes and management of cervical intraepithelial neoplasia. *Cancer* 1987; 60: 1951-1959.

[90] Ambros, RA; Kurman, RJ. Current concepts in the relationship of human papillomavirus infection to the pathogenesis and classification of precancerous squamous lesions of the uterine cervix. *Semin. Diagn. Pathol.* 1990; 7:158-172.

[91] Robert, ME; Fu, YS. Squamous cell carcinoma of the uterine cervix – A review with emphasis on prognostic factors and unusual variants. *Semin. Diagn. Pathol.* 1990; 7: 173-189.

[92] Smedts, F; Ramaekers, FC; Vooijs, PG. The dynamics of keratin expression in malignant transformation of cervical epithelium: a review. *Obstet. Gynecol.* 1993; 82: 465.

[93] Young, RH; Scully, RE. Invasive adenocarcinoma and related tumors of the uterine cervix. *Semin. Diagn. Pathol.*, 1990; 7: 205-227.

[94] Yeh, IT; LiVolsi, VA; Noumoff, JS. Endocervical carcinoma. *Pathol. Res. Pract.* 1991; 187: 129-144.

[95] Nayar, R; Tabbara, SO. Atypical squamous cells: update on current concepts. *Clin. Lab. Med.* 2003; 23: 605-632.

[96] McCann, GA; Boutsicaris, CE; Preston, MM; Backes, FJ; Eisenhauer, EL; Fowler, JM; Cohn, DE; Copeland, LJ; Salani, R; O'Malley, DM. Neuroendocrine carcinoma of the uterine cervix: the role of multimodality therapy in early-stage disease. *Gynecol. Oncol.* 2013; 129: 135-139.

[97] McCoy, JP Jr, Haines HG. The antigenicity and immunology of human cervical squamous cell carcinoma: a review. *Am. J. Obstet. Gynecol.* 1981; 140: 329-336.

[98] Puts, JJ; Moesker, O; Kenemans, P; Vooijs, GP; Ramaekers, FC. Expression of cytokeratins in early neoplastic epithelial lesions of the uterine cervix. *Int. J. Gynecol. Pathol.* 1985; 4: 300-313.

[99] Serra, V; Ramirez, A; Marzo, MC; Valcuende, F; Lara, C; Castells, A; Bonilla-Musoles, F. Distribution of epithelial antigens in the human uterine cervix: a review. *Arch. Gynecol. Obstet.* 1989; 246: 61-84.

[100] Kato, H. Studies on the special tumor marker of cervical cancer of the uterus. *Semin. Surg. Oncol.* 1987; 3: 55-63.

[101] Roche, JK; Crum, CP. Local immunity and the uterine cervix: implications for cancer-associated viruses. *Cancer Immunol. Immunother.* 1991; 33: 203-209.

[102] Stubbe Teglbjaerg, C; Ravn, V; Mandel, U; Dabelsteen, E. Distribution of histo-blood group antigens in cervical and uterine endometrium. *APMIS Suppl.* 1991; 23: 100-106.

[103] Jenson, AB; Kurman, RJ; Lancaster, WD. Tissue effects of and host response to human papillomavirus infection. *Dermatol. Clin.* 1991; 9: 203-209.

[104] Shah, KV. Human papillomaviruses and other biological markers in cervical cancer. *IARC Sci. Publ.* 1992; 119: 209-218.

[105] Evans, CH; Flugelman, AA; DiPaolo, JA. Cytokine modulation of immune defenses in cervical cancer. *Oncology* 1993; 50: 245-251.

[106] Einstein, MH; Schiller, JT; Viscidi, RP; Strickler, HD; Coursaget, P; Tan, T; Halsey, N; Jenkins, D. Clinician's guide to human papillomavirus immunology: knowns and unknowns. *Lancet Infect. Dis.* 2009; 9: 347-356.

[107] Doorbar, J; Quint, W; Banks, L; Bravo, IG; Stoler, M; Broker, TR; Stanley, MA. The biology and life-cycle of human papillomaviruses. *Vaccine* 2012; 30 Suppl 5: F55-F70.

[108] Palefsky, J. Human papillomavirus infection among HIV-infected individuals. Implications for development of malignant tumors. *Hematol. Oncol. Clin. North Am.* 1991; 5: 357-370.

[109] Palefsky, JM. Human papillomavirus-associated anogenital neoplasia and other solid tumors in human immunodeficiency virus-infected individuals. *Curr. Opin. Oncol.* 1991; 3: 881-885.

[110] Judson, FN. Interactions between human papillomavirus and human immunodeficiency virus infections. *IARC Sci. Publ.* 1992; 119: 199-207.

[111] Mandelblatt, JS; Fahs, M; Garibaldi, K; Senie, RT; Peterson, HB. Association between HIV infection and cervical neoplasia: implications for clinical care of women at risk for both conditions. *AIDS* 1992; 6: 173-178.

[112] Vernon, SD; Icenogle, JP; Johnson, PR; Reeves, WC. Human papillomavirus, human immunodeficiency virus, and cervical cancer: newly recognized associations? *Infect. Agents Dis.* 1992; 1: 319-324.

[113] Stratton, P; Ciacco, KH. Cervical neoplasia in the patient with HIV infection. *Curr. Opin. Obstet. Gynecol.* 1994; 6: 86-91.

[114] Northfelt, DW. Cervical and anal neoplasia and HPV infection in persons with HIV infection. *Oncology* (Williston Park) 1994; 8: 33-37.

[115] Braun, L. Role of human immunodeficiency virus infection in the pathogenesis of human papillomavirus-associated cervical neoplasia. *Am. J. Pathol.* 1994; 144: 209-214.

[116] Boccalon, M; Tirelli, U; Sopracordevole, F; Vaccher, E. Intra-epithelial and invasive cervical neoplasia during HIV infection. *Eur. J. Cancer* 1996; 32A: 2212-2217.

[117] Palefsky, J. Human papillomavirus-related disease in people with HIV. *Curr. Opin. HIV AIDS* 2009; 4: 52-56.

[118] Denny, LA; Franceschi, S; de Sanjosé, S; Heard, I; Moscicki, AB; Palefsky, J. Human papillomavirus, human immunodeficiency virus and immunosuppression. *Vaccine* 2012; 30 Suppl 5: F168-F174.

[119] Falkenberry, SS. Cancer in pregnancy. *Surg. Oncol. Clin. N. Am.* 1998 7, 375-397.

[120] Method, MW; Brost, BC. Management of cervical cancer in pregnancy. *Semin. Surg. Oncol.* 1999; 16: 251-260.

[121] Nevin, J; Soeters, R; Dehaeck, K; Bloch, B; van Wyk, L. Cervical carcinoma associated with pregnancy. *Obstet. Gynecol. Surv.* 1995; 50: 228-239.

[122] Campion, MJ; Sedlacek, TV. Colposcopy in pregnancy. *Obstet. Gynecol. Clin. North Am.* 1993; 20: 153-163.

[123] Sood, AK; Sorosky, JI. Invasive cervical cancer complicating pregnancy. How to manage the dilemma. *Obstet. Gynecol. Clin. North Am.* 1998; 25: 343-352.

[124] Lewandowski, GS; Vaccarello, L; Copeland, LJ. Surgical issues in the management of carcinoma of the cervix in pregnancy. *Surg. Clin. North Am.* 1995; 75: 89-100.

[125] Magrina, JF. Primary surgery for stage IB-IIA cervical cancer, including short-term and long-term morbidity and treatment in pregnancy. *J. Natl. Cancer Inst. Monogr.* 1996; 21: 53-59.

[126] Shivvers, SA; Miller, DS. Preinvasive and invasive breast and cervical cancer prior to or during pregnancy. *Clin. Perinatol.* 1997; 24: 369-389.

[127] Apgar, BS; Zoschnick, LB. Triage of the abnormal Papanicolaou smear in pregnancy. *Prim. Care* 1998; 25: 483-503.

[128] Connor, JP. Noninvasive cervical cancer complicating pregnancy. *Obstet. Gynecol. Clin. North Am.* 1998; 25: 331-342.

[129] Selleret, L; Mathevet, P. Precancerous cervical lesions during pregnancy: diagnostic and treatment. *J. Gynecol. Obstet. Biol. Reprod.* (Paris) 2008; 37 Suppl 1: S131-S138.

[130] Zagouri, F; Sergentanis, TN; Chrysikos, D; Bartsch, R. Platinum derivatives during pregnancy in cervical cancer: a systematic review and meta-analysis. *Obstet. Gynecol.* 2013; 121: 337-343.

[131] Foltz, AM; Kelsey, JL. The annual Pap test: a dubious policy success. *Milbank Mem. Fund Q. Health Soc.* 1978; 56: 426-462.

[132] Shield, PW; Daunter, B; Wright, RG. The Pap smear revisited. *Aust. N. Z. J. Obstet. Gynaecol.* 1987; 27: 269-283.

[133] Noller, KL. Cervical cytology and the evaluation of the abnormal Papanicolaou smear. *Prim. Care* 1988; 15: 461-471.

[134] Lynge, E. Screening for cancer of the cervix uteri. *World J. Surg.* 1989; 13: 71-78.

[135] Koss, LG. The Papanicolaou test for cervical cancer detection. A triumph and a tragedy. *JAMA* 1989; 261: 737-743.

[136] Mandelblatt, J. Cervical cancer screening in primary care: issues and recommendations. *Prim. Care* 1989; 16: 133-155.

[137] Singh, P; Ilancheran, A. The "Pap" or cervical smear and the role of colposcopy in screening for carcinoma of the cervix. *Singapore Med. J.,* 1989; 30: 302-305.

[138] Eddy, DM. Screening for cervical cancer. *Ann. Intern. Med.* 1990; 113: 214-226.

[139] Pettersson, F. Efficacy of cervical cancer screening. *Med. Oncol. Tumor Pharmacother.* 1991; 8: 175-181.

[140] Davey-Sullivan, BJ; Gearhart, JG. The use of the Pap smear in Mississippi. *J. Miss State Med. Assoc.* 1991; 32: 167-171.

[141] Paul, C; Bagshaw, S; Bonita, R; Durham, G; Fitzgerald, NW; Jones, RW; Marshall, B; McAvoy, BR. 1991 cervical screening recommendations: a working group report. *N. Z. Med. J.* 1991; 104: 291-295.

[142] Gillam, SJ. Understanding the uptake of cervical cancer screening: the contribution of the health belief model. *Br. J. Gen. Pract.* 1991; 41: 510-513.

[143] King, CS. Carcinoma of the cervix and cervical cytology – Short epidemiological review. *Cent. Afr. J. Med.* 1992; 38: 198-202.

[144] Coyne, CA; Hohman, K; Levinson, A. Reaching special populations with breast and cervical cancer public education. *J. Cancer Educ.* 1992; 7: 293-303.

[145] Stoler, MH. Advances in cervical screening technology. *Mod. Pathol.* 2000; 13: 275-284.

[146] Fowler, J. Screening for cervical cancer. Current terminology, classification, and technique. *Postgrad. Med.* 1993; 93: 57-64.

[147] Banda-Gamboa, H; Ricketts, I; Cairns, A; Hussein, K; Tucker, JH; Husain, N. Automation in cervical cytology: an overview. *Anal. Cell Pathol.,* 1992; 4: 25-48.

[148] Spitzer, M. Cervical screening adjuncts: recent advances. *Am. J. Obstet. Gynecol.* 1998; 179: 544-556.

[149] Greenberg, MD; Campion, MJ; Rutledge, LH. Cervicography as an adjunct to cytologic screening. *Obstet. Gynecol. Clin. North Am.* 1993; 20: 13-29.

[150] Beral, V; Day, NE. Screening for cervical cancer: is there a place for incorporating tests for the human papillomavirus? *IARC Sci. Publ.* 1992; 119: 263-269.

[151] Melchers, WJ; Claas, HC; Quint, WG. Use of the polymerase chain reaction to study the relationship between human papillomavirus infections and cervical cancer. *Eur. J. Clin. Microbiol. Infect. Dis.* 1991; 10: 714-727.

[152] Miller, KE; Losh, DP; Folley, A. Evaluation and follow-up of abnormal Pap smears. *Am. Fam. Physician* 1992; 45: 143-150.

[153] Dewar, MA; Hall, K; Perchalski, J. Cervical cancer screening. Past success and future challenge. *Prim. Care* 1992; 19: 589-606.

[154] Soler, ME; Blumenthal, PD. New technologies in cervical cancer precursor detection. *Curr. Opin. Oncol.* 2000; 12: 460-465.

[155] Nuovo, J; Melnikow, J; Howell, LP. New tests for cervical cancer screening. *Am. Fam. Physician* 2001; 64: 780-786.

[156] Wright, TC Jr. Cervical cancer screening in the 21st century: is it time to retire the PAP smear? *Clin. Obstet. Gynecol.* 2007; 50: 313-323.

[157] Arbyn, M; Ronco, G; Anttila, A; Meijer, CJ; Poljak, M; Ogilvie, G; Koliopoulos, G; Naucler, P; Sankaranarayanan, R; Peto, J. Evidence regarding human papillomavirus testing in secondary prevention of cervical cancer. *Vaccine* 2012; 30 Suppl 5: F88-F99.

[158] Javaheri, G. Microinvasive carcinoma of the uterine cervix. *Int. J. Gynaecol. Obstet.* 1978-1979; 16: 106-114.

[159] Lang, WR. The respective roles of cytology and colposcopy in obstetric and gynaecologic practice. *J. Reprod. Med.* 1976; 1: 249-252.

[160] Ramzy, I; Mody, DR. Gynecologic cytology. Practical considerations and limitations. *Clin. Lab. Med.* 1991; 11: 271-292.

[161] Husain, OA; Butler, EB; Evans, DM; Macgregor, JE; Yule, R. Quality control in cervical cytology. *J. Clin. Pathol.* 1974; 27: 935-944.

[162] Bengtsson, EW; Nordin, B. Image analysis in cytology: DNA-histogramming versus cervical smear prescreening. *Ann. Biol. Clin.* (Paris) 1993; 51: 27-38.

[163] Wickenden, C; Malcolm, AD; Coleman, DV. DNA hybridization of cervical tissues. *Crit. Rev. Clin. Lab. Sci.* 1987; 25: 1-18.

[164] Gissmann, L. Human papillomavirus DNA in genital tumours. *IARC Sci. Publ.* 1984; 63: 405-411.

[165] Gissmann, L; Boshart, M; Dürst, M; Ikenberg, H; Wagner, D; zur Hausen, H. Presence of human papillomavirus in genital tumors. *J. Invest. Dermatol.* 1984; 83: 26s-28s.

[166] Schiffman, MH. Validation of hybridization assays: correlation of filter in situ, dot blot and PCR with Southern blot. *IARC Sci. Publ.* 1992; 119: 169-179.

[167] de Sanjosé, S; Santamaria, M; Alonso de Ruiz, P; Aristizabal, N; Guerrero, E; Castellsagué, X; Bosch, FX. HPV types in women with normal cervical cytology. *IARC Sci. Publ.* 1992; 119: 75-84.

[168] Roman, A; Fife, KH. Human papillomaviruses: are we ready to type? *Clin. Microbiol. Rev.* 1989; 2: 166-190.

[169] Crum, CP; Barber, S; Roche, JK. Pathobiology of papillomavirus-related cervical diseases: prospects for immunodiagnosis. *Clin. Microbiol. Rev.* 1991; 4: 270-285.

[170] Galloway, DA. Serological assays for the detection of HPV antibodies. *IARC Sci. Publ.* 1992; 119: 147-161.

[171] Wilkinson, EJ; Smith, LJ. Cervical neoplasia. Its association with human papillomavirus infection. *J. Fla. Med. Assoc.* 1993; 80: 106-111.

[172] van Niekerk, WA; Dunton, CJ; Richart, RM; Hilgarth, M; Kato, H; Kaufman, RH; Mango, LJ; Nozawa, S; Robinowitz, M. Colposcopy, cervicography, speculoscopy and endoscopy. International Academy of Cytology Task Force summary. Diagnostic

Cytology Towards the 21st Century: An International Expert Conference and Tutorial. *Acta Cytol.* 1998; 42: 33-49.

[173] Ebner, F; Tamussino, K; Kressel, HY. Magnetic resonance imaging in cervical carcinoma: diagnosis, staging, and follow-up. *Magn. Reson Q.* 1994; 10: 22-42.

[174] Waggenspack, GA; Amparo, EG; Hannigan, EV; O'Neal, MF. MRI of cervical carcinoma. *Semin. Ultrasound CT MR* 1988; 9: 158-166.

[175] Breitenecker, G; Gitsch, G. What's new in diagnosis and treatment of HPV-associated cervical lesions. *Pathol. Res. Pract.* 1992; 188: 242-247.

[176] Mitrani-Rosenbaum, S. Human papillomaviruses and the diagnosis of genital microorganisms. *Isr. J. Med. Sci.* 1994; 30: 443-447.

[177] Apgar, BS; Brotzman, G. HPV testing in the evaluation of the minimally abnormal Papanicolaou smear. *Am. Fam. Physician* 1999; 59: 2794-2801.

[178] Bishop, JW; Marshall, CJ; Bentz, JS. New technologies in gynecologic cytology. *J. Reprod. Med.* 2000; 45: 701-719.

[179] Coutlée, F; Mayrand, MH; Roger, M; Franco, EL. Detection and typing of human papillomavirus nucleic acids in biological fluids. *Public Health Genomics* 2009; 12: 308-318.

[180] Booth, CN; Bashleben, C; Filomena, CA; Means, MM; Wasserman, PG; Souers, RJ; Henry, MR. Monitoring and ordering practices for human papillomavirus in cervical cytology: findings from the College of American Pathologists Gynecologic Cytopathology Quality Consensus Conference working group 5. *Arch. Pathol. Lab. Med.* 2013; 137: 214-219.

[181] Hricak, H. Cancer of the uterus: the value of MRI pre- and post-irradiation. *Int. J. Radiat. Oncol. Biol. Phys.* 1991; 21: 1089-1094.

[182] Monaghan, JM. Management decision making using clinical and operative staging in cervical cancer. *Baillieres Clin. Obstet. Gynaecol.* 1988; 2: 737-746.

[183] Onnis, A; Marchetti, M. Adequate staging for an adequate management in uterine cancers. Clinical experience. *Eur. J. Gynaecol. Oncol.* 1991; 12: 99-102.

[184] Hacker, NF. Clinical and operative staging of cervical cancer. *Baillieres Clin. Obstet. Gynaecol.* 1988; 2: 747-759.

[185] Sevin, BU; Averette, HE. Staging laparotomy and radical hysterectomy for cancer of the cervix. *Baillieres Clin. Obstet. Gynaecol.* 1988; 2: 761-768.

[186] Heaps, JM; Berek, JS. Surgical staging of cervical cancer. *Clin. Obstet. Gynecol.* 1990; 33: 852-862.

[187] Shingleton, HM. Surgical treatment of cancer of the cervix. *Eur. J. Gynaecol. Oncol.* 1992; 13: 45-52.

[188] McGonigle, KF; Berek, JS. Early-stage squamous cell and adenocarcinoma of the cervix. *Curr. Opin. Obstet. Gynecol.* 1992; 4: 109-119.

[189] Sala, E; Rockall, AG; Freeman, SJ; Mitchell, DG; Reinhold, C. The added role of MR imaging in treatment stratification of patients with gynecologic malignancies: what the radiologist needs to know. *Radiology* 2013; 266: 717-740.

[190] Runowicz, CD; Smith, HO; Goldberg, GL. Multimodality therapy in locally advanced cervical cancer. *Curr. Opin. Obstet. Gynecol.* 1993; 5: 92-98.

[191] Orr, JW Jr; Holloway, RW. Surgical aspects of cervical cancer. *Surg. Clin. North Am.* 1991; 71: 1067-1083.

[192] Richart, RM; Wright, TC Jr. Controversies in the management of low-grade cervical intraepithelial neoplasia. *Cancer* 1993; 71: 1413-1421.

[193] Townsend, DE; Marks, EJ. Cryosurgery and the CO_2 laser. *Cancer* 1981; 48: 632-637.

[194] Dorsey, JH. Laser surgery for cervical intraepithelial neoplasia. *Obstet. Gynecol. Clin. North Am.* 1991; 18: 475-489.

[195] Creasman, WT; Weed, JC Jr. Conservative management of cervical intraepithelial neoplasia. *Clin. Obstet. Gynecol.* 1980; 23: 281-291.

[196] DiSaia, PJ. Surgical aspects of cervical carcinoma. *Cancer* 1981; 48: 548-559.

[197] Lichtenegger, W; Anderhuber, F; Ralph, G. Operative anatomy and technique of radical parametrial resection in the surgical treatment of cervical cancer. *Baillieres Clin. Obstet. Gynaecol.* 1988; 2: 841-856.

[198] Johnson, N; Lilford, RJ; Jones, SE; McKenzie, L; Billingsley, P; Songane, FF. Using decision analysis to calculate the optimum treatment for microinvasive cervical cancer. *Br. J. Cancer* 1992; 65: 717-722.

[199] Johnson, N. Computer-aided clinical management: microscopic cancer of the ectocervix. *Baillieres Clin. Obstet. Gynaecol.* 1990; 4: 885-904.

[200] Smit, BM. Prospects for proton therapy in carcinoma of the cervix. *Int. J. Radiat. Oncol. Biol. Phys.* 1992; 22: 349-353.

[201] Perez, CA. Radiation therapy in the management of cancer of the cervix. *Oncology* (Williston Park) 1993; 7: 61-69.

[202] Jones, WB. Surgical approaches for advanced or recurrent cancer of the cervix. *Cancer* 1987; 60: 2094-2103.

[203] Barber, HR. Pelvic exenteration. *Cancer Invest.* 1987; 5: 331-338.

[204] Arterbery, VE. High-dose rate brachytherapy for carcinoma of the cervix. *Curr. Opin. Oncol.* 1993; 5: 1005-1009.

[205] Guthrie, D. Chemotherapy of cervical cancer. *Clin. Obstet. Gynaecol.* 1985; 12: 229-246.

[206] Alberts, DS; Mason-Liddil, N. The role of cisplatin in the management of advanced squamous cell cancer of the cervix. *Semin. Oncol.* 1989; 16: 66-78.

[207] Alberts, DS; Garcia, D; Mason-Liddil, N. Cisplatin in advanced cancer of the cervix: an update. *Semin. Oncol.* 1991; 18: 11-24.

[208] Muggia, FM; Gill, I. Role of carboplatin in endometrial and cervical carcinomas. *Semin. Oncol.* 1992; 19: 90-93.

[209] Stehman, FB. Concurrent chemoradiation in carcinoma of the uterine cervix. *Semin. Oncol.* 1992; 19: 88-91.

[210] Omura, GA. Current status of chemotherapy for cancer of the cervix. *Oncology* (Williston Park) 1992; 6: 27-32.

[211] Park, RC; Thigpen, JT. Chemotherapy in advanced and recurrent cervical cancer. A review. *Cancer* 1993; 71: 1446-1450.

[212] Jones, WB. New approaches to high-risk cervical cancer. Advanced cervical cancer. *Cancer* 1993; 71: 1451-1459.

[213] Muggia, FM; Muderspach, L. Platinum compounds in cervical and endometrial cancers: focus on carboplatin. *Semin. Oncol.* 1994; 21: 35-41.

[214] Angioli, R; Sevin, BU; Perras, JP; Untch, M; Hightower, RD; Nguyen, HN; Steren, A; Villani, C; Averette, HE. Rationale of combining radiation and interferon for the treatment of cervical cancer. *Oncology* 1992; 49: 445-449.

[215] Gallup, DG; Stock, RJ; Talledo, OE. Current management of non-squamous carcinoma of the cervix. *Oncology* (Williston Park) 1989; 3: 95-102.

[216] Rogo, KO; Stendahl, U. Management of recurrent cervical cancer: the place of ultra-radical surgery. *East Afr. Med. J.* 1993; 70: 380-385.

[217] Estape, R; Angioli, R. Surgical management of advanced and recurrent cervical cancer. *Semin. Surg. Oncol.* 1999; 16: 236-241.

[218] Photopulos, GJ. Surgery or radiation for early cervical cancer. *Clin. Obstet. Gynecol.* 1990; 33: 872-882.

[219] Sedlacek, TV; Owens, KJ. Cervical malignancies. *Curr. Opin. Obstet. Gynecol.* 1991; 3: 49-57.

[220] Barber, HR. Cervical cancer: pelvic and para-aortic lymph node sampling and its consequences. *Baillieres Clin. Obstet. Gynaecol.* 1988; 2: 769-777.

[221] Kim, MK; Kim, HS; Kim, SH; Oh, JM; Han, JY; Lim, JM; Juhnn, YS; Song, YS. Human papillomavirus type 16 E5 oncoprotein as a new target for cervical cancer treatment. *Biochem. Pharmacol.* 2010; 80: 1930-1935.

[222] Baalbergen, A; Veenstra, Y; Stalpers, L. Primary surgery versus primary radiotherapy with or without chemotherapy for early adenocarcinoma of the uterine cervix. *Cochrane Database Syst. Rev.* 2013; 1. CD006248.

[223] Berget, A; Lenstrup, C. Cervical intraepithelial neoplasia. Examination, treatment and follow-up. *Obstet. Gynecol. Surv.* 1985; 40: 545-552.

[224] Shield, PW; Daunter, B; Wright, RG. Post-irradiation cytology of cervical cancer patients. *Cytopathology* 1992; 3: 167-182.

[225] Mergui, JL; Levêque, J. What kind of follow-up after surgical treatment for high-grade cervix lesion? *Gynecol. Obstet. Fertil.* 2008; 36: 441-447.

[226] Chan, PK; Picconi, MA; Cheung, TH; Giovannelli, L; Park, JS. Laboratory and clinical aspects of human papillomavirus testing.*Crit. Rev. Clin. Lab. Sci.* 2012; 49: 117-136.

[227] Pillai, R. Oncogene expression and prognosis in cervical cancer. *Cancer Lett.* 1991; 59: 171-175.

[228] Pillai, R; Balaram, P; Nair, MK. Role of immune response in the prognosis of carcinoma of the uterine cervix: can in vitro analysis provide a better framework for more effective management? *Tumori* 1992; 78: 87-93.

[229] Riou, GF. Proto-oncogenes and prognosis in early carcinoma of the uterine cervix. *Cancer Surv.* 1988; 7: 441-456.

[230] Burke, TW. Factors affecting recurrence and survival in stage I carcinoma of the uterine cervix. *Oncology* (Williston Park) 1992; 6: 111-116.

[231] Schink, JC; Lurain, JR. Microinvasive cervix cancer. *Int. J. Gynaecol. Obstet.* 1991; 36: 5-11.

[232] Hoskins, WJ. Prognostic factors for risk of recurrence in stages Ib and IIa cervical cancer. *Baillieres Clin. Obstet. Gynaecol.* 1988; 2: 817-828.

[233] van Bommel, PF; van Lindert, AC; Kock, HC; Leers, WH; Neijt, JP. A review of prognostic factors in early-stage carcinoma of the cervix (FIGO I B and II A) and implications for treatment strategy. *Eur. J. Obstet. Gynecol. Reprod. Biol.* 1987; 26: 69-84.

[234] Franco, EL. Prognostic value of human papillomavirus in the survival of cervical cancer patients: an overview of the evidence. *Cancer Epidemiol. Biomarkers Prev.* 1992; 1: 499-504.

[235] Burger, RA; Monk, BJ; Kurosaki, T; Anton-Culver, H; Vasilev, SA; Berman, ML; Wilczynski, SP. Human papillomavirus type 18: association with poor prognosis in early stage cervical cancer. *J. Natl. Cancer Inst.* 1996; 88: 1361-1368.

[236] Schmid, MP; Mansmann, B; Federico, M; Dimopoulous, JC; Georg, P; Fidarova, E; Dörr, W; Pötter, R. Residual tumour volumes and grey zones after external beam radiotherapy (with or without chemotherapy) in cervical cancer patients. A low-field MRI study. *Strahlenther. Onkol.* 2013; 189: 238-244.

[237] Spitzer, M; Krumholz, BA. Human papillomavirus-related diseases in the female patient. *Urol. Clin. North Am.* 1992; 19: 71-82.

[238] Crum, CP; Roche, JK. Papillomavirus-related genital neoplasia: present and future prevention. *Cancer Detect. Prev.* 1990; 14: 465-469.

[239] Hudson, E. The prevention of cervical cancer: the place of the cytological smear test. *Clin. Obstet. Gynaecol.* 1985; 12: 33-51.

[240] Hasson, HM. Cervical removal at hysterectomy for benign disease. Risks and benefits. *J. Reprod. Med.* 1993; 38: 781-790.

[241] Jones, DE; Shackelford, DP; Brame, RG. Supracervical hysterectomy: back to the future? *Am. J. Obstet. Gynecol.* 1999; 180: 513-515.

[242] Arbyn, M; Cuzick, J. International agreement to join forces in synthesizing evidence on new methods for cervical cancer prevention. *Cancer Lett.* 2009; 278: 1-2.

[243] Ciesielska, U; Nowińska, K; Podhorska-Okołów, M; Dziegiel, P. The role of human papillomavirus in the malignant transformation of cervix epithelial cells and the importance of vaccination against this virus. *Adv. Clin. Exp. Med.* 2012; 21: 235-244.

[244] Campo, MS; Jarrett, WF. Vaccination against cutaneous and mucosal papillomavirus in cattle. *Ciba Found Symp.* 1994; 187: 61-73.

[245] Campo, MS. Vaccination against papillomavirus. *Cancer Cells* 1991; 3: 421-426.

[246] Khan, SA. Cervical cancer, human papillomavirus and vaccines. *Clin. Oncol.* (R Coll Radiol) 1993; 5: 386-390.

[247] Cason, J; Khan, SA; Best, JM. Towards vaccines against human papillomavirus type-16 genital infections. *Vaccine,* 1993; 11: 603-611.

[248] Crawford, L. Prospects for cervical cancer vaccines. *Cancer Surv.* 1993; 16: 215-229.

[249] Lowy, DR; Kirnbauer, R; Schiller, JT. Genital human papillomavirus infection. *Proc. Natl. Acad. Sci. U S A* 1994; 91: 2436-2340.

[250] Lowy, DR; Schiller, JT. Papillomaviruses: prophylactic vaccine prospects. *Biochim. Biophys. Acta* 1999; 1423: M1-M8.

[251] Schiller, JT. Papillomavirus-like particle vaccines for cervical cancer. *Mol. Med. Today* 1999; 5: 209-215.

[252] Duggan-Keen, MF; Brown, MD; Stacey, SN; Stern, PL. Papillomavirus vaccines. *Front Biosci.* 1998; 3: D1192-D1208.

[253] Gariglio, P; Benitez-Bribiesca, L; Berumen, J; Alcocer, JM; Tamez, R; Madrid, V. Therapeutic uterine-cervix cancer vaccines in humans. *Arch. Med. Res.* 1998; 29: 279-284.

[254] Hilleman, MR. Overview of vaccinology with special reference to papillomavirus vaccines. *J. Clin. Virol.* 2000; 19: 79-90.

[255] Gissmann, L; Osen, W; Müller, M; Jochmus, I. Therapeutic vaccines for human papillomaviruses. *Intervirology* 2001; 44: 167-175.

[256] Murakami, M; Gurski, KJ; Steller, MA. Human papillomavirus vaccines for cervical cancer. *J. Immunother.* 1999; 22: 212-218.

[257] Herzog, TJ; Huh, WK; Einstein, MH. How does public policy impact cervical screening and vaccination strategies? *Gynecol. Oncol.* 2010; 119: 175-180.

[258] Kane, MA; Serrano, B; de Sanjosé, S; Wittet, S. Implementation of human papillomavirus immunization in the developing world. *Vaccine* 2012; 30 Suppl 5: F192-F200.

[259] Fahs, MC; Plichta, SB; Mandelblatt, JS. Cost-effective policies for cervical cancer screening. An international review. *Pharmacoeconomics* 1996; 9: 211-230.

[260] Celentano, DD; deLissovoy, G. Assessment of cervical cancer screening and follow-up programs. *Public Health Rev.* 1989-1990; 17: 173-240.

[261] Wilson, S; Woodman, C. Assessing the effectiveness of cervical screening. *Clin. Obstet. Gynecol.* 1995; 38: 577-584.

[262] Wagner, JL. Cost-effectiveness of screening for common cancers. *Cancer Metastasis Rev.* 1997; 16: 281-294.

[263] Myers, ER; McCrory, DC; Subramanian, S; McCall, N; Nanda, K; Datta, S; Matchar, DB. Setting the target for a better cervical screening test: characteristics of a cost-effective test for cervical neoplasia screening. *Obstet. Gynecol.* 2000; 96: 645-652.

[264] Brown, AD; Raab, SS; Suba, EJ; Wright, RG; International Consensus Conference on the Fight Against Cervical Cancer, IAC Task Force 15 Summary, Chicago, Illinois, USA. Cost-effectiveness studies on cervical cancer. *Acta Cytol.* 2001; 45: 509-514.

[265] Marra, F; Cloutier, K; Oteng, B; Marra, C; Ogilvie, G. Effectiveness and cost effectiveness of human papillomavirus vaccine: a systematic review. *Pharmacoeconomics* 2009; 27: 127-147.

[266] Canfell, K; Chesson, H; Kulasingam, SL; Berkhof, J; Diaz, M; Kim, JJ. Modeling preventative strategies against human papillomavirus-related disease in developed countries. *Vaccine* 2012; 30 Suppl 5: F157-F167.

[267] Fernández-Esquer, ME; Ross, MW; Torres, I. The importance of psychosocial factors in the prevention of HPV infection and cervical cancer. *Int. J. STD AIDS* 2000; 11: 701-713.

[268] Lambley, P. The role of psychological processes in the aetiology and treatment of cervical cancer: a biopsychological perspective. Br J Med Psychol 1993; 66: 43-60.

[269] Andersen, BL. Stress and quality of life following cervical cancer. *J. Natl. Cancer Inst. Monogr.* 1996; 21: 65-70.

[270] Sevin, BU. Social implications of sexually transmitted cancer. *J. Womens Health Gend. Based Med.* 1999; 8: 759-766.

[271] Fylan, F. Screening for cervical cancer: a review of women's attitudes, knowledge, and behaviour. *Br. J. Gen. Pract.* 1998; 48: 1509-1514.

[272] Lester, H; Wilson, S. Is default from colposcopy a problem, and if so what can we do? A systematic review of the literature. *Br. J. Gen. Pract.* 1999; 49: 223-229.

[273] Goodkin, K; Antoni, MH; Helder, L; Sevin, B. Psychoneuroimmunological aspects of disease progression among women with human papillomavirus-associated cervical dysplasia and human immunodeficiency virus type 1 co-infection. *Int. J. Psychiatry Med.* 1993; 23: 119-148.

[274] Graziottin, A; Serafini, A. HPV infection in women: psychosexual impact of genital warts and intraepithelial lesions. *J. Sex Med.* 2009; 6: 633-645.

[275] Williams-Brennan, L; Gastaldo, D; Cole, DC; Paszat, L. Social determinants of health associated with cervical cancer screening among women living in developing countries: a scoping review. *Arch. Gynecol. Obstet.* 2012; 286: 1487-1505.

[276] Bowling, A. Implications of preventive health behaviour for cervical and breast cancer screening programmes: a review. *Fam. Pract.* 1989; 6: 224-231.

[277] Verhoeven, V; Baay, M; Baay, P. People seeking health information about human papillomavirus via the internet have a very high level of anxiety. *Sex Health* 2009; 6: 258-259.

[278] Galaal, K; Bryant, A; Deane, KH; Al-Khaduri, M; Lopes, AD. Interventions for reducing anxiety in women undergoing colposcopy. *Cochrane Database Syst. Rev.* 2011; 12: CD006013.

[279] Frable, WJ. Does a zero error standard exist for the Papanicolaou smear? A pathologist's perspective. *Arch. Pathol. Lab. Med.* 1997; 121: 301-310.

[280] Mitchell, H. Report disclaimers and informed expectations about Papanicolaou smears: an Australian view. *Arch. Pathol. Lab. Med.* 1997; 121: 327-330.

[281] Skoumal, SM; Florell, SR; Bydalek, MK; Hunter, WJ 3rd. Malpractice protection: communication of diagnostic uncertainty. *Diagn. Cytopathol.* 1996; 14: 385-389.

[282] Greening, SE. Errors in cervical smears: minimizing the risk of medicolegal consequences. *Monogr. Pathol.* 1997; 39: 16-39.

[283] Freedman, LF. Implications of mandating amended reports following retrospective review of Papanicolaou smears. *Arch. Pathol. Lab. Med.* 1997; 121: 299-300.

[284] Krieger, PA; McGoogan, E; Vooijs, GP; Amma, NS; Cochand-Priollet, B; Colgan, TJ; Davey, DD; Geyer, JW; Goodell, RM; Grohs, DH; Gupta, SK; Jones, BA; Koss, LG; Mango, LJ; McCallum, SM; Nielsen, M; Robinowitz, M; Sauer, T; Schumann, JL; Syrjänen, KJ; Suprun, HZ; Topalidis, T; Wertlake, PT; Whittaker, J. Quality assurance/control issues. International Academy of Cytology Task Force summary. Diagnostic Cytology Towards the 21st Century: An International Expert Conference and Tutorial. *Acta Cytol.* 1998; 42: 133-140.

[285] Frable, WJ; Austin, RM; Greening, SE; Collins, RJ; Hillman, RL; Kobler, TP; Koss, LG; Mitchell, H; Perey, R; Rosenthal, DL; Sidoti, MS; Somrak, TM. Medicolegal affairs. International Academy of Cytology Task Force summary. Diagnostic Cytology Towards the 21st Century: An International Expert Conference and Tutorial. *Acta Cytol.* 1998; 42: 76-119.

[286] Benítez-Bribiesca, L. Ethical dilemmas and great expectations for human papilloma virus vaccination. *Arch. Med. Res.* 2009; 40: 499-502.

[287] Freckelton, I. Gynaecological cytopathology and the search for perfection: civil liability and regulatory ramifications. *J. Law Med.* 2003; 11: 185-200.

[288] Larsen, PM; Vetner, M; Hansen, K; Fey, SJ. Future trends in cervical cancer. *Cancer Lett.* 1988; 41: 123-137.

[289] Koutsky, LA; Wølner-Hanssen, P. Genital papillomavirus infections: current knowledge and future prospects. *Obstet. Gynecol. Clin. North Am.,* 1989; 16: 541-564.

[290] Richart, RM. Screening. The next century. *Cancer* 1995; 76: 1919-1927.

[291] Coutlée, F; Mayrand, MH; Provencher, D; Franco, E. The future of HPV testing in clinical laboratories and applied virology research. *Clin. Diagn. Virol.* 1997; 8: 123-141.

[292] Thigpen, T; Vance, RB; Khansur, T. Carcinoma of the uterine cervix: current status and future directions. *Semin. Oncol.* 1994; 21: 43-54.

[293] Monsonego, J. Prevention of cervical cancer: screening, progress and perspectives. *Presse Med.* 2007; 36: 92-111.

[294] Monsonego, J. Prevention of cervical cancer (II): prophylactic HPV vaccination, current knowledge, practical procedures and new issues. *Presse Med.* 2007; 36: 640-666.

[295] Markman, M. Chemoradiation in the management of cervix cancer: current status and future directions.*Oncology* 2013; 84: 246-250.

Index

D

E

F

G

H

I

O

P

S

T